Sarcopenia

Sarcopenia

Editors

Alfonso J. Cruz-Jentoft
*Servicio de Geriatría, Hospital Universitario Ramón y Cajal,
Madrid, Spain*

John E. Morley
*Division of Geriatric Medicine and Division of Endocrinology,
Saint Louis University School of Medicine, St. Louis, MO, USA*

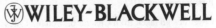

WILEY-BLACKWELL

A John Wiley & Sons, Ltd., Publication

Library of Congress Cataloging-in-Publication Data

Sarcopenia / editors, Alfonso J. Cruz-Jentoft and John Morley.
   p. ; cm.
 Includes bibliographical references and index.
 ISBN 978-1-119-97587-8 (cloth)
 I. Cruz-Jentoft, Alfonso J.   II. Morley, John E.
 [DNLM: 1. Sarcopenia–physiopathology.   2. Aging–physiology.   WE 550]
 612.6′7–dc23

                                             2012022792

A catalogue record for this book is available from the British Library.

Wiley also publishes its books in a variety of electronic formats. Some content that appears in print may not be available in electronic books.

Set in 10/12pt Times by Aptara Inc., New Delhi, India
Printed and bound in Malaysia by Vivar Printing Sdn Bhd

First Impression 2012

Cover design taken from Chapter 6: 'Potential sites and physiological mechanisms that regulate strength'. Courtesy of Danette Pratt, a Biomedical Illustrator in the Office of Communication at the Ohio University Heritage College of Osteopathic Medicine, who developed the figure in collaboration with Brian Clark and Todd Manini.

Contents

List of Contributors

Gabor Abellan van Kan, MD, PhD
INSERM Unit 1027, Toulouse, France; Université de Toulouse, Toulouse, France; Gérontopôle, Centre Hospitalier Universitaire de Toulouse, Toulouse, France.

Jürgen M. Bauer, MD, PhD
Institute for Biomedicine of Aging, Friedrich-Alexander Universität Erlangen-Nürnberg, Germany; Geriatrics Center Oldenburg, Germany.

Ivan Bautmans, PhD
Frailty in Ageing Research Department (FRIA), University of Brussels, Brussels, Belgium.

Minal Bhanushali, MD
National Institute of Neurological Disorders and Stroke and National Institute of Health, Rockville, MD, USA.

Yves Boirie, MD, PhD
Clermont Université, Université d'Auvergne, Unité de Nutrition Humaine, Clermont-Ferrand, France; INRA, UNH, CRNH Auvergne, Clermont-Ferrand, France; CHU Clermont-Ferrand, Service de Nutrition Clinique, Clermont-Ferrand, France.

Tommy Cederholm, MD, PhD
Clinical Nutrition and Metabolism, Department of Public Health and Caring Sciences, Uppsala University, Department of Geriatric Medicine, Uppsala University Hospital, Uppsala, Sweden.

Matteo Cesari, MD, PhD
INSERM Unit 1027, Toulouse, France; Université de Toulouse, Toulouse, France; Gérontopôle, Centre Hospitalier Universitaire de Toulouse, Toulouse, France.

Brian C. Clark, PhD
Ohio Musculoskeletal and Neurological Institute (OMNI); Department of Biomedical Sciences, Ohio University, Athens, OH, USA.

Robin Conwit, MD
National Institute of Neurological Disorders and Stroke and National Institute of Health, Rockville, MD, USA.

Alfonso J. Cruz-Jentoft, MD, PhD
Servicio de Geriatría, Hospital Universitario Ramón y Cajal, Madrid, Spain.

Michael Drey, MD
Institute for Biomedicine of Aging, Friedrich-Alexander Universität Erlangen-Nürnberg, Germany.

Filippo Rossi Fanelli, MD
Department of Clinical Medicine, Sapienza, University of Rome, Italy.

Luigi Ferrucci, MD, PhD
National Institute of Aging, Clinical Research Branch, Harbor Hospital, Baltimore, USA.

Christelle Guillet, PhD
Clermont Université, Université d'Auvergne, Unité de Nutrition Humaine, Clermont-Ferrand, France; INRA, UNH, CRNH Auvergne, Clermont-Ferrand, France.

Francesco Landi, MD, PhD
Department of Geriatrics – Policlinico A. Gemelli, Catholic University of the Sacred Heart, Rome, Italy.

Thomas F. Lang PhD
University of California San Francisco, San Francisco, CA, USA.

Simone Lucia, MD
Department of Clinical Medicine, Sapienza, University of Rome, Italy.

Todd M. Manini, PhD
Institute on Aging & The Department of Aging and Geriatric Research, University of Florida, Gainesville, FL, USA.

Jeffrey Metter, MD
National Institute of Aging, Clinical Research Branch, Harbor Hospital, Baltimore, USA.

Jean-Pierre Michel, MD
Honorary Professor of Medicine, Geneva University, Switzerland.

John E. Morley, MB, BCh
Division of Geriatric Medicine, Saint Louis University School of Medicine, St. Louis, MO, USA.

Maurizio Muscaritoli, MD FACN
Department of Clinical Medicine, Sapienza, University of Rome, Italy.

Graziano Onder, MD, PhD
Department of Geriatrics – Policlinico A. Gemelli, Catholic University of the Sacred Heart, Rome, Italy.

Douglas Paddon-Jones, PhD
Department of Nutrition and Metabolism, University of Texas Medical Branch, Galveston, TX, USA.

Mark D. Peterson, PhD
Department of Physical Medicine and Rehabilitation, University of Michigan, Ann Arbor, MI, USA.

Blake B. Rasmussen, PhD
Department of Nutrition & Metabolism, Sealy Center on Aging, University of TX Medical Branch, Galveston, TX, USA.

Yves Rolland, MD, PhD
INSERM Unit 1027, Toulouse, France; Université de Toulouse, Toulouse, France; Gérontopôle, Centre Hospitalier Universitaire de Toulouse, Toulouse, France.

Andrea P. Rossi, MD, PhD
Department of Medicine, Geriatric Division, University of Verona, Verona, Italy.

David W. Russ, PhD
Ohio Musculoskeletal and Neurological Institute (OMNI); School of Rehabilitation and Communication Sciences, Ohio University, Athens, OH USA.

Avan Aihie Sayer, BSc, MBBS, MSc, PhD, FRCP
Academic Geriatric Medicine, MRC Lifecourse Epidemiology Unit, University of Southampton, Southampton, UK.

Laura Schaap, PhD
Department of Epidemiology and Biostatistics, VU University Medical Center, Amsterdam, The Netherlands.

José A. Serra-Rexach, MD, PhD
Geriatric Department, Hospital General Universitario Gregorio Marañón, Universidad Complutense, Madrid, Spain.

Cornel C. Sieber, MD
Institute for Biomedicine of Ageing, Friedrich-Alexander-University Erlangen-Nürnberg, Germany.

David R. Thomas, MD, FACP, AGSF, GSAF
Division of Geriatric Medicine, Saint Louis University, Saint Louis, MO, USA.

Maurits Vandewoude, MD, PhD
Medical School, Department of Geriatrics, University of Antwerp, Antwerp, Belgium.

Luc van Loon, PhD
Department of Human Movement Sciences, Maastricht University Medical Centre, Maastricht, The Netherlands.

Marjolein Visser, PhD
Department of Health Sciences, Faculty of Earth and Life Sciences, VU University Amsterdam, The Netherlands; Department of Epidemiology and Biostatistics, VU University Medical Center, Amsterdam, The Netherlands.

Elena Volpi, MD, PhD
Department of Internal Medicine, Division of Geriatrics, Sealy Center on Aging, University of TX Medical Branch, Galveston, TX, USA.

Stéphane Walrand, PhD
Clermont Université, Université d'Auvergne, Unité de Nutrition Humaine, Clermont-Ferrand, France; INRA, UNH, CRNH Auvergne, Clermont-Ferrand, France.

Mauro Zamboni, MD
Department of Medicine, Geriatric Division, University of Verona, Verona, Italy.

Elena Zoico, MD, PhD
Department of Medicine, Geriatric Division, University of Verona, Verona, Italy.

Preface

Over the past few years, sarcopenia has moved rapidly from being a concept used by a couple of academics to one that is widely explored in journals and scientific meetings. All aspects of sarcopenia, from basic science to clinical applicability, are now an extremely active area of research and clinical practice for those working in geriatric medicine, nutrition, epidemiology, basic biological research and many other disciplines. Its recent emergence, together with the conceptualization of frailty, is a step forward in the quest to identify and prevent the unwelcome disabilities that accompany many people in their last years of life.

Thus, the moment has come to summarize, to define where we are and where we are going, to stand on solid ground for the next step – or jump. This book is intended to be a clear and precise reference work for those physicians or researchers interested in having a global, yet detailed understanding of such a complex topic. Rooted in basic science and in the critical use of diagnostic tools, the book also covers clinical aspects, trying to identify the role of sarcopenia in the complex arena of age, disease, and physical disability.

To accomplish this task, we have carefully selected authors from both Europe and the United States, as the approach to sarcopenia differs slightly in each continent. This wide range of authors allows the reader a clearer picture of the issues involved. Of course, all of the authors, with no exception, are leading experts in the field. As editors we are extremely grateful for their enthusiastic acceptance to contribute to this book, the high quality of their submissions, and their patience in adapting their chapters to fit the book.

After describing the epidemiological challenge that sarcopenia brings to current geriatric care, and reviewing the definitions of the word, the first chapters, explore the biological aspects of muscle and the central nervous system and their relation with movement and function. Sarcopenia is then explored in the context of the individual, from a lifetime and a syndromic approach, looking at the adverse effects it has on health and function. An analysis of the intimate relations between sarcopenia, cachexia, frailty and bones opens the door to a description of the complexity of measuring different parameters linked to muscle mass and function. Finally, the door opens to intervention, from nutrition and exercise to drugs, ending with a difficult question: can sarcopenia (and thus disability) really be prevented?

We believe that we have produced a state-of-the-art textbook with a comprehensive approach to sarcopenia. We hope that it will be a valuable reference tool, not only for experts, but also for those who are interested in starting their own research in this area and those who wish to develop their own criteria about such a promising field within geriatric medicine.

CHAPTER 1

Epidemiology of Muscle Mass Loss with Age

Marjolein Visser

Department of Health Sciences, Faculty of Earth and Life Sciences, VU University Amsterdam, The Netherlands; Department of Epidemiology and Biostatistics, VU University Medical Center, Amsterdam, The Netherlands

INTRODUCTION

The development of new body composition methods in the early 1970s and 1980s led to more research on this topic, including the study of differences in body composition between young and older persons. These initial studies were followed by much larger studies covering a wide age range investigating how body composition varied across the life span. Variations in lean body mass and fat-free mass were described between age groups. These studies served as the important scientific basis for developing the concept Sarcopenia. Sarcopenia was defined as the age-related loss of muscle mass [1]. The term is derived from the Greek words *sarx* (flesh) and *penia* (loss). The development of this concept further stimulated research in this specific body composition area. More recently, large-scale studies among older persons have included accurate and precise measurements of skeletal muscle mass. Moreover, these measurements have been repeated over time, enabling the sarcopenia process to be studied.

This chapter will discuss the results of epidemiological studies investigating the age-related loss of skeletal muscle mass. First, several cross-sectional studies will be presented comparing the body composition between younger and older persons. Then prospective studies will be discussed investigating the change in body composition with aging. The chapter will conclude with the results of more recent, prospective studies that precisely measured change in skeletal muscle mass in large samples of older persons.

MUSCLE MASS DIFFERENCES BETWEEN AGE GROUPS

Comparisons between young and older men and women with regard to muscle size have been made in several small studies. The results showed that healthy women in their 70s had a

Sarcopenia, First Edition. Edited by Alfonso J. Cruz-Jentoft and John E. Morley.
© 2012 John Wiley & Sons, Ltd. Published 2012 by John Wiley & Sons, Ltd.

33% smaller quadriceps cross-sectional area as obtained by compound ultrasound imaging compared to women in their 20s [2]. Using the same methodology and age groups, healthy older men had a 25% smaller quadriceps cross-sectional area [3]. In a study investigating thigh composition using five computed tomography scans of the total thigh, smaller muscle cross-sectional areas were observed in older men compared to younger men even though their total thigh cross-sectional area was similar. The older men had a 13% smaller total muscle cross-sectional area, 25.4% smaller quadriceps and 17.9% smaller hamstring cross-sectional area [4]. Using magnetic resonance imaging of the leg anterior compartment, muscle area was measured in young and older men and women [5]. The older persons had a smaller area of contractile tissue; 11.5% less in women and 19.2% less in men; compared to the young persons. These data, obtained by different body composition technologies, clearly showed a smaller muscle size in older persons compared to young persons. The observed differences in muscle size between age 20 and age 70 suggested a loss of skeletal muscle mass of about 0.26% to 0.56% per year.

The amount of non-muscle tissue within the muscle was also assessed using five computed tomography scans of the thigh in 11 elderly men and 13 young men [4]. Older men had 59.4% more non-muscle tissue within the quadriceps and 127.3% within the hamstring muscle. In a similar study, the amount of non-muscle tissue in older men was 81% higher in the plantar flexors as compared to young men [6]. Thus, apart from the smaller muscle size in old age, these studies suggested that the composition of the muscle also changed with aging, leading to less 'lean' muscle tissue in old age.

With the greater availability of body composition methods such as bioelectrical impedance and dual-energy x-ray absorptiometry over time, cross-sectional data on muscle size in large study samples including a broad age range have been collected. Examples of these studies using lean mass from DXA (the non-bone, non-fat soft tissue mass) and fat-free mass from bioelectrical impedance, presented by 10-year age groups of men, are presented in Figure 1.1 [7,8]. Older age groups had a lower total body fat-free mass, lower

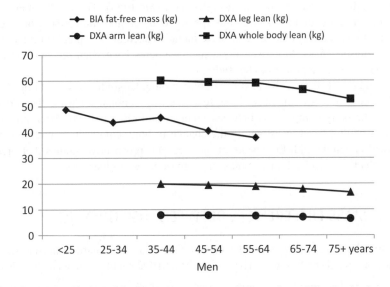

Figure 1.1 Differences in fat-free mass and lean mass using different body composition methodologies between men of different age groups. BIA = bioelectrical impedance. DXA = dual-energy x-ray absorptiometry. Based on references 7 and 8.

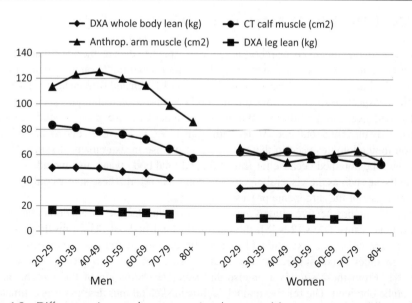

Figure 1.2 Differences in muscle cross-sectional area and lean mass using different body composition methodologies between men and women of different age groups. DXA = dual-energy x-ray absorptiometry. CT = computed tomography. Anthrop. = anthropometry, using arm circumference and triceps skinfold. Based on references 9–11.

total body lean mass, and lower arm and leg lean mass. Figure 1.2 presents the differences in muscle size between 10-year age groups in men and women. With increasing age group, the data suggested a lower whole body lean mass and leg lean mass as assessed by DXA [9], a smaller arm muscle cross-sectional area (from anthropometric measures [10]) and a smaller calf muscle cross-sectional area (from peripheral qualitative computed tomography [11]). These cross-sectional data derived from samples from Italy, Australia, India, Japan, and the USA consistently suggested a decline in muscle size with aging. These data also suggested a steeper decline in muscle size with aging in men compared to women.

Cross-sectional data from a sample of 72 women aged 18 years to 69 years suggested a strong correlation between age and the amount of low density lean tissue as assessed by a computed tomography scan of the mid-thigh. The density of muscle tissue as assessed by computed tomography is indicative of the amount of fat infiltration into the muscle [12]. Higher age was associated with greater amounts of low density lean tissue (correlation coefficient = 0.52 [13]). This result again suggested a greater fat infiltration into the muscle with increasing age.

These cross-sectional data, however, should be interpreted carefully as cohort and period effects, and not aging per se, may have caused the observed differences in muscle size and muscle composition between the age groups. For example, well-known cohort differences in body height, a strong determinant of muscle size, may partly explain the lower muscle mass in older persons compared to younger persons. In addition, period differences in lifestyle (e.g. sports participation and diet) and job demands may have differentially affected muscle size and muscle composition between age groups. Therefore, prospective data are preferred to investigate the change in muscle mass with aging.

CHANGE IN MUSCLE MASS WITH AGING

Forbes was among the first researchers to report prospective data on the age-related decrease in lean body mass in a small group of adults using potassium[40] counting data [14]. The reported decline was −0.41% per year as obtained in 13 men and women aged 22–48 years.

Many prospective studies followed using body composition techniques such as bioelectrical impedance, isotope dilution, skinfolds and underwater weighing to study change in fat-free body mass and total body water with aging [15–21]. However, due to the body composition methodologies used in these studies, no precise measurement of skeletal muscle mass could be obtained because fat-free mass and total body water also include lean, non-muscle tissue such as the visceral organs and bone. Therefore, these studies only provide a crude estimate of the sarcopenia process with aging.

More recent prospective studies have measured the decline in appendicular skeletal muscle mass using DXA [22–25], the decline in total body skeletal muscle mass using 24-h urinary creatinine excretion [26], and the decline in muscle cross-sectional area by CT in older persons [27,28]. The characteristics of these studies are presented in Table 1.1. From these studies a precise and accurate estimation of the sarcopenia process can be obtained. The relative annual decline in skeletal muscle mass was estimated to be between −0.64 and −1.29 % per year for older men and between −0.53 and −0.84 % per year for older women (Figure 1.3). In older persons the absolute as well as the relative decline of skeletal muscle mass with aging was larger in men compared to women.

Table 1.1 Characteristics of prospective studies investigating the age-related change in skeletal muscle mass in older men and women

Reference	N and sex	Age (mean (SD)) or range (y)	Mean follow-up time (y)	Body composition method	Muscle measurement
27	12 men	71.1 (5.4)	8.9	CT	Mid-thigh total anterior muscle cross-sectional area
28	813 men 865 women	70–79	5	CT	Mid-thigh muscle cross-sectional area
25	26 women	75.5 (5.1)	2.0	DXA	Leg skeletal muscle mass
24	1129 men 1178 women	70–90	5	DXA	Leg skeletal muscle mass
22	24 men 54 women	60–90	4.7	DXA	Appendicular skeletal muscle mass
23	62 men 97 women	71.6 (2.2) 71.4 (2.2)	5.5	DXA	Appendicular skeletal muscle mass
26	52 men 68 women	60.4 (7.9) 60.4 (7.4)	9.7	24-h urinary creatinine excretion	Total body skeletal muscle mass

SD = standard deviation, CT = computed tomography, DXA = dual-energy x-ray absorptiometry

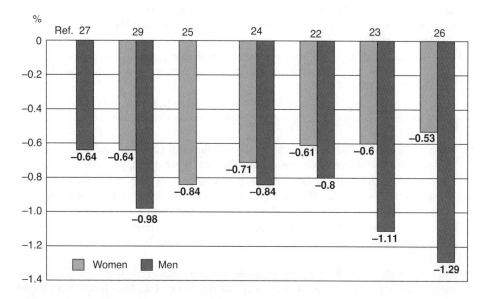

Figure 1.3 Annual decline (%) in skeletal muscle mass in older men and women from prospective studies with follow-up times from 2 to 9.7 years.

Limited data are available on the prospective change in muscle fat with aging. Data from the Health, Aging and Body Composition Study showed an increase in intermuscular fat at the mid-thigh of 3.1 cm^2 in older men and 1.7 cm^2 in older women during the 5-year follow-up [28]. This translated to an annual increase of 9.7% in men and 5.8% in women. This increase was paralleled by a decline in subcutaneous fat at the mid-thigh and shows specifically the increasing fat infiltration into muscle tissue with increasing age.

From these body composition studies it can be concluded that the amount of skeletal muscle mass declines substantially with aging. At the same time, the composition of the muscle changes and a greater fat infiltration into the muscle occurs. It is important to understand the potential impact of these changes on healthy aging.

REFERENCES

1. Rosenberg IH (1997) Sarcopenia: origins and clinical relevance. J Nutr 127(5 Suppl): 990S–991S.
2. Young A, Stokes M, Crowe M (1984) Size and strength of the quadriceps muscles of old and young women. Eur J Clin Invest 14, 282–287.
3. Young A, Stokes M, Crowe M (1985) The size and strength of the quadriceps muscles of old and young men. Clin Physiol 5, 145–154.
4. Overend TJ, Cunningham DA, Paterson DH, Lefcou MS (1992) Thigh composition in young and elderly men determined by computed tomography. Clin Physiol 12, 629–640.
5. Kent-Braun JA, Ng AV, Young K (2000) Skeletal muscle contractile and noncontractile components in young and older women and women. J Appl Physiol 88, 662–668.
6. Rice CL, Cunningham DA, Paterson DH, Lefcoe MS (1989) Arm and leg composition determined by computed tomography in young and elderly men. Clin Physiol 9, 207–220.

7. Atlantis E, Martin SA, Haren MT, Taylor AW, Wittert GA (2008) Lifestyle factors associated with age-related differences in body composition: the Florey Adelaide Male Aging Study. Am J Clin Nutr 88, 95–104.

8. Das BM, Roy SK (2010) Age changes in the anthropometric and body composition characteristics of the Bishnupriya Maniopuris of Cachar district, Assam. Advances in Bioscience and Biotechnology 1, 122–130.

9. Ito H, Ohshima A, Ohto N, Ogasawara M, Tsuzuki M, Takao K, Hijii C, Tanaka H, Nishioka K (2001) Relation between body composition and age in healthy Japanese subjects. Eur J Clin Nutr 55, 462–470.

10. Metter EJ, Lynch N, Conwit R, Lindle R, Tobin J, Hurley B (1999) Muscle quality and age: cross-sectional and longitudinal comparisons. J Gerontol Biol Sci 54A, B207–18.

11. Lauretani F, Russo CR, Bandinelli S, Bartali B, Cavazzini C, Di Iorio A, Corsi AM, Rantanen T, Guralnik JM, Ferrucci L (2003) Age-associated changes in skeletal muscles and their effect on mobility: an operational diagnosis of sarcopenia. J Appl Physiol 95, 1851–1860.

12. Goodpaster BH, Kelley DE, Thaete FL, et al. (2000) Skeletal muscle attenuation determined by computed tomography is associated with skeletal muscle lipid content. J Appl Physiol 89, 104–110.

13. Ryan AS, Nicklas BJ (1999) Age-related changes in fat deposition in mid-thigh muscle in women: relationships with metabolic cardiovascular disease risk factors. Int J Obes Relat Metab Disord 23, 126–132.

14. Forbes GB, Reina JC (1970) Adults lean body mass declines with age: some longitudinal observations. Metabolism 19, 653–663.

15. Noppa H, Anderson M, Bengtsson C, Bruce Å, Isaksson B (1980) Longitudinal studies of anthropometric data and body composition. Am J Clin Nutr 33, 155–262.

16. Murray LA, Reilly JJ, Choudhry M, Durnin JVGA (1996) A longitudinal study of changes in body composition and basal metabolism in physically active elderly men. Eur J Appl Physiol 72, 215–218.

17. Guo SS, Zeller C, Chumlea WC, Siervogel RM (1999) Aging, body composition, and lifestyle: the Fels Longitudinal Study. Am J Clin Nutr 70, 405–411.

18. Hughes VA, Frontera WR, Roubenoff R, Evans WJ, Singh MA (2002) Longitudinal changes in body composition in older men and women: role of body weight change and physical activity. Am J Clin Nutr 76, 473–481.

19. Kyle UG, Zhang FF, Morabia A, Pichard C (2006) Longitudinal study of body composition changes associated with weight change and physical activity. Nutrition 22, 1103–1111.

20. Dey DK, Bosaeus I, Lissner L, Steen B (2009) Changes in body composition and its relation to muscle strength in 75-year-old men and women: a 5-year prospective follow-up study of the NORA cohort in Göteborg, Sweden. Nutrition 25, 613–619.

21. Genton L, Karsegard VL, Chevalley T, Kossovsky MP, Darmon P, Pichard C (2011) Body composition changes over 9 years in healthy elderly subjects and impact of physical activity. Clin Nutr 30, 436–442.

22. Gallagher D, Ruts E, Visser M, Heshka S, Baumgartner RN, Wang J, Pierson RN, Pi-Sunyer FX, Heymsfield SB (2000) Weight stability masks sarcopenia in elderly men and women. Am J Physiol 279, E366–75.

23. Fantin F, Di Francesco V, Fontanan G, Zivelonghi A, Bissoli L, Zoico E, Rossi A, Micciolo R, Bosello O, Zamboni M (2007) Longitudinal body composition changes in old men and women: interrelationships with worsening disability. J Gerontol Med Sci 62A, 1375–1381.

24. Koster A, Ding J, Stenholm S, Caserotti P, Houston DK, Nicklas BJ, You T, Lee JS, Visser M, Newman AB, Schwartz AV, Cauley JA, Tylavsky FA, Goodpaster BH, Kritchevsky SB, Harris

TB; Health ABC study (2011) Does the amount of fat mass predict age-related loss of lean mass, muscle strength, and muscle quality in older adults? J Gerontol A Biol Sci Med Sci 66, 888–895.

25. Song M, Ruts E, Kim J, Jamumala I, Heymsfield S, Gallagher D (2004) Sarcopenia and increased adipose tissue infiltration of muscle in elderly African American women. Am J Clin Nutr 79, 874–880.

26. Hughes VA, Frontera WR, Wood M, Evans WJ, Dallal GE, Roubenoff R, Fiatarone Singh MA (2001) Longitudinal muscle strength changes in older adults: influence of muscle mass, physical activity, and health. J Gerontol Biol Sci 56A, B209–17.

27. Frontera WR, Reid KF, Phillips EM, Krivickas LS, Highes VA, Roubenoff R, Fielding RA (2008) Muscle fiber size and function in elderly humans: a longitudinal study. J Appl Physiol 105, 637–642.

28. Delmonico MJ, Harris TB, Visser M, Park SW, Conroy MB, Velasquez-Mieyer P, Boudreau R, Manini TM, Nevitt M, Newman AB, Goodpaster BH (2009) Longitudinal study of muscle strength, quality, and adipose tissue infiltration. Am J Clin Nutr 90, 1579–1585.

CHAPTER 2

Definitions of Sarcopenia

John E. Morley

*Division of Geriatric Medicine, Saint Louis University School of Medicine,
St. Louis, Missouri, USA*

Alfonso J. Cruz-Jentoft

Servicio de Geriatría, Hospital Universitario Ramón y Cajal, Madrid, Spain

THE ORIGINS OF THE WORD 'SARCOPENIA'

Sarcopenia has rapidly become a common term in geriatrics and gerontology, both in academic forums and in clinical practice. This is somehow surprising, as the word sarcopenia was introduced quite recently, trying to improve understanding of a previously eluding concept. In fact, while sarcopenia seems to be common and has huge personal and societal costs, sarcopenia still has no broadly accepted definition, diagnostic criteria, ICD-9 codes, or treatment guidelines. This chapter will review the still changing concept of sarcopenia, and recent efforts that are trying to agree on a definition that may reach wide consensus and be useful both for research and clinical practice.

In 1988, a meeting was convened in Albuquerque (USA) to discuss the assessment of health and nutrition in older populations. Rosenberg, who is accredited for the first use of the word, noted that 'no decline with age is more dramatic or potentially more functionally significant than the decline in muscle mass' and suggested that to provide recognition by the scientific community this phenomenon needed a name. He proposed a name derived from the Greek roots *sarx* for flesh and *penia* for loss [1].

Although the word chosen only described muscle mass, from the very beginning it was acknowledged that the consequences of muscle mass loss affected ambulation, mobility, nutrient intake and status, and functional independence.

DEFINITIONS BASED ON MUSCLE MASS

Availability and standards on techniques that measure muscle mass (or lean body mass) were initially far more advanced than measures of other parameters involved in sarcopenia. It is thus not surprising that most major epidemiological studies fixed to a strict definition of sarcopenia as loss of muscle mass.

Sarcopenia, First Edition. Edited by Alfonso J. Cruz-Jentoft and John E. Morley.
© 2012 John Wiley & Sons, Ltd. Published 2012 by John Wiley & Sons, Ltd.

The first epidemiological studies to determine the prevalence of sarcopenia measured muscle mass (lean body mass) either using BIA or DXA. For instance, Baumgartner used a definition based on appendicular skeletal muscle mass measured by DXA, corrected for height, and defined sarcopenia as being two standard deviations below sex specific means of healthy young persons (18-40 years) of a reference population [2].

Many studies performed in recent years use the word sarcopenia as synonymous of muscle wasting or muscle mass loss (as reviewed in Chapter 1). From them we have learned that muscle mass declines at approximately 1-2% per year after the age of 50 years. If sarcopenia is defined using only severe muscle mass (two standard deviations below healthy young) it is present in 5 to 13% of 60 to 70 year olds and 11 to 50% of those 80 and older [3]. Over a thousand publications have used this definition of sarcopenia, and the term is still used as a surrogate for muscle mass.

LIMITS OF ONLY USING MUSCLE MASS

While the definition of sarcopenia based on loss of muscle mass alone has served the scientific community fairly well, it has been less satisfying for clinicians, the pharmaceutical industry, and regulatory agencies. Unlike the measurements of bone mineral density, the measurement of muscle mass has not been widely adopted by clinicians. Regulatory agencies have failed to accept that restoration of muscle mass is, of itself, a sufficient reason to allow a drug to be approved for use. It should be noted that this is not different from the situation with osteoporosis wherein reduced bone mineral density is recognized as a legitimate indication for treatment, but for regulatory considerations, drugs have had to show a reduction in fracture incidence before approval [4].

There are many crucial aspects of sarcopenia that are missed by the simplistic use of muscle mass. Relevant patient outcomes of sarcopenia include mortality and physical disability (i.e. the inability to walk or perform activities of daily living). A number of studies have shown that reduced muscle mass is predictive of disability and mortality. However, muscle mass by itself has shown to be a weak predictor of outcomes [5–10]. It has also been shown that the link between muscle mass, muscle function (strength and power), physical performance and other downstream outcomes is not linear [10;11]. These relationships are better explored in Chapters 6 and 8.

Some reasons for this inconsistency related to muscle quality are: 1) The infiltration into muscle by fat, which is a powerful predictor of future disability and mortality [6]. The percent of body fat (obesity) to muscle mass may be a confounding factor in understanding the link between muscle mass and physical function [12]. 2) Infiltration of collagen into muscle with aging can also lead to a dichotomy in the relationship between muscle mass and strength [13]. 3) Age-associated changes in neuromuscular activation that are superimposed on changes in muscle mass may further explain the dichotomy between mass and strength/power losses [14]. Other changes in muscle that may lead to a loss of strength include deposition of abnormal proteins, contractile and structural protein misfolding, mitochondrial dysfunction, neuromuscular and plaque dysfunction.

A final problem with the definition of sarcopenia by muscle mass are the variety of measures available to measure muscle mass, even within the same technique, each based on some assumptions that may be true or not. This happens even for the gold standards based on radiology (see Chapter 14). Each measure leads to different cut-offs for muscle mass and are indirect measures [15]. As such, they can be influenced by adiposity and total

Table 2.1   Alternative names proposed for sarcopenia and related disorders

Dynapenia [14]	Age related loss of strength
Kratopenia [19]	Age related loss of strength
Myopenia [46]	Clinically relevant muscle wasting due to any illness and at any age
Frailty	See Chapter 11

body water. Different equations and assumptions in measurements may also yield different results. For instance, some authors sum up the muscle mass of the four limbs from a DXA scan to define appendicular skeletal muscle mass (ASM), and define a skeletal muscle mass index (SMI) as ASM/height^2 (as kg/m^2) [2]. Other describe a skeletal muscle index (SMI), where SMI = (skeletal muscle mass/body mass) × 100 [16], and use a two tier approach (class I and II sarcopenia, depending on the number of standard deviations below mean values for young adults. Other approaches have also been explored [17].

The evidence that the isolated measure of muscle mass has practical limitations has boosted a debate, and many authors have being looking for an alternative term to sarcopenia that better describes the complexity of the problem of mass and function (Table 2.1). However, if one looks at other widely used medical terms used to define common diseases (diabetes in Greek comes from 'siphon', dementia in Latin means 'out of mind'), they seem to be very limited compared to the wide range of problems each disease carries. Thus, using a word that is now in common use, such as sarcopenia, and improving its definition seems to be wiser than wasting time in arguments about the best word to describe each element of a complex condition.

RECENT CONSENSUS DEFINITIONS

Two international consensus definitions have been published recently, supported by different scientific societies and with some common authors, which may be a step forward in our understanding of sarcopenia [18;19]. They share some common ideas, and both open the door to further refinements when evidence allows.

European Working Group on Sarcopenia in Older People

The first definition, published in 2010, was promoted by the European Union Geriatric Medicine Society (EUGMS) and endorsed by the European Society of Clinical Nutrition and Metabolism (ESPEN), the International Academy of Nutrition and Aging (IANA) and the International Association of Gerontology and Geriatrics – European Region (IAGG-ER) [18]. An international Working Group was convened, with the task of developing an operational definition and diagnostic criteria for sarcopenia that could be used in clinical practice as well as in research studies. The following questions were discussed:

- What is sarcopenia?
- What parameters define sarcopenia?
- What variables will measure them, and what measurement tools and cut-off points will be used?
- How does sarcopenia relate to other diseases/conditions?

Table 2.2 Criteria for the diagnosis of sarcopenia

Diagnosis is based on documentation of criterion 1 plus (criterion 2 or criterion 3).
1. Low muscle mass
2. Low muscle strength
3. Low physical performance

EWGSOP defines sarcopenia *as a syndrome characterized by progressive and generalized loss of skeletal muscle mass and strength with a risk of adverse outcomes, such as physical disability, poor quality of life, and death.* The operational definition recommends using the presence of both low muscle mass + low muscle function (strength or performance) for the diagnosis of sarcopenia. Thus diagnosis requires documentation of criterion 1 plus documentation of either criterion 2 or criterion 3 (Table 2.2).

Although this definition intends to be inclusive, it is acknowledged that sarcopenia is a geriatric syndrome, and the cause or causes that lead into it are complex and interacting. Thus, EWGSOP suggests that dividing sarcopenia into categories may be helpful in clinical practice, and proposes the use of the terms primary sarcopenia and secondary sarcopenia. Sarcopenia can be considered *primary* (or age-related) when no other cause is evident but aging itself, while sarcopenia can be considered *secondary* when one or more other causes are evident (Table 2.3). In many older people, the aetiology of sarcopenia is multifactorial so that it may not be possible to characterize each individual as having a primary or secondary condition.

Sarcopenia staging, which reflects the severity of the condition, is also considered here as a concept that can help guide clinical management of the condition. EWGSOP suggests a conceptual staging as *presarcopenia, sarcopenia*, and *severe sarcopenia* (Table 2.4). The *presarcopenia* stage is characterized by low muscle mass without impact on muscle strength or physical performance. This stage can only be identified by techniques that measure muscle mass accurately and in reference to standard populations. The *sarcopenia* stage is characterized by low muscle mass, plus low muscle strength *or* low physical performance. *Severe sarcopenia* is the stage identified when all three criteria of the definition are met

Table 2.3 Sarcopenia categories by cause

Primary sarcopenia	Examples
Age-related sarcopenia	No other cause evident except aging
Secondary sarcopenia	
Activity-related sarcopenia	Can result from bed rest, sedentary lifestyle, deconditioning, or zero-gravity conditions
Disease-related sarcopenia	Associated with advanced organ failure (heart, lung, liver, kidney, brain), inflammatory disease, malignancy, or endocrine disease
Nutrition-related sarcopenia	Results from inadequate dietary intake of energy and/or protein, as with malabsorption, gastrointestinal disorders, or use of medications that cause anorexia

Table 2.4 EWGSOP conceptual stages of sarcopenia

Stage	Muscle mass	Muscle strength		Performance
Presarcopenia	↓			
Sarcopenia	↓	↓	Or	↓
Severe sarcopenia	↓	↓		↓

(low muscle mass, low muscle strength, and low physical performance). Recognizing stages of sarcopenia may help in selecting treatments and setting appropriate recovery goals, and staging may be a link with the following definition.

Society for Sarcopenia, Cachexia and Wasting Disorders

The Society for Sarcopenia, Cachexia and Wasting Disorders published its consensus definition in 2011 [19], after a meeting with the stated purpose to find a definition or set of definitions that are universally acceptable and can lead to easily definable endpoints for clinical trials. The definition developed would:

- be a meaningful surrogate for clinically useful endpoints (decline in activities of daily living, hospitalization, nursing home residence, injurious falls or mortality);
- allow for treatments that worked in ways different from increasing muscle mass;
- include only measurements that have been demonstrated to lead longitudinally to clinically meaningful outcomes and have definable cut points based on data;
- be independent of the molecular target(s) for drug development.

It was decided that 'sarcopenia with limited mobility' would be an acceptable term to define persons with a need for therapeutic interventions. This is a specific syndrome with clear loss of muscle mass and a clear target for intervention.

Sarcopenia with limited mobility is defined as a person with muscle loss whose walking speed is equal to or less than 1 m/s or who walks less than 400 m during a 6 minute walk. The person should also have a lean appendicular mass corrected for height squared of more than two standard deviations below that of healthy persons between 20 to 30 years of age of the same ethnic group. The limitation in mobility should not be clearly attributable to the direct effect of specific disease such as peripheral vascular disease, or central or peripheral nervous system disorders, dementia, or cachexia.

This definition also tried to define targets for interventions: interventions are considered clinically significant if they increase the 6 minute walk by 50 meters or they increase gait speed by 0.1 m/sec.

Although the EWGSOP looks mainly to sarcopenia as an age-related condition, this group leaves open the question of whether sarcopenia as a term should be limited to use in older persons or used as a general term for adults of any age. Thus, while emphasizing that this is a common condition in older age, the panel was not comfortable in limiting the definition to only older persons.

COMMON ASPECTS OF RECENT DEFINITIONS

Although both definitions are clearly different, probably due to a different focus or objective of each of the panels, they both seem to reach a high level of agreement in some aspects of sarcopenia. Reviewing these aspects may lead into a better insight in the concept of sarcopenia.

Sarcopenia as a syndrome

Sarcopenia can be considered an age-related process of normative ageing, a disease or a syndrome. Both definitions consider that sarcopenia (or sarcopenia with limited mobility) is a syndrome, not a disease or normal aging. Moreover, sarcopenia can be best viewed as a geriatric syndrome [20].

Geriatric syndromes are common, complex, and costly states of impaired health in older individuals, that result from incompletely understood interactions of disease and age on multiple systems, producing a constellation of signs and symptoms. Sarcopenia is prevalent in older populations, has multiple contributing factors – the aging process over the life course, early life developmental influences, less-than-optimal diet, bed rest or sedentary lifestyle, chronic diseases, and certain drug treatments – and is linked with other comorbid disorders, impaired mobility, increased risk of falls and fractures, impaired ability to perform activities of daily living and increased risk of death [21–23].

Considering sarcopenia as a syndrome mandates a multidimensional approach to understand its pathophysiology, to investigate its aetiology in affected individuals, to define the molecular targets for intervention, and probably to successfully treat it.

Not only muscle mass

Although muscle mass is a constitutive part of sarcopenia, the concept of using muscle mass alone in definitions of sarcopenia has probably been stretched to its limits. Measurement of muscle mass is quite straight (although many problems persist, as described in Chapters 14 and 15), easy to understand and amenable to be used in big epidemiological studies. However, muscle mass is not enough.

One of the definitions has opted to define sarcopenia by adding reduced muscle function and/or physical performance to the loss of muscle mass. The second has opted to add poor physical performance (not due to other conditions) to the loss of muscle mass. In both cases, it seems evident that clinical consequences of muscle wasting have to be considered if sarcopenia wants to have a place in clinical practice.

Physical performance

The clinical relevance of sarcopenia depends on its being a marker of impaired outcomes, mortality being the most striking, but perhaps not the most relevant. Disability is a major concern in older people, and sarcopenia and frailty are emerging as stepping stones in the path from good health and function to disability and death. The earliest identification of the impairments that may push a subject to fall down the slope of disability would theoretically allow for an early, more effective intervention to avoid disability or reduce its speed.

The EWGSOP opted to use two dimensions that may help identify those individuals with sarcopenia that are in the highest need of intervention (muscle strength and physical performance), and to propose a wide range of methods to measure these dimensions. The SSCWD opted for a more practical approach, choosing two single measurements of physical performance (gait speed and 6 minute walk). In both cases, physical performance (not established disability [24]) emerges as a key parameter to be measured in sarcopenia.

Sarcopenia and cachexia

Sarcopenia is only one in a list of conditions associated with prominent muscle wasting, malnutrition and cachexia being perhaps the most evident. These conditions interact so deeply, that defining them as different entities is a complex task [25,26]. The main reasons to differentiate between these conditions are to encourage research into age related mechanisms and to guide targeted and appropriate therapy for each of them.

Cachexia is widely recognized in older adults as severe wasting accompanying disease states. Definitions of cachexia are also evolving in the last decade, but in most cases it includes the concept of inflammation [27–31] as a leading mechanism into muscle wasting. Thus, most cachectic individuals are also sarcopenic, but most sarcopenic individuals are not considered cachectic. Sarcopenia is one of the elements of some proposed definition for cachexia [27]. Both new definitions of sarcopenia agree with the concept that cachexia and sarcopenia are different. However, while the SSCWD definition excludes cachectic individuals from the definition of sarcopenia, the EWGSOP accepts that cachexia may be part of disease induced sarcopenia.

OPEN AREAS FOR DISCUSSION

Research and scientific discussion in sarcopenia are blooming, so many key elements of the definitions of sarcopenia are still waiting for more evidence to support before they settle down. A brief review of these open aspects may also help to gain some insight into this ongoing debate.

Case finding and populations at risk

Identifying subjects with sarcopenia, both for clinical practice, and for selection of individuals for clinical trials, seems to be an important task. Obviously, this case finding is directly linked with the definition used. However, case finding may be started in the general population, or by identifying some risk groups.

EWGSOP chooses a population approach, by suggesting screening all patients over 65 years. However, it proposes a gradual approach, starting with the measure of gait speed, and using a cutoff of less than 0.8 meters per second to identify the risk for sarcopenia [32]. Those with low gait speed will go on with further testing to determine if they reach full diagnostic criteria for sarcopenia. This approach is now being tested [33].

SSCWD uses a lower age threshold (60 years), but recommends screening for sarcopenia with limited mobility only in those who are falling, who feel that their walking speed has decreased, who have had a recent hospitalization, who have been on a prolonged bed rest, have problems arising from a chair or need to use an assistive device for walking. This approach of looking for risk factors, clinical suspicion or functional impact to detect populations at risk has also been proposed by others [20].

Relevant outcomes

While reduced mobility and functionality are increasingly prevalent in older people, only a handful of clinical trials are under way to test potential sarcopenia treatments. The absence of standardized primary outcomes is a major challenge for the design of such studies. A very active debate is ongoing as of what outcomes should be used in sarcopenia research [34–37].

For intervention trials, EWGSOP recommends three primary outcome variables—muscle mass, muscle strength and physical performance. Other outcomes (ADL, quality of life, metabolic and biochemical markers, falls or admission to nursing home or hospital) are considered secondary by this group and of particular interest in specific research areas and intervention trials.

SSCWD opts again for a more practical approach. It states that at present there is no clear consensus pertaining to the magnitude of change in muscle mass that is predictive of clinically meaningful outcomes, and recommends that gait speeds equal or less than 1 m/s are predictive of poor outcomes, with a clinically significant improvement in gait speed of at least 0.1 m/sec as being useful. For the 6 minute walking test, which has already been utilized as a measure for drug approval by several regulatory agencies in peripheral vascular disease and pulmonary hypertension, it is recommended that, in persons who can walk at least 100m, a clinically significant change would be >50 meters.

Reference populations and cutoff values

For any given parameter included in a definition, there is a need to identify cutoff points that separate normal from abnormal values. Except in the rare occasion where disease and health are extremely separate, the choice of cutoff values is arbitrary by nature, as it depends upon the measurement technique chosen and availability of reference studies and populations. In sarcopenia research, the cutoffs determined are usually arbitrary, as the associations between variables and outcomes are usually continuous in nature. The choice of the right reference populations may also influence cutoff points [18].

Both definitions recommend the use of normative (healthy young adult) rather than other predictive reference populations, with cutoff points at two standard deviations below the mean of healthy persons between 20 to 30 years of age of the same ethnic group. However, high quality reference populations are still lacking for most groups. More research is urgently needed in order to obtain good reference values for populations around the world.

Muscle fat and sarcopenic obesity

The problem posed by the infiltration of muscle by fat and other qualitative aspects that define muscle quality is only starting to be understood [38–40]. One reason for this

Table 2.5   Comparison of three definitions of frailty

Cardiovascular Health Study	Study of Osteoporotic Fractures	International Association of Nutrition and Aging
• Unintentional weight loss • Poor grip strength • Reduced energy level • Slow walking speed • Low level of physical activity	• Weight loss • Inability to raise from a chair 5 times without using arms • Reduced energy level	• Fatigue • Resistance (climb one flight of stairs) • Aerobic (walk one block) • Illnesses (>5) • Loss of weight

inconsistency is the infiltration into muscle by fat which is a powerful predictor of future disability and mortality [6]. This seems to be an important aspect of the definition of sarcopenia. However, measurement is complex and expensive, and its relative weight compared with other parameters still waits to be known.

Some definitions of muscle mass, related to other anthropometric parameters, may miss the importance of the relative amount of muscle and fat in body composition. Sarcopenic obesity (obesity associated with low muscle mass) may be promoted by excess energy intake, physical inactivity, low-grade inflammation, insulin resistance and changes in hormonal milieu [12]. Considering both obesity and muscle mass and function may be a better predictor of outcomes than using only muscle related parameters [41]. No definition of sarcopenia has yet been able to disentangle the relation between muscle mass and body fat in a clear way (see Chapter 13).

Sarcopenia and frailty

Like sarcopenia and cachexia, frailty is a developing concept, and a number of different definitions for frailty have been developed (Table 2.5) [42;43]. Generally speaking, frailty is the consequence of age-related cumulative declines across multiple physiologic systems, with impaired homeostatic reserve and a reduced capacity of the organism to withstand stress, thus increasing vulnerability to adverse health outcomes including falls, hospitalization, institutionalization and mortality [44]. The conditions of frailty and sarcopenia overlap; most frail older people exhibit sarcopenia, and some older people with sarcopenia are also frail. The general concept of frailty, however, goes beyond physical factors to encompass psychological and social dimensions as well, including cognitive status, social support and other environmental factors. These complex relations are further explored in Chapter 11.

SUMMARY

Sarcopenia was originally defined as age-related muscle mass. More recent definitions have extended this to include muscle strength, function and limited mobility. These definitions seem more likely to be predictors of poor outcome and to be useful for clinical trials of drugs used to treat sarcopenia (muscle loss). The evolving process of refining the definition of sarcopenia in accordance with the clinical needs and improved understanding of the complex etiology of this condition will continue [45].

REFERENCES

1. Rosenberg IH (1997) Sarcopenia: origins and clinical relevance. J Nutr 127: 990S-991S.

2. Baumgartner RN, Koehler KM, Gallagher D, Romero L, Heymsfield SB, Ross RR, Garry PJ, Lindeman RD (1998) Epidemiology of sarcopenia among the elderly in New Mexico. Am J Epidemiol 147: 755–763.

3. von HS, Morley JE, Anker SD (2010) An overview of sarcopenia: facts and numbers on prevalence and clinical impact. J Cachex Sarcopenia Muscle 1: 129–133.

4. Cummings SR, Bates D, Black DM (2002) Clinical use of bone densitometry: scientific review. JAMA 288: 1889–1897.

5. Visser M, Deeg DJ, Lips P, Harris TB, Bouter LM (2000) Skeletal muscle mass and muscle strength in relation to lower-extremity performance in older men and women. J Am Geriatr Soc 48: 381–386.

6. Visser M, Goodpaster BH, Kritchevsky SB, Newman AB, Nevitt M, Rubin SM, Simonsick EM, Harris TB (2005) Muscle mass, muscle strength, and muscle fat infiltration as predictors of incident mobility limitations in well-functioning older persons. J Gerontol A Biol Sci Med Sci 60: 324–333.

7. Newman AB, Kupelian V, Visser M, Simonsick EM, Goodpaster BH, Kritchevsky SB, Tylavsky FA, Rubin SM, Harris TB (2006) Strength, but not muscle mass, is associated with mortality in the health, aging and body composition study cohort. J Gerontol A Biol Sci Med Sci 61: 72–7.

8. Gale CR, Martyn CN, Cooper C, Sayer AA (2007) Grip strength, body composition, and mortality. Int J Epidemiol 36: 228–235.

9. Hairi NN, Cumming RG, Naganathan V, Handelsman DJ, Le Couteur DG, Creasey H, Waite LM, Seibel MJ, Sambrook PN (2010) Loss of muscle strength, mass (sarcopenia), and quality (specific force) and its relationship with functional limitation and physical disability: the Concord Health and Ageing in Men Project. J Am Geriatr Soc 58: 2055–2062.

10. Goodpaster BH, Park SW, Harris TB, Kritchevsky SB, Nevitt M, Schwartz AV, Simonsick EM, Tylavsky FA, Visser M, Newman AB (2006) The loss of skeletal muscle strength, mass, and quality in older adults: the health, aging and body composition study. J Gerontol A Biol Sci Med Sci 61: 1059–1064.

11. Janssen I, Baumgartner RN, Rss RR, Rosenberg IH, Roubenoff R (2004) Skeletal muscle cut-points associated with elevated physical disability risk in older men and women. Am J Epidemiol 159: 413–421.

12. Stenholm S, Harris TB, Rantanen T, Visser M, Kritchevsky SB, Ferrucci L (2008) Sarcopenic obesity: definition, cause and consequences. Curr Opin Clin Nutr Metab Care 11: 693–700.

13. Lawler JM, Hindle A (2011) Living in a Box or Call of the Wild? Revisiting Lifetime Inactivity and Sarcopenia. Antioxid Redox Signal.

14. Clark BC, Manini TM (2008) Sarcopenia $= / =$ dynapenia. J Gerontol A Biol Sci Med Sci 63: 829–34.

15. Lupoli L, Sergi G, Coin A, Perissinotto E, Volpato S, Busetto L, Inelmen EM, Enzi G (2004) Body composition in underweight elderly subjects: reliability of bioelectrical impedence analysis. Clin Nutr 23: 1371–1380.

16. Janssen I, Heymsfield SB, Ross R (2002) Low relative skeletal muscle mass (sarcopenia) in older persons is associated with functional impairment and physical disability. J Am Geriatr Soc 50: 889–896.

17. Newman AB, Kupelian V, Visser M, Simonsick EM, Goodpaster B, Nevitt M, Kritchevsky SB, Tylavsky FA, Rubin SM, Harris B, Health AS (2003) Sarcopenia: alternative definitions and association with lower extremity function. J Am Geriatr Soc 51: 1602–1609.

18. Cruz-Jentoft AJ, Baeyens JP, Bauer JM, Boirie Y, Cederholm T, Landi F, Martin FC, Michel JP, Rolland Y, Schneider SM, Topinkova E, Vandewoude M, Zamboni M (2010) Sarcopenia: European consensus on definition and diagnosis: Report of the European Working Group on Sarcopenia in Older People. Age Ageing 39: 412–423.

19. Morley JE, Abbatecola AM, Argiles JM, Baracos V, Bauer J, Bhasin S, Cederholm T, Coats AJ, Cummings SR, Evans WJ, Fearon K, Ferrucci L, Fielding RA, Guralnik JM, Harris TB, Inui A, Kalantar-Zadeh K, Kirwan BA, Mantovani G, Muscaritoli M, Newman AB, Rossi-Fanelli F, Rosano GM, Roubenoff R, Schambelan M, Sokol GH, Storer TW, Vellas B, von HS, Yeh SS, Anker SD (2011) Sarcopenia with limited mobility: an international consensus. J Am Med Dir Assoc 12: 403–409.

20. Cruz-Jentoft AJ, Landi F, TopinkovÃi E, Michel JP (2010) Understanding sarcopenia as a geriatric syndrome. Curr Opin Clin Nutr Metab Care 13: 1–7.

21. Sayer AA, Syddall H, Martin H, Patel H, Baylis D, Cooper C (2008) The developmental origins of sarcopenia. J Nutr Health Aging 12: 427–432.

22. Laurentani F, Russo CR, Bandinelli S, Bartali B, Cavazzini C, DiIorio A, Corsi AM, Rantanen T, Guralnik JM, Ferruci L (2003) Age-associated changes in skeletal muscles and their effect on mobility: an operational diagnosis of sarcopenia. J Appl Physiol 95: 1851–1860.

23. Rolland Y, Czerwinski S, Bellan van Kan G, Morley JE, Cesari M, Onder G, Woo J, Baumgartner R, Pillard F, Boirie Y, Chumlea WM, Vellas B (2008) Sarcopenia: its assessment, etiology, pathogenesis, consequences and future perspectives. J Nutr Health Aging 12: 433–450.

24. Working Group on Functional Outcome Measures for Clinical Trials (2008) Functional outcomes for clinical trials in frail older persons: time to be moving. J Gerontol A Biol Sci Med Sci 63: 160–164.

25. Thomas DR (2007) Loss of skeletal muscle mass in aging: examining the relationship of starvation, sarcopenia and cachexia. Clin Nutr 26: 389–399.

26. Evans WJ (2010) Skeletal muscle loss: cachexia, sarcopenia, and inactivity. Am J Clin Nutr 91: 1123S–1127S.

27. Muscaritoli M, Anker SD, Argiles J, Aversa Z, Bauer JM, Biolo G, Boirie Y, Bosaeus I, Cederholm T, Costelli P, Fearon KC, Laviano A, Maggio M, Fanelli FR, Schneider SM, Schols A, Sieber CC (2010) Consensus definition of sarcopenia, cachexia and pre-cachexia: Joint document elaborated by Special Interest Groups (SIG) 'cachexia-anorexia in chronic wasting diseases' and 'nutrition in geriatrics. Clin NutrEpub

28. Fearon K, Strasser F, Anker SD, Bosaeus I, Bruera E, Fainsinger RL, Jatoi A, Loprinzi C, MacDonald N, Mantovani G, Davis M, Muscaritoli M, Ottery F, Radbruch L, Ravasco P, Walsh D, Wilcock A, Kaasa S, Baracos VE (2011) Definition and classification of cancer cachexia: an international consensus. Lancet Oncol 12: 489–495.

29. Rolland Y, Van Kan GA, Gillette-Guyonnet S, Vellas B (2011) Cachexia versus sarcopenia. Curr Opin Clin Nutr Metab Care 14: 15–21.

30. Evans WJ, Morley JE, Argiles J, Bales C, Baracos V, Guttridge D, Jatoi A, Kalantar-Zadeh K, Lochs H, Mantovani G, Marks D, Mitch WE, Muscaritoli M, Najand A, Ponikowski P, Rossi Fanelli F, Schambelan M, Schols A, Schuster M, Thomas D, Wolfe R, Anker SD (2008) Cachexia: a new definition. Clin Nutr 27: 793–799.

31. Morley JE, Anker SD, Evans WJ (2009) Cachexia and aging: an update based on the Fourth International Cachexia Meeting. J Nutr Health Aging 13: 47–55.

32. Abellan van Kan G, Rolland Y, Onder G (2009) Gait speed as a marker of adverse outcomes. J Nutr Health and Aging 13: 881–889.

33. Landi F, Liperoti R, Fusco D, Mastropaolo S, Quattrociocchi D, Proia A, Russo A, Bernabei R, Onder G (2011) Prevalence and Risk Factors of Sarcopenia Among Nursing Home Older Residents. J Gerontol A Biol Sci Med Sci.

34. Vandewoude MF, Cederholm T, Cruz-Jentoft AJ (2011) Relevant outcomes in intervention trials for sarcopenia. J Am Geriatr Soc 59: 1566–1567.

35. Abellan van Kan G, Cameron CW, Gillette-Guyonet S, Houles M, Dupuy C, Rolland Y, Vellas B (2011) Clinical trials on sarcopenia: methodological issues regarding phase 3 trials. Clin Geriatr Med 27: 471–482.

36. Brass EP, Sietsema KE (2011) Considerations in the development of drugs to treat sarcopenia. J Am Geriatr Soc 59: 530–535.

37. Evans CJ, Chiou CF, Fitzgerald KA, Evans WJ, Ferrell BR, Dale W, Fried LP, Gandra SR, nee-Sommers B, Patrick DL (2011) Development of a new patient-reported outcome measure in sarcopenia. J Am Med Dir Assoc 12: 226–233.

38. Song MY, Ruts E, Kim J, Janumala I, Heymsfield S, Gallagher D (2004) Sarcopenia and increased adipose tissue infiltration of muscle in elderly African American women. Am J Clin Nutr 79: 874–880.

39. Delmonico MJ, Harris TB, Visser M, Park SW, Conroy MB, Velasquez-Mieyer P, Boudreau R, Manini TM, Nevitt M, Newman AB, Goodpaster BH (2009) Longitudinal study of muscle strength, quality, and adipose tissue infiltration. Am J Clin Nutr 90: 1579–1585.

40. Koster A, Ding J, Stenholm S, Caserotti P, Houston DK, Nicklas BJ, You T, Lee JS, Visser M, Newman AB, Schwartz AV, Cauley JA, Tylavsky FA, Goodpaster BH, Kritchevsky SB, Harris TB (2011) Does the Amount of Fat Mass Predict Age-Related Loss of Lean Mass, Muscle Strength, and Muscle Quality in Older Adults? J Gerontol A Biol Sci Med Sci 66A: 888–895.

41. Visser M (2011) Obesity, sarcopenia and their functional consequences in old age. Proc Nutr Soc 70: 114–118.

42. Fried LP, Tangen CM, Walston J, Newman AB, Hirsch C, Gottdiener J, Seeman T, Tracy R, Kop WJ, Burke G, McBurnie MA (2001) Frailty in older adults: evidence for a phenotype. J Gerontol A Biol Sci Med Sci 56: M146-M156.

43. Abellan van KG, Rolland YM, Morley JE, Vellas B (2008) Frailty: toward a clinical definition. J Am Med Dir Assoc 9: 71–72.

44. Bauer JM, Sieber CC (2008) Sarcopenia and frailty: a clinician's controversial point of view. Exp Gerontol 43: 674–678.

45. Cederholm TE, Bauer JM, Boirie Y, Schneider SM, Sieber CC, Rolland Y (2011) Toward a definition of sarcopenia. Clin Geriatr Med 27: 341–353.

46. Fearon K, Evans WJ, Anker SD (2011) Myopenia-a new universal term for muscle wasting. J Cachex Sarcopenia Muscle 2: 1–3.

CHAPTER 3

Muscle Biology and mTORC1 Signaling in Aging

Blake B. Rasmussen

Department of Nutrition & Metabolism, Sealy Center on Aging, University of TX Medical Branch, Galveston, TX, USA

Elena Volpi

Department of Internal Medicine, Division of Geriatrics, Sealy Center on Aging, University of TX Medical Branch, Galveston, TX, USA

INTRODUCTION

Aging is accompanied by an involuntary loss of skeletal muscle mass, strength and function, termed sarcopenia. This loss of muscle occurs at a rate of 3-8% per decade after the age of thirty with a higher rate of muscle loss with advanced age [1–2]. Sarcopenia is associated with a decreased metabolic rate [3], decreased strength [4,5], increased risk of falls and fractures [6], greater chance of disability and a loss of functionality in older individuals [7–13], leading to increased morbidity [14,15], and eventually the loss of independence [8]. Recent estimates show that one-quarter to one-half of men and women aged 65 and older are likely sarcopenic as defined by an appendicular skeletal muscle mass/height^2 less than two standard deviations below the mean for young, healthy adults [14,15]. The population of individuals over 60 years of age is expected to triple in the next fifty years, such that the resulting significant impact on health care systems will increase the focus on the necessity to maintain good health during aging not only to prevent many chronic diseases but also to remain independent. A pivotal factor in the ability to remain healthy and functionally independent is the capacity to preserve skeletal muscle mass and strength.

Skeletal muscle in humans contains 50-75% of all proteins and is the body's primary amino acid reservoir [16,17]. The functions of skeletal muscle include control of movement and posture, regulation of metabolism, storage of energy and nitrogen, a main source of amino acids for the brain and immune system, and a substrate for malnutrition/starvation, injury/wound healing and disease [16–18]. Maintaining body protein mass is critical not only for remaining physically independent, but also for survival. An excessive loss of body proteins results in impaired respiration and circulation due to muscle weakness, reduced

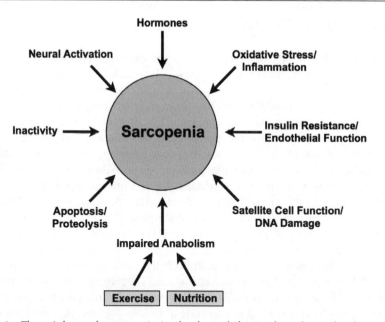

Figure 3.1 The etiology of sarcopenia is clearly multifactorial as shown by the numerous factors known to contribute to sarcopenia. However, the control of overall muscle mass is ultimately due to an imbalance between the rates of muscle protein synthesis and breakdown. Exercise and nutrition are potent stimulators of muscle protein synthesis and can be utilized in the development of clinical interventions designed to prevent sarcopenia.

immune function due to lack of nutrients, and an inadequate barrier effect of the epithelia, which eventually will result in death [17]. In support of the importance of maintaining skeletal muscle mass, strength and function, a recent study has demonstrated that all cause, as well as cancer based, mortality was lowest for men in the highest tertile of strength, an indicator of high muscle mass [19].

The mechanisms underlying the development of sarcopenia are not completely understood and most likely multifactorial, but significant progress has been made over the past few years to identify some of the major contributors. On a muscle-specific level, sarcopenia is characterized by muscle fiber necrosis, grouping of fiber types, atrophy of type II muscle fibers and a loss of satellite cell content in type II fibers [20–27]. Another consequence of aging on skeletal muscle is reduced muscle specific and whole body oxidative capacity [28,29]. These changes place older individuals at a greater risk of developing chronic diseases such as insulin resistance, hyperlipidemia and hypertension. Figure 3.1 provides a summary of the physiological changes and potential mechanisms that contribute to sarcopenia, although a basic understanding of the underlying mechanisms driving these changes is still somewhat elusive. A better understanding of the cellular mechanisms leading to sarcopenia is required to establish evidence-based interventions to prevent the onset of symptoms associated with sarcopenia and to promote the independent living of older adults. This chapter focuses on the basic mechanisms that primarily impact muscle protein homeostasis.

MUSCLE PROTEIN TURNOVER IN AGING

Although the mechanisms leading to sarcopenia are likely numerous, a major result will be a disproportionately higher rate of muscle protein breakdown relative to muscle protein synthesis. Such an imbalance between breakdown and synthesis is smaller in size than that observed in wasting conditions, such as bed rest, immobilization or trauma; however, over time it can lead to gradual and significant loss of muscle. In fact, studies show a different basal gene and protein expression of molecules associated with protein synthesis and breakdown in older adults [30–34] leading one to predict that aging alters basal muscle protein turnover. However, basal rates of muscle protein breakdown are not altered by aging [35–39], and while some studies have reported a decrease in basal muscle protein synthesis rate with age [40,41], others [35–39,42] could not confirm those findings in older adults. It is also possible that very small differences in muscle protein synthesis and/or breakdown in the basal postabsorptive state may be undetectable. For example, if a difference as little as 10% in basal muscle protein synthesis were detected between young and older adults with no differences in breakdown (assuming an individual is in the basal state for approximately 16 hr/d and the response to feeding and other stimuli are constant with aging), this would result in a $\sim$17% net loss of skeletal muscle in one year. This clearly does not occur, as sarcopenia results in a gradual loss in skeletal muscle over decades and such changes in basal muscle protein turnover would be too small to detect even with current mass spectrometry methodologies. With no detectable age-related differences in basal muscle protein net balance, it must be inferred that the role of protein turnover in the development of sarcopenia is most likely due to alterations during other metabolic conditions, such as during muscle contraction or nutrient intake. Recent studies suggest that aging is associated with an impaired ability of skeletal muscle to properly respond to anabolic stimuli (i.e., exercise, feeding, insulin). The next sections will examine how muscle protein turnover is regulated at the cellular level and whether aging alters the protein anabolic response to nutrients and physical activity.

REGULATION OF MUSCLE PROTEIN TURNOVER BY THE mTORC1 SIGNALING PATHWAY

The regulation of skeletal muscle protein turnover is multifaceted and involves the coordination of several processes including gene transcription, protein translation and proteolysis (as well as various pre- and post-transcriptional modifications). However, recent work in humans has identified the mammalian target of rapamycin complex 1 (mTORC1) signaling pathway as being required to stimulate muscle protein synthesis in humans in response to muscle contraction and nutrition [43,44]. The control of the mTORC1 pathway is displayed in Figure 3.2. Nutrient, hormonal and exercise stimuli can signal through mTORC1 to control the rate of muscle protein synthesis, an important modulator of muscle growth. The first study to demonstrate the importance of the mTORC1 signaling pathway in the control of in vivo muscle hypertrophy found a positive correlation between the acute phosphorylation of the downstream mTORC1 effector, p70 ribosomal S6 kinase 1 (S6K1), and the increase in muscle mass over 6 weeks of electrical stimulation in rodent hindlimb muscles [45]. This association has also been reported in human subjects after 12 weeks of resistance

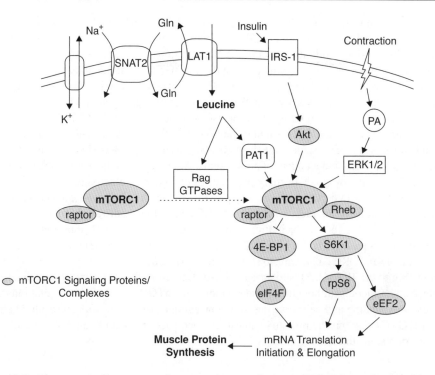

Figure 3.2 The mammalian target of rapamycin complex 1 (mTORC1) signaling pathway plays a central role in the control of muscle protein synthesis in human skeletal muscle. Insulin, essential amino acids and muscle contraction can activate mTORC1 signaling independent of each other. Insulin activates mTORC1 through the well-known insulin signaling pathway (IRS-1/Akt). Amino acids such as leucine enter the muscle cell via amino acid transporters (e.g., SNAT2 and LAT1) and activate mTORC1 via a Rag GTPase mechanism. Muscle contraction from exercise is thought to activate mTORC1 directly by phosphatidic acid (PA) or indirectly via ERK1/2. Aging is associated with an impaired ability to activate mTORC1 signaling and muscle protein synthesis in response to insulin, insufficient amounts of protein/amino acids, or exercise. The combination of a sufficient amount of protein or amino acid supplementation following exercise is capable of restoring both mTORC1 signaling and muscle protein synthesis.

exercise training [46]. The first mechanistic study to demonstrate the key regulatory role of mTORC1 in muscle hypertrophy used rapamycin, a direct inhibitor of mTORC1, to block muscle hypertrophy following functional overload in rodents [47], further suggesting an important role for the mTOR pathway in controlling skeletal muscle growth.

The mTOR protein is a large molecule with many regulatory domains and exists in two protein complexes: mTORC1 and mTORC2. The mTORC1 complex is sensitive to rapamycin and is directly involved in the control of muscle protein synthesis and hypertrophy [47]. Two downstream targets of mTORC1 stimulate translation initiation and elongation: S6K1 and eukaryotic initiation factor 4E-binding protein (4E-BP1). S6K1 is activated upon phosphorylation, enabling the kinase to phosphorylate several targets [48], including ribosomal protein S6 (rpS6) [49] and eukaryotic elongation factor 2 (eEF2) kinase [50]. Phosphorylation of rpS6 enhances cell size and proliferation [51], although its precise role is somewhat uncertain. The phosphorylation of 4E-BP1 by mTORC1 inhibits the binding of eIF4E to 4E-BP1, which promotes eIF4E to complex with eIF4G and promotes the formation of the translation initiation complex [52]. Inhibition of eEF2 kinase by mTORC1 causes a dephosphorylation of eEF2, which facilitates the mediation of the ribosome to the mRNA following the addition of each amino acid [53]. For example, insulin activation of Akt (protein kinase B) can directly activate mTORC1 through phosphorylation [54] or indirectly by phosphorylating (and inhibiting) tuberous sclerosis complex 2 (TSC2) [55,56]. Proteins, and essential amino acids in particular, can also directly activate mTORC1 signaling, most likely through a Rag dependent mechanism as shown in Figure 3.2. Muscle contraction also activates mTORC1 independent of amino acids, Akt and growth factors [57–59]. Although the mTORC1 pathway is a primary regulator of cell growth, other signaling pathways are also involved in hypertrophy. For example, the extracellular signal-regulated kinase 1/2 (ERK1/2) pathway interacts with the mTORC1 signaling pathway through direct interaction with TSC2 [60,61] or indirectly by phosphorylation of p90 ribosomal protein S6 kinase polypeptide 1 (RSK1) [62]. ERK1/2 can also enhance protein synthesis independent of the mTORC1 pathway [63], through MAP kinase-interacting kinase 1 (MNK1) signaling to eIF4E [64]. Most data on mTORC1 control of muscle size are obtained from non-human models, although our understanding of mTORC1 in human skeletal muscle is rapidly expanding and below we describe how aging is associated with an impaired ability of mTORC1 and muscle protein synthesis to adequately respond to anabolic stimuli such as nutrients, insulin and physical exercise.

AGING AND THE IMPAIRED MUSCLE PROTEIN RESPONSE TO ANABOLIC STIMULI

Nutrient intake. Nutrition is a fundamental anabolic stimulus for skeletal muscle proteins as it allows for replenishing the essential amino acids lost with oxidation during fasting. A number of studies have shown that amino acids can stimulate muscle protein synthesis and improve net protein balance in young and older persons [42–69]. Essential amino acids, leucine in particular, can directly stimulate muscle protein synthesis in the elderly, while non-essential amino acids do not appear to provide any additional anabolic advantage for muscle proteins [69]. Among the essential amino acids, the branched-chain amino acid leucine has been shown to be a key regulator of muscle protein synthesis in both humans and rats [70–72]. Leucine activates mTORC1 signaling which stimulates translation initiation in the skeletal muscle cells by increasing the phosphorylation of several signaling proteins including S6K1 and 4E-BP1 [70,71,73,74].

However, although large amounts of essential amino acids exert similar effects in young and older persons [42,68], there are age-related differences in the muscle anabolic response to submaximal doses of essential amino acids. Specifically, older subjects had significantly less muscle protein accretion than younger subjects following the ingestion of a 7 g EAA bolus [75,76]. In addition, while in young men a 7 g essential amino acid bolus containing 26% (1.7 g) of leucine stimulated muscle protein synthesis to the same extent as a 7 g essential amino acid bolus containing 41% (2.8 g) of leucine, in older men only the 41% leucine EAA bolus was able to effectively increase protein synthesis in older adults. These data are consistent with data demonstrating that the isocaloric ingestion of an essential amino acid mixture containing 2.79 g of leucine increased muscle protein synthesis to a significantly greater degree in older adults than did ingestion of the same amount of a whole protein supplement, whey protein, containing only 1.75 g leucine [77]. It has also been found that leucine supplementation improved the muscle protein anabolic response in older adults independent of hyperaminoacidemia [78].

On the other hand, no major differences have been reported between young and older adults with regards to the essential amino acid dose capable of maximally stimulating muscle protein synthesis and metabolism [67–69,79–81]. Based on these studies it appears that aged muscle may be less sensitive to the anabolic effects of low doses of leucine and protein than younger muscle, while it maintains an adequate responsiveness to higher amino acid doses. However, it is also becoming evident that a ceiling effect likely exists, beyond which acute exposure of skeletal muscle to excess amino acids will not exert any additional benefit. While adequate doses of amino acids can still stimulate the activation of skeletal muscle protein synthesis in older adults, there is evidence that the protein anabolic response of muscle to mixed nutrients including carbohydrate is blunted with aging [82,83] due to reduced mTORC1 signaling [82]. These observations have led researchers to explore the potential role that insulin plays in the development of sarcopenia.

Insulin. Insulin stimulates muscle protein synthesis and anabolism in young adults regardless of glucose tolerance, and provided that amino acid delivery to the muscle is not decreased [84–92]. However, a series of studies have shown that aging is associated with an inability of insulin to stimulate muscle protein synthesis and net amino acid uptake in healthy, glucose tolerant persons [91–93] which is associated with reduced mTORC1 signaling [91,94,95]. This is a true insulin resistance of skeletal muscle proteins because supraphysiological doses of insulin can overcome this problem and induce an increase in mTORC1 signaling, muscle protein synthesis and net anabolism [95]. The decline in the muscle protein anabolic response to insulin is likely responsible for the observed reduction in muscle protein anabolism following mixed feeding in elders [36,82], and may contribute to the development of sarcopenia. Recent studies (see below) have also highlighted that in addition to a blunted mTORC1 signaling, the age-related insulin resistance of muscle protein metabolism is associated with endothelial dysfunction and a consequent impairment in muscle vasodilation [91,93,–95].

Exercise. Physical activity is essential in reducing physical disability [96–98]. An excellent protection against the effects of age-related muscle loss is resistance exercise training. Resistance exercise training increases muscle protein synthesis [99,100], skeletal muscle mass [101–104] and strength [105–107] in older adults and even in frail elders [107]. However, resistance exercise training studies typically show an attenuated muscle protein anabolic response in older compared to younger adults [101,104,108] or, in the case of older women (>85y), protein anabolic responses are blunted [109]. Furthermore, many researchers have repeatedly indicated that older adults have an altered anabolic response at the gene and protein level during the early recovery hours following a single bout of resistance exercise [30,31,110–114]. A recent study reported no change in muscle protein synthesis 3h after a single bout of resistance exercise in older adults [115]. This was later confirmed in a study that found blunted muscle protein synthesis and mTORC1 signaling in older adults (versus younger adults) following a single bout of resistance exercise at intensities of 60-90% 1RM [116]. In another study older adults had an unresponsive muscle protein synthesis response while mTORC1 signaling was dysregulated 24h following a single bout of resistance exercise [117]. These data are in stark contrast to young muscle, which responds robustly with an increase in muscle protein synthesis and mTORC1 signaling 1-48h following an acute bout of resistance exercise [116–118. More recently, a study performed in a larger number of subjects has confirmed that mTORC1 signaling, MAPK signaling and muscle protein synthesis are all impaired in older adults following an acute bout of resistance exercise [119]. One hypothesis for the impairment is that older adults have an increase in markers of cellular stress that may affect the remodeling response following resistance exercise [112,120,121]. Perhaps AMP-activated protein kinase, a negative regulator of muscle protein synthesis, plays a role as it was seen to be elevated in older (but not in the young) subjects following resistance exercise [112]. Although older adults do experience improvement in muscle mass and strength following resistance exercise training [101,104,122], these responses are less than those seen in young healthy subjects. Together, these data suggest that older adults have an impaired anabolic response to both acute and chronic resistance exercise training as compared to their younger counterparts.

OTHER CONTRIBUTORS TO IMPAIRED MUSCLE PROTEIN ANABOLISM

Endothelial Dysfunction. The insulin studies mentioned above have raised the question as to whether the age-related insulin resistance of muscle proteins is in fact only the product of endothelial dysfunction. One of the effects of insulin is to increase muscle perfusion by inducing a nitric oxide-dependent vasodilation of the precapillary arterioles in skeletal muscle [123,124]. Insulin-induced vasodilation may or may not be followed by increases in total blood flow, but is accompanied by capillary recruitment resulting in an increased and more homogenous tissue perfusion [125–127]. This mechanism increases capillary exchange of substrates and hormones in skeletal muscle. The insulin-stimulated changes in protein synthesis appear to be dependent upon changes in blood flow and amino acid delivery to the muscle, rather than to changes in amino acid or insulin concentrations [65,93,128]. Recent studies have confirmed the rather important role of vasodilation in the determination of skeletal muscle protein anabolism both in young and older adults. In one study, the insulin stimulation of endothelial-dependent vasodilation was blocked using L-monomethyl-L-arginine (L-NMMA), a nitric-oxide synthase inhibitor [128]. As a result, the physiological increase in skeletal muscle anabolic signaling and muscle protein synthesis with insulin was blocked, effectively rendering the young subjects "metabolically old" [128]. In another experiment, nitric oxide-dependent vasodilation was induced using sodium nitroprusside during physiological hyperinsulinemia in older adults [129]. The result was a normalization of skeletal muscle protein synthesis and anabolism to youthful levels [129]. The mechanisms responsible for endothelial dysfunction with aging are still unclear. However, it is likely that they involve a dysregulation of nitric-oxide synthase rather than sensitivity to nitric oxide, because the vasodilatory response to acetylcholine is blunted in older adults and is not inhibited by L-NMMA, while the vasculature still responds well to sodium nitroprusside [130] such that aging was associated with a blunted endothelial-dependent dilatory response to acetylcholine, but not SNP, a direct NO donor and endothelium-independent vasodilator. In addition, increased endothelin-1 concentration with aging could contribute to the alterations in capillary recruitment by insulin [93,131], as this endothelial-derived peptide is a powerful vasoconstrictor that regulated vascular tone along with nitric oxide.

Inflammation Inflammation, along with oxidative stress, increases with aging [132,133] and both may be significant contributors to endothelial dysfunction and sarcopenia [134]. TNF-α in particular may reduce endothelial-dependent dilation by disrupting intercellular communication [135], thereby disrupting the coordination of the vasodilatory response. Recent studies further suggest that inhibition of TNF-α may return vascular perfusion to youthful levels in older animals [136]. Increased oxidative stress, can also inactivate tetrahydrobiopterin, a cofactor for the production of nitric oxide, reducing nitric oxide production [137]. Reduced antioxidant status can also aggravate oxidative stress and endothelial-dependent vasodilation, and several studies have shown that treatment with antioxidants may improve endothelial-dependent vasodilation. Altogether, these studies highlight the potential contribution of inflammation and oxidative stress to an impaired endothelial responsiveness [131–138]. In addition to a role in the development of endothelial dysfunction, and, consequently, of the insulin-resistance of skeletal muscle protein anabolism, inflammation may directly impact skeletal muscle by activating skeletal muscle protein breakdown [139].

MicroRNA dysregulation The mechanisms responsible for the reduced ability of older muscle cells to respond to anabolic stimuli are not completely understood. It has recently been discovered that microRNA (miRNA) expression is dramatically different in the skeletal muscles of young and older men [140]. Specifically, the study identified the Let-7 family of miRNAs to be significantly increased in older men. One role of miRNAs is to regulate protein translation by targeting specific mRNAs for inhibition or degradation. In addition they are important regulators of several key cellular processes. In this recent study a miRNA array analyses was performed on muscle biopsies obtained from older and younger men. A functional and network analysis using the Ingenuity Pathway Analysis Software identified the cellular processes that were being targeted by the differential miRNA expression with aging. Interestingly, the increased expression of Let-7 miRNAs was associated with the inhibition of cell cycle, growth, proliferation, differentiation, and post-translational modification. All are cellular processes likely involved in regulating muscle protein turnover and ultimately sarcopenia. In agreement with the miRNA data, skeletal muscle satellite cell content increased only in young men 24 hr following exercise indicating an impaired ability of older men to activate these cellular processes [141]. Future work is necessary to determine the role of miRNA expression in the impaired anabolic response in older adults.

CLINICAL INTERVENTIONS TO COUNTERACT SARCOPENIA

Combination of nutritional supplementation and exercise. Inadequate protein intake and a reduced anabolic response to nutrients may be contributing factors to age-related loss in skeletal muscle [142,143]. Therefore, protein quantity must be considered to maximize muscle protein anabolic responses. Reports show that the muscle protein synthesis response is the same for young and older adults when the amino acid or protein dosage is of sufficient amount (10-15g of essential amino acids) [42,144]. For this reason, some have suggested that the protein intake for older adults be increased from the recommended daily allowance of 0.8g/kg/day [145,146]. Another useful strategy may be to optimize the specific amino acid profile, such as increasing the amount of leucine. As mentioned previously, an amino acid mixture containing 41% leucine (2.79g) was more effective at eliciting an increase in muscle protein synthesis than about half the dose (26%) in older subjects [76]. Leucine is a key branched chain amino acid that stimulates muscle protein synthesis through the mTORC1 pathway [147] while simultaneously slightly reducing muscle protein breakdown [148], with the overall effect of improving muscle protein turnover. There also appears to be a maximal muscle protein synthesis response to a given amount of ingested protein. For example, one study found that 30g of protein was sufficient to stimulate muscle protein synthesis in older subjects, but a dosage of 90g did not increase muscle protein synthesis [144]. Therefore, utilizing the correct amino acid or protein dose (~30g protein; 10-15g of essential amino acids) and supplementing meals with extra leucine may stimulate muscle protein synthesis and intracellular signaling in older human skeletal muscle.

Few data are available on chronic protein supplementation to improve the muscle protein synthesis response in older adults. Rieu et al. showed that when meals are supplemented with leucine over a single day, the protein anabolic response to feeding is improved in older adults [78]. However, the therapeutic potential of supplementing with leucine is suspect. Recently, Verheven and colleagues performed a 12-week intervention in older adults in which they supplemented leucine (2.5g) with each meal (7.5g/day) [149]. Unfortunately, muscle mass or strength was not improved over that of a group that received a placebo. It is unclear if a longer period of leucine supplementation (i.e., 1yr) is needed or perhaps in persons such as the frail elderly or other muscle wasting condition chronic leucine supplementation would be of significant benefit. Furthermore, supplementing with high quantities of protein in older adults may impair renal function [150]. Leucine supplementation may be less of a physiological concern in older adults if supplementation is intermittent (i.e., one day on, one day off). Whatever the case, supplementation with leucine may prove to be a noteworthy intervention for age-related muscle loss.

As mentioned previously, following an acute bout of resistance exercise, muscle protein synthesis rapidly increases within 1h [118] and can remain elevated up to 24-48h post exercise in young, healthy adults [151,152]. When resistance exercise is performed independently of nutrient intake, protein breakdown exceeds synthesis and protein balance is negative [153,154]. However, when nutrients in the form of amino acids or protein are given shortly after a bout of resistance exercise, muscle protein balance is positive [147,155]. Research from our laboratory and others have shown that nutrition given after exercise, whether in the form of amino acids or protein, augments the acute muscle protein synthesis response [147,156,157,158]. Furthermore, resistance exercise training combined with protein supplementation has been shown to increase muscle mass [102,159–164] and muscle growth markers [163,164] beyond that of resistance exercise alone.

When nutrition in the form of essential amino acids is given to older adults after a traditional bout of high-intensity resistance exercise, muscle protein synthesis increases to a similar extent, albeit in a delayed manner, compared to young adults [112]. However, if muscle protein synthesis is calculated over the entire 6h post resistance exercise period, the response was similar between age groups [112] and confirmed by another group of researchers [79]. It remains unknown if muscle protein synthesis in the old continues to be elevated beyond 6h post resistance exercise and protein ingestion, or if it then diverges from the anabolic response found in young subjects. There also appears to be a critical time period in which to ingest amino acids following a resistance exercise bout. After a 12-week resistance exercise training program, older subjects who consumed a 10g protein mixture immediately after the exercise bout experienced muscle hypertrophy, but not in those that consumed protein at a later time point [102]. Therefore, providing nutritional supplementation (e.g., essential amino acids, protein) in combination with each resistance exercise session may maximize muscle size following a resistance exercise training program in older adults [165]. Some disagree on the effectiveness of combining protein supplementation with resistance exercise. Verdiik et al. found that protein supplementation taken before and after each resistance exercise session during a 12 week resistance exercise training program in healthy, older adults did not further enhance muscle anabolic responses in comparison to a placebo group [166]. However, the authors may not have seen an effect since the total amount of essential amino acids consumed was rather low and protein synthesis is not enhanced when amino acids are consumed prior to resistance exercise [167]. Future interventions in sarcopenic populations should utilize a larger amount of essential amino acids consumed during the postexercise recovery period. We have recently shown that this approach is successful in older men following an acute bout of traditional high-intensity resistance exercise [112].

Blood flow restriction exercise. It is generally accepted that a resistance exercise program must be of sufficient intensity to increase muscle mass. The American College of Sports Medicine recommends that exercise intensity be at least 70% of the individual's one repetition maximum (1RM) to achieve maximum muscle hypertrophy [168]. However, for most older adults, such resistance exercise intensity is too great to complete or perform, especially in those with osteoarthritis, frailty or following surgery during a rehabilitation program. Recent attention has focused on resistance exercise that requires intensities ranging around 20-50% 1RM. In normal circumstances, resistance exercise at a low load is more useful for improving muscular endurance [168] with little improvement in muscle size [169]. Low intensity resistance exercise (20-50% 1RM) combined with moderate blood flow restriction (BFR) increases both muscle mass and strength, even to an extent similar to traditional resistance exercise [170–175]. Low intensity BFR exercise is characterized by a high number of repetitions (15-45) of each set performed to fatigue, while blood flow is restricted (predominately venous blood flow) typically through a pressurized cuff around the proximal thigh. Only after completion of several sets is the pressure released from the cuff [175–177].

The metabolic and molecular mechanisms of BFR exercise are currently not well described. However, a recent study has found that translation initiation through the mTORC1 pathway is acutely enhanced following BFR [177], while gene transcription is unaffected [178]. In young adults, phosphorylation of S6K1 and muscle protein synthesis were increased within hours of a single bout of BFR exercise (20% 1RM), while these changes were not observed following low intensity resistance exercise without BFR [177]. An exciting and recent finding was that BFR exercise in older adults was capable of restoring mTORC1 signaling and muscle protein synthesis in older men [179]. Since mTORC1 signaling and muscle protein synthesis are impaired following traditional high-intensity resistance exercise [119], the possibility of using BFR exercise as a countermeasure for sarcopenia is promising and future clinical trials are needed to determine the effectiveness of this novel intervention.

SUMMARY

The loss of skeletal muscle mass as we age is essentially due to an imbalance between the rates of muscle protein synthesis and muscle protein breakdown. The etiology of sarcopenia is clearly multifactorial and includes genetic and epigenetic changes in skeletal muscle, physical inactivity, decreased number of motor units, oxidative stress, inflammation, mitochondrial dysfunction, insulin resistance, dysregulated microRNA expression, decreased hormones, decreased capillary blood flow and malnutrition. The ultimate end result is change in the cellular processes of muscle protein turnover that determine overall muscle mass. However, two well-known interventions can directly activate muscle protein synthesis in humans: nutrition (primarily protein/essential amino acids) and exercise. Recent work in humans has also determined that the ability of exercise and amino acids to stimulate muscle protein synthesis requires activation of the mTORC1 signaling pathway. Aging is associated with an impaired ability to fully activate mTORC1 and muscle protein synthesis in response to nutrients, insulin or exercise. However, aerobic exercise prior to receiving an insulin infusion restores the ability of insulin to stimulate muscle protein synthesis in older adults. In addition, providing protein or essential amino acids following exercise is also capable of overcoming the impaired protein anabolic response to exercise with aging. One novel exercise treatment, blood flow restriction during low-intensity resistance exercise, may prove to be an effective rehabilitation strategy to prevent sarcopenia. Clinical interventions to overcome the impairment, utilizing exercise and nutrition to activate mTORC1 signaling and muscle protein synthesis, should result in an improved ability to counteract sarcopenia.

ACKNOWLEDGEMENTS

The experiments described in this review that were performed in the authors laboratories were supported by NIH grants R01 AR049877, R01 AG018311, R01 AG030070, P30 AG024832 (UTMB Claude D. Pepper Older Americans Independence Center) and 1UL1RR029876-01 (UTMB CTSA). We also thank Dr. Sarah Toombs-Smith for editing the chapter and Drs. Jared M. Dickinson, Micah J. Drummond and Kyle L. Timmerman for their assistance with both the chapter and figures.

REFERENCES

1. Holloszy JO. (2000) The biology of aging. Mayo Clin Proc 75 Suppl: S3–S8.
2. Melton LJ, III, Khosla S, Riggs BL. (2000) Epidemiology of sarcopenia. Mayo Clin Proc 75 Suppl: S10-S12.
3. Karakelides H, Sreekumaran NK. (2005) Sarcopenia of aging and its metabolic impact. Curr Top Dev Biol 68: 123–148.
4. Janssen I, Heymsfield SB, Ross R. (2002) Low relative skeletal muscle mass (sarcopenia) in older persons is associated with functional impairment and physical disability. J Am Geriatr Soc 50: 889–896.
5. Iannuzzi-Sucich M, Prestwood KM, Kenny AM. (2002) Prevalence of sarcopenia and predictors of skeletal muscle mass in healthy, older men and women. J Gerontol A Biol Sci Med Sci 57: M772-M777.
6. Sayer AA, Syddall HE, Martin HJ, Dennison EM, Anderson FH, Cooper C. (2006) Falls, sarcopenia, and growth in early life: findings from the Hertfordshire cohort study. Am J Epidemiol 164: 665–671.

7. Wolfson L, Judge J, Whipple R and King M. (1995) Strength is a major factor in balance, gait, and the occurrence of falls. J Gerontol A Biol Sci Med Sci 50: 64–67.

8. Landers KA, Hunter GR, Wetzstein CJ, Bamman MM and Weinsier RL. (2001) The interrelationship among muscle mass, strength, and the ability to perform physical tasks of daily living in younger and older women. J Gerontol A Biol Sci Med Sci 56: B443–B48.

9. Bean JF, Kiely DK, Herman S, Leveille SG, Mizer K, Frontera WR, Fielding RA. (2002) The relationship between leg power and physical performance in mobility-limited older people. J Am Geriatr Soc 50: 461–470.

10. Bassey EJ, Fiatarone MA, Oneill EF, Kelly M, Evans WJ and Lipsitz LA. (1992) Leg extensor power and functional performance in very old men and women. Clin Sci 82: 321–27.

11. Vandervoort AA and Symons TB. (2001) Functional and metabolic consequences of sarcopenia. Can J Appl Physiol 26: 90–101.

12. Brown M, Sinacore DR and Host HH. (1995) The relationship of strength to function in the older adult. J Gerontol A Biol Sci Med Sci 50: 55–59.

13. Larsson L and Karlsson J. (1978) Isometric and dynamic endurance as a function of age and skeletal-muscle characteristics. Acta Physiol Scand 104: 129–136.

14. Janssen I, Baumgartner RN, Ross R, Rosenberg IH, Roubenoff R. (2004) Skeletal muscle cutpoints associated with elevated physical disability risk in older men and women. Am J Epidemiol 159: 413–421.

15. Baumgartner RN, Koehler KM, Gallagher D, Romero L, Heymsfield SB, Ross RR et al. (1998) Epidemiology of sarcopenia among the elderly in New Mexico. Am J Epidemiol 147: 755–763.

16. Welle S. (1999) Human Protein Metabolism. New York, NY: Springer.

17. Matthews DE. (1999) Proteins and amino acids. In: Shils ME (ed). Modern Nutrition in Health and Disease. Williams and Wilkins, Baltimore, MD, pp. 11–48.

18. Reeds PJ, Fjeld CR, Jahoor F. (1994) Do the differences between the amino acid compositions of acute-phase and muscle proteins have a bearing on nitrogen loss in traumatic states? J Nutr 124: 906–910.

19. Ruiz, JR, X Sui, F Lobelo, JR Morrow, AW Jackson, M Sjostrom, et al. (2008) Association between muscular strength and mortality in men: Prospective cohort study. Br Med J; 337: a439. doi: 10.1136/bmj.a439.

20. Verdijk LB, Koopman R, Schaart G, Meijer K, Savelberg H and van Loon LJC. (2007) Satellite cell content is specifically reduced in type II skeletal muscle fibers in the elderly. Am J Physiol Endocrinol Metab 292: E151–E57.

21. Verdijk LB, Gleeson BG, Jonkers RAM, Meijer K, Savelberg H, Dendale P, et al. (2009) Skeletal muscle hypertrophy following resistance training is accompanied by a fiber type-specific increase in satellite cell content in elderly men. J Gerontol A Biol Sci Med Sci 64: 332–339.

22. Kadi F, Charifi N, Denis C and Lexell J. (2004) Satellite cells and myonuclei in young and elderly women and men. Muscle Nerve 29: 120–127.

23. Larsson L, Sjodin B and Karlsson J. (1978) Histochemical and biochemical changes in human skeletal-muscle with age in sedentary males, age 22–65 years. Acta Physiol Scand 103: 31–39.

24. Larsson L. (1978) Morphological and functional characteristics of aging skeletal-muscle in man cross-sectional study. Acta Physiol Scand 457: 5–36.

25. Lexell J, Henrikssonlarsen K, Winblad B and Sjostrom M. (1983) Distribution of different fiber types in human skeletal muscles - effects of aging studied in whole muscle cross-sections. Muscle Nerve 6: 588–595.

26. Lexell J, Henrikssonlarsen K and Sjostrom M. (1983) Distribution of different fiber types in human skeletal muscles. 2. A study of cross-sections of whole m-vastus lateralis. Acta Physiol Scand 117: 115–122.

27. Lexell J. (1995) Human aging, muscle mass, and fiber-type composition. J Gerontol A Biol Sci Med Sci 50: 11–16.

28. Nair KS. (1995) Muscle protein-turnover - methodological issues and the effect of aging. J Gerontol A Biol Sci Med Sci 50: 107–112.

29. Nair KS. (2005) Aging muscle. Am J Clin Nutr 81: 953–963.

30. Jozsi AC, Dupont-Versteegden EE, Taylor-Jones JM, et al. (2000) Aged human muscle demonstrates an altered gene expression profile consistent with an impaired response to exercise. Mech Ageing Dev 120: 45–56.

31. Drummond MJ, Miyazaki M, Dreyer HC, et al. (2009) Expression of growth-related genes in young and older human skeletal muscle following an acute stimulation of protein synthesis. J Appl Physiol 106: 1403–1411.

32. Raue U, Slivka D, Jemiolo B, et al. (2006) Myogenic gene expression at rest and after a bout of resistance exercise in young (18–30 yr) and old (80–89 yr) women. J Appl Physiol 101: 53–59.

33. Welle S, Brooks AI, Delehanty JM, et al. (2004) Skeletal muscle gene expression profiles in 20–29 year old and 65–71 year old women. Exp Gerontol 39, 369–377.

34. Welle S, Brooks AI, Delehanty JM, et al. (2003) Gene expression profile of aging in human muscle. Physiol Genomics 14: 149 159.

35. Hasten DL, Pak-Loduca J, Obert KA, Yarasheski KE. (2000) Resistance exercise acutely increases MHC and mixed muscle protein synthesis rates in 78–84 and 23–32 yr olds. Am J Physiol Endocrinol Metab 278: E620–E626.

36. Volpi E, Mittendorfer B, Rasmussen BB, Wolfe RR. (2000) The response of muscle protein anabolism to combined hyperaminoacidemia and glucose-induced hyperinsulinemia is impaired in the elderly. J Clin Endocrinol Metab 85: 4481–4490.

37. Volpi E, Sheffield-Moore M, Rasmussen BB, Wolfe RR. (2001) Basal muscle amino acid kinetics and protein synthesis in healthy young and older men. JAMA 286: 1206–1212.

38. Welle S, Thornton C, Statt M. (1995) Myofibrillar protein synthesis in young and old human subjects after three months of resistance training. Am J Physiol 268: E422-E427.

39. Yarasheski KE, Zachwieja JJ, Bier DM. (1993) Acute effects of resistance exercise on muscle protein synthesis rate in young and elderly men and women. Am J Physiol 265: E210-E214.

40. Balagopal P, Rooyackers OE, Adey DB, Ades PA, Nair KS. (1997) Effects of aging on in vivo synthesis of skeletal muscle myosin heavy-chain and sarcoplasmic protein in humans. Am J Physiol 273: E790-E800.

41. Welle S, Thornton C, Jozefowicz R, Statt M. (1993) Myofibrillar protein synthesis in young and old men. Am J Physiol 264: E693-E698.

42. Paddon-Jones D, Sheffield-Moore M, Zhang XJ, Volpi E, Wolf SE, Aarsland A et al. (2004) Amino acid ingestion improves muscle protein synthesis in the young and elderly. Am J Physiol Endocrinol Metab 286: E321-E328.

43. Drummond MJ, Fry CS, Glynn EL, Dreyer HC, Dhanani S, Timmerman KL, Volpi E, and Rasmussen BB. (2009) Rapamycin administration in humans blocks the contraction-induced increase in skeletal muscle protein synthesis. J Physiol 587: 1535–1546.

44. Dickinson JM, Fry CS, Drummond MJ, Gundermann DM, Walker DK, Glynn EL, Timmerman KL, Dhanani S, Volpi E, and Rasmussen BB. (2011) Mammalian target of rapamycin complex 1 activation is required for the stimulation of human skeletal muscle protein synthesis by essential amino acids. J Nutr 141: 856–862.

45. Baar K and Esser K. (1999) Phosphorylation of p70(S6k) correlates with increased skeletal muscle mass following resistance exercise. Am J Physiol 276: C120–127.

46. Terzis G, Georgiadis G, Stratakos G, Vogiatzis I, Kavouras S, Manta P, Mascher H and Blomstrand E. (2008) Resistance exercise-induced increase in muscle mass correlates with p70S6 kinase phosphorylation in human subjects. Eur J Appl Physiol 102: 145–152.

47. Bodine SC, Stitt TN, Gonzalez M, Kline WO, Stover GL, Bauerlein R, Zlotchenko E, Scrimgeour A, Lawrence JC, Glass DJ and Yancopoulos GD. (2001) Akt/mTOR pathway is a crucial regulator of skeletal muscle hypertrophy and can prevent muscle atrophy in vivo. Nat Cell Biol 3: 1014–1019.

48. Ruvinsky I and Meyuhas O. (2006) Ribosomal protein S6 phosphorylation: from protein synthesis to cell size. Trends Biochem Sci 31: 342–348.

49. Roux PP, Shahbazian D, Vu H, Holz MK, Cohen MS, Taunton J, Sonenberg N and Blenis J. (2007) RAS/ERK signaling promotes site-specific ribosomal protein S6 phosphorylation via RSK and stimulates cap-dependent translation. J Biol Chem 282: 14056–14064.

50. Wang X, Li W, Williams M, Terada N, Alessi DR and Proud CG. (2001) Regulation of elongation factor 2 kinase by p90(RSK1) and p70 S6 kinase. Embo J 20: 4370–4379.

51. Ruvinsky I, Sharon N, Lerer T, Cohen H, Stolovich-Rain M, Nir T, Dor Y, Zisman P and Meyuhas O. (2005) Ribosomal protein S6 phosphorylation is a determinant of cell size and glucose homeostasis. Genes Dev 19: 2199–2211.

52. Wang X and Proud CG. (2006) The mTOR pathway in the control of protein synthesis. Physiology (Bethesda) 21: 362–369.

53. Browne GJ and Proud CG. (2002) Regulation of peptide-chain elongation in mammalian cells. Eur J Biochem 269: 5360–5368.

54. Nave BT, Ouwens M, Withers DJ, Alessi DR and Shepherd PR. (1999) Mammalian target of rapamycin is a direct target for protein kinase B: identification of a convergence point for opposing effects of insulin and amino-acid deficiency on protein translation. Biochem J 344: 427–431.

55. Inoki K, Li Y, Zhu T, Wu J and Guan KL. (2002) TSC2 is phosphorylated and inhibited by Akt and suppresses mTOR signalling. Nat Cell Biol 4: 648–657.

56. Manning BD, Tee AR, Logsdon MN, Blenis J and Cantley LC. (2002) Identification of the tuberous sclerosis complex-2 tumor suppressor gene product tuberin as a target of the phosphoinositide 3-kinase/akt pathway. Mol Cell 10: 151–162.

57. Hornberger TA, Stuppard R, Conley KE, Fedele MJ, Fiorotto ML, Chin ER and Esser KA. (2004) Mechanical stimuli regulate rapamycin-sensitive signalling by a phosphoinositide 3-kinase-, protein kinase B- and growth factor-independent mechanism. Biochem J 380: 795–804.

58. Hornberger TA and Chien S. (2006) Mechanical stimuli and nutrients regulate rapamycin-sensitive signaling through distinct mechanisms in skeletal muscle. J Cell Biochem 97: 1207–1216.

59. Hornberger TA, Chu WK, Mak YW, Hsiung JW, Huang SA and Chien S. (2006) The role of phospholipase D and phosphatidic acid in the mechanical activation of mTOR signaling in skeletal muscle. Proc Natl Acad Sci U S A 103: 4741–4746.

60. Ma L, Chen Z, Erdjument-Bromage H, Tempst P and Pandolfi PP. (2005) Phosphorylation and functional inactivation of TSC2 by Erk implications for tuberous sclerosis and cancer pathogenesis. Cell 121: 179–193.

61. Rolfe M, McLeod LE, Pratt PF and Proud CG. (2005) Activation of protein synthesis in cardiomyocytes by the hypertrophic agent phenylephrine requires the activation of ERK and involves phosphorylation of tuberous sclerosis complex 2 (TSC2). Biochem J 388: 973–984.

62. Roux PP, Shahbazian D, Vu H, Holz MK, Cohen MS, Taunton J, Sonenberg N and Blenis J. (2007) RAS/ERK signaling promotes site-specific ribosomal protein S6 phosphorylation via RSK and stimulates cap-dependent translation. J Biol Chem 282: 14056–14064.

63. Fluckey JD, Knox M, Smith L, Dupont-Versteegden EE, Gaddy D, Tesch PA and Peterson CA. (2006) Insulin-facilitated increase of muscle protein synthesis after resistance exercise involves a MAP kinase pathway. Am J Physiol Endocrinol Metab 290: E1205–1211.

64. Wang X, Yue P, Chan CB, Ye K, Ueda T, Watanabe-Fukunaga R, Fukunaga R, Fu H, Khuri FR and Sun SY. (2007) Inhibition of mammalian target of rapamycin induces phosphatidylinositol 3-kinase-dependent and Mnk-mediated eukaryotic translation initiation factor 4E phosphorylation. Mol Cell Biol 27: 7405–7413.

65. Fujita S, Rasmussen BB, Cadenas JG, Grady JJ, Volpi E. (2006) Effect of insulin on human skeletal muscle protein synthesis is modulated by insulin-induced changes in muscle blood flow and amino acid availability. Am J Physiol Endocrinol Metab; 291: E745-E754.

66. Rasmussen BB, Wolfe RR, Volpi E. (2002) Oral and intravenously administered amino acids produce similar effects on muscle protein synthesis in the elderly. J Nutr Health Aging 6: 358–362.

67. Volpi E, Ferrando AA, Yeckel CW, Tipton KD, Wolfe RR. (1998) Exogenous amino acids stimulate net muscle protein synthesis in the elderly. J Clin Invest 101: 2000–2007.

68. Volpi E, Mittendorfer B, Wolf SE, Wolfe RR. (1999) Oral amino acids stimulate muscle protein anabolism in the elderly despite higher first-pass splanchnic extraction. Am J Physiol 277: E513-E520.

69. Volpi E, Kobayashi H, Sheffield-Moore M, Mittendorfer B, Wolfe RR. (2003) Essential amino acids are primarily responsible for the amino acid stimulation of muscle protein anabolism in healthy elderly adults. Am J Clin Nutr 78: 250–258.

70. Anthony JC, Yoshizawa F, Anthony TG, Vary TC, Jefferson LS, Kimball SR. (2000) Leucine stimulates translation initiation in skeletal muscle of post-absorptive rats via a rapamycin-sensitive pathway. J Nutr 130: 2413–2419.

71. Anthony JC, Anthony TG, Kimball SR, Vary TC, Jefferson LS. (2000) Orally administered leucine stimulates protein synthesis in skeletal muscle of postabsorptive rats in association with increased eIF4F formation. J Nutr 130: 139–145.

72. Garlick PJ. (2005) The role of leucine in the regulation of protein metabolism. J Nutr 135 (6 Suppl): 1553S–1556S.

73. Anthony TG, Anthony JC, Yoshizawa F, Kimball SR, Jefferson LS. (2001) Oral administration of leucine stimulates ribosomal protein mRNA translation but not global rates of protein synthesis in the liver of rats. J Nutr 131: 1171–1176.

74. Fujita S, Dreyer HC, Drummond MJ, Glynn EL, Cadenas JG, Yoshizawa F et al. (2007) Nutrient signalling in the regulation of human muscle protein synthesis. J Physiol 582: 813–823.

75. Katsanos CS, Kobayashi H, Sheffield-Moore M, Aarsland A, Wolfe RR (2005). Aging is associated with diminished accretion of muscle proteins after the ingestion of a small bolus of essential amino acids. Am J Clin Nutr 82: 1065–1073.

76. Katsanos CS, Kobayashi H, Sheffield-Moore M, Aarsland A, Wolfe RR. (2006) A high proportion of leucine is required for optimal stimulation of the rate of muscle protein synthesis by essential amino acids in the elderly. Am J Physiol Endocrinol Metab 291: E381–E387.

77. Paddon-Jones D, Sheffield-Moore M, Katsanos CS, Zhang XJ, Wolfe RR. (2006) Differential stimulation of muscle protein synthesis in elderly humans following isocaloric ingestion of amino acids or whey protein. Exp Gerontol; 41: 215–219.

78. Rieu I, Balage M, Sornet C, et al. (2006) Leucine supplementation improves muscle protein synthesis in elderly men independently of hyperaminoacidaemia. J Physiol 575: 1–15.

79. Koopman R, Verdijk L, Manders RJ, Gijsen AP, Gorselink M, Pijpers E et al. (2006) Co-ingestion of protein and leucine stimulates muscle protein synthesis rates to the same extent in young and elderly lean men. Am J Clin Nutr 84: 623–632.

80. Symons TB, Sheffield-Moore M, Wolfe RR, Paddon-Jones D. (2009) A moderate serving of high-quality protein maximally stimulates skeletal muscle protein synthesis in young and elderly subjects. J Am Diet Assoc 109: 1582–1586.

81. Koopman R, Walrand S, Beelen M et al. (2009) Dietary protein digestion and absorption rates and the subsequent postprandial muscle protein synthetic response do not differ between young and elderly men. J Nutr 139: 1707–1713.

82. Guillet C, Prod'homme M, Balage M, Gachon P, Giraudet C, Morin L et al. (2004) Impaired anabolic response of muscle protein synthesis is associated with S6K1 dysregulation in elderly humans. FASEB J 18: 1586–1587.

83. Boirie Y, Gachon P, Beaufrere B. (1997) Splanchnic and whole-body leucine kinetics in young and elderly men. Am J Clin Nutr 65: 489–495.

84. Fujita S, Rasmussen BB, Cadenas JG, Grady JJ, Volpi E (2006) The effect of insulin on human skeletal muscle protein synthesis is modulated by insulin-induced changes in muscle blood flow and amino acid availability. Am J Physiol Endocrinol Metab 291: E745–E754.

85. Bennet WM, Connacher AA, Scrimgeour CM, Jung RT, Rennie MJ (1990) Euglycemic hyperinsulinemia augments amino acid uptake by leg tissues during hyperaminoacidemia. Am J Physiol 259: E185-E194.

86. Biolo G, Declan Fleming RY, Wolfe RR (1995) Physiologic hyperinsulinemia stimulates protein synthesis and enhances transport of selected amino acids in human skeletal muscle. J Clin Invest 95: 811–819.

87. Newman E, Heslin MJ, Wolf RF, Pisters PW, Brennan MF (1994) The effect of systemic hyperinsulinemia with concomitant amino acid infusion on skeletal muscle protein turnover in the human forearm. Metabolism 43: 70–78.

88. Wolf RF, Heslin MJ, Newman E, Pearlstone DB, Gonenne A, Brennan MF (1992) Growth hormone and insulin combine to improve whole-body and skeletal muscle protein kinetics. Surgery 112: 284–291.

89. Hillier TA, Fryburg DA, Jahn LA, Barrett EJ (1998) Extreme hyperinsulinemia unmasks insulin's effect to stimulate protein synthesis in the human forearm. Am J Physiol 274: E1067–E1074.

90. Nygren J, Nair KS (2003) Differential regulation of protein dynamics in splanchnic and skeletal muscle beds by insulin and amino acids in healthy human subjects. Diabetes 52: 1377–1385.

91. Guillet C, Prod'homme M, Balage M, et al. (2004) Impaired anabolic response of muscle protein synthesis is associated with S6K1 dysregulation in elderly humans. FASEB Journal 18: 1586–1587.

92. Bell JA, Volpi E, Fujita S, Cadenas JG, Sheffield-Moore M, Rasmussen BB (2006) Skeletal muscle protein anabolic response to increased energy and insulin is preserved in poorly controlled type 2 diabetes. J Nutr 136: 1249–1255.

93. Rasmussen BB, Fujita S, Wolfe RR, et al. (2006) Insulin resistance of muscle protein metabolism in aging. FASEB Journal 20: 768–769.

94. Fujita S, Rasmussen BB, Cadenas JG, et al. (2007) Aerobic exercise overcomes the age-related insulin resistance of muscle protein metabolism by improving endothelial function and akt/mammalian target of rapamycin signaling. Diabetes 56: 1615–1622.

95. Fujita S, Glynn EL, Timmerman KL, Rasmussen BB, Volpi E. (2009) Supraphysiological hyperinsulinaemia is necessary to stimulate skeletal muscle protein anabolism in older adults:

evidence of a true age-related insulin resistance of muscle protein metabolism. Diabetologia 52: 1889–1898.

96. Ferrucci L, Izmirlian G, Leveille S, et al. (1999) Smoking, physical activity, and active life expectancy. Am J Epidemiol. 149: 645–653.

97. Leveille SG, Guralnik JM, Ferrucci L, et al. (1999) Aging successfully until death in old age: opportunities for increasing active life expectancy. Am J Epidemiol. 149: 654–664.

98. Ruiz JR, Sui X, Lobelo F, et al. (2008) Association between muscular strength and mortality in men: prospective cohort study. BMJ 337: a439.

99. Yarasheski KE, Zachwieja JJ, and Bier DM. (1993) Acute effects of resistance exercise on muscle protein synthesis rate in young and elderly men and women. Am J Physiol. 265: E210–4.

100. Yarasheski KE, Pak-Loduca J, Hasten DL, et al. (1999) Resistance exercise training increases mixed muscle protein synthesis rate in frail women and men >/ = 76 yr old. Am J Physiol. 277: E118–25.

101. Welle S, Thornton C, and Statt M. (1995) Myofibrillar protein synthesis in young and old human subjects after three months of resistance training. Am J Physiol. 268: E422–7.

102. Esmarck B, Andersen JL, Olsen S, et al. (2001) Timing of postexercise protein intake is important for muscle hypertrophy with resistance training in elderly humans. J Physiol. 535: 301–311.

103. Frontera WR, Meredith CN, O'Reilly KP, et al. (1988) Strength conditioning in older men: skeletal muscle hypertrophy and improved function. J Appl Physiol. 64: 1038–1044.

104. Kosek DJ, Kim JS, Petrella JK, et al. (2006) Efficacy of 3 days/wk resistance training on myofiber hypertrophy and myogenic mechanisms in young vs. older adults. J Appl Physiol. 101: 531–544.

105. Brown AB, McCartney N, and Sale DG. (1990) Positive adaptations to weight-lifting training in the elderly. J Appl Physiol. 69: 1725–1733.

106. McCartney N, Hicks AL, Martin J, et al. (1996) A longitudinal trial of weight training in the elderly: continued improvements in year 2. J Gerontol A Biol Sci Med Sci. 51: B425–33.

107. Fiatarone MA, Marks EC, Ryan ND, et al. (1990) High-intensity strength training in nonagenarians. Effects on skeletal muscle. JAMA. 263: 3029–3034.

108. Slivka D, Raue U, Hollon C, et al. (2008) Single muscle fiber adaptations to resistance training in old (>80 yr) men: evidence for limited skeletal muscle plasticity. Am J Physiol Regul Integr Comp Physiol. 295: R273–80.

109. Raue U, Slivka D, Minchev K, et al. (2009) Improvements in whole muscle and myocellular function are limited with high-intensity resistance training in octogenarian women. J Appl Physiol. 106: 1611–1617.

110. Carey KA, Farnfield MM, Tarquinio SD, et al. (2007) Impaired expression of Notch signaling genes in aged human skeletal muscle. J Gerontol A Biol Sci Med Sci. 62: 9–17.

111. Dennis RA, Przybyla B, Gurley C, et al. (2008) Aging alters gene expression of growth and remodeling factors in human skeletal muscle both at rest and in response to acute resistance exercise. Physiol Genomics. 32: 393–400.

112. Drummond MJ, Dreyer HC, Pennings B, et al. (2008) Skeletal muscle protein anabolic response to resistance exercise and essential amino acids is delayed with aging. J Appl Physiol. 104: 1452–1461.

113. Kim JS, Cross JM, and Bamman MM. (2005) Impact of resistance loading on myostatin expression and cell cycle regulation in young and older men and women. Am J Physiol Endocrinol Metab. 288: E1110–9.

114. Williamson D, Gallagher P, Harber M, et al. (2003) Mitogen-activated protein kinase (MAPK) pathway activation: effects of age and acute exercise on human skeletal muscle. J Physiol. 547: 977–987.

115. Sheffield-Moore M, Paddon-Jones D, Sanford AP, et al. (2005) Mixed muscle and hepatic derived plasma protein metabolism is differentially regulated in older and younger men following resistance exercise. Am J Physiol Endocrinol Metab. 288: E922–9.

116. Kumar V, Selby A, Rankin D, et al. (2008) Age-related differences in the dose-response of muscle protein synthesis to resistance exercise in young and old men. J Physiol 587: 211–217.

117. Mayhew DL, Kim JS, Cross JM, et al. (2009) Translational signaling responses preceding resistance training-mediated myofiber hypertrophy in young and old humans. J Appl Physiol. 107: 1655–1662.

118. Dreyer HC, Fujita S, Cadenas JG, et al. (2006) Resistance exercise increases AMPK activity and reduces 4E-BP1 phosphorylation and protein synthesis in human skeletal muscle. J Physiol. 576: 613–624.

119. Fry CS, Drummond MJ, Glynn EL, Dickinson JM, Gundermann DM, Timmerman KL, Walker DK, Dhanani S, Volpi E, and Rasmussen BB. (2011) Aging impairs contraction-induced human skeletal muscle mTORC1 signaling and protein synthesis. Skelet Muscle 1: 11.

120. Thalacker-Mercer A, Dell'italia LJ, Cui X, et al. (2009) Differential Genomic Responses in Old Vs. Young Humans Despite Similar Levels of Modest Muscle Damage after Resistance Loading. Physiol Genomics 40: 141–149.

121. Kim JS, Kosek DJ, Petrella JK, et al. (2005) Resting and load-induced levels of myogenic gene transcripts differ between older adults with demonstrable sarcopenia and young men and women. J Appl Physiol. 99: 2149–2158.

122. Melov S, Tarnopolsky MA, Beckman K, et al. (2007) Resistance exercise reverses aging in human skeletal muscle. PLoS One 2: e465.

123. Scherrer U, Randin D, Vollenweider P, Vollenweider L, Nicod P. (1994) Nitric oxide release accounts for insulin's vascular effects in humans. J Clin Invest 94: 2511–2515.

124. Steinberg HO, Brechtel G, Johnson A, Fineberg N, Baron AD. (1994) Insulin-mediated skeletal muscle vasodilation is nitric oxide dependent. A novel action of insulin to increase nitric oxide release. J Clin Invest 94: 1172–1179.

125. Baron AD, Tarshoby M, Hook G, Lazaridis EN, Cronin J, Johnson A, Steinberg HO. (2000) Interaction between insulin sensitivity and muscle perfusion on glucose uptake in human skeletal muscle: evidence for capillary recruitment. Diabetes 49: 768–774.

126. Coggins M, Lindner J, Rattigan S, Jahn L, Fasy E, Kaul S, Barrett EJ. (2001) Physiologic hyperinsulinemia enhances human skeletal muscle perfusion by capillary recruitment. Diabetes 50: 2682–2690.

127. Vincent MA, Dawson D, Clark AD, Lindner JR, Rattigan S, Clark MG, Barrett EJ. (2002) Skeletal muscle microvascular recruitment by physiological hyperinsulinemia precedes increases in total blood flow. Diabetes 51: 42–48.

128. Timmerman KL, Lee JL, Dreyer HC, Dhanani S, Glynn EL, Fry CS, Drummond MJ, Sheffield-Moore M, Rasmussen BB, and Volpi E. (2010) Insulin stimulates human skeletal muscle protein synthesis via an indirect mechanism involving endothelial-dependent vasodilation and mammalian target of rapamycin complex 1 signaling. J Clin Endocrinol Metab 95: 3848–3857.

129. Timmerman KL, Lee JL, Fujita S et al. (2010) Pharmacological vasodilation improves insulin-stimulated muscle protein anabolism but not glucose utilization in older adults. Diabetes 59: 2764–2771.

130. Taddei S, Virdis A, Ghiadoni L et al. (2001) Age-related reduction of NO availability and oxidative stress in humans. Hypertension 38: 274–279.

131. Donato AJ, Gano LB, Eskurza I et al. (2009) Vascular endothelial dysfunction with aging: endothelin-1 and endothelial nitric oxide synthase. Am J Physiol Heart Circ Physiol 297: H425–H432.

132. Bruunsgaard H, Pedersen AN, Schroll M, Skinhoj P, Pedersen BK. (2001) Decreased natural killer cell activity is associated with atherosclerosis in elderly humans. Exp Gerontol 37: 127–136.

133. Zanni F, Vescovini R, Biasini C et al. (2003) Marked increase with age of type 1 cytokines within memory and effector/cytotoxic CD8+ T cells in humans: a contribution to understand the relationship between inflammation and immunosenescence. Exp Gerontol 38: 981–987.

134. Bruunsgaard H, Pedersen BK. (2003) Age-related inflammatory cytokines and disease. Immunol Allergy Clin North Am 23: 15–39.

135. Payne GW. (2006) Effect of inflammation on the aging microcirculation: impact on skeletal muscle blood flow control. Microcirculation 13: 343–352.

136. Csiszar A, Labinskyy N, Smith K, Rivera A, Orosz Z, Ungvari Z. (2007) Vasculoprotective effects of anti-tumor necrosis factor-alpha treatment in aging. Am J Pathol 170: 388–398.

137. Landmesser U, Dikalov S, Price SR et al. (2003) Oxidation of tetrahydrobiopterin leads to uncoupling of endothelial cell nitric oxide synthase in hypertension. J Clin Invest 111: 1201–1209.

138. Tatchum-Talom R, Martin DS. (2004) Tempol improves vascular function in the mesenteric vascular bed of senescent rats. Can J Physiol Pharmacol 82: 200–207.

139. Li YP, Chen Y, John J et al. (2005) TNF-alpha acts via p38 MAPK to stimulate expression of the ubiquitin ligase atrogin1/MAFbx in skeletal muscle. FASEB J. 19: 362–370.

140. Drummond MJ, McCarthy JJ, Sinha M, Spratt HM, Volpi E, Esser KA, and Rasmussen BB. (2011) Aging and microRNA expression in human skeletal muscle: a microarray and bioinformatics analysis. Physiol Genomics 43: 595–603.

141. Walker DK, Fry CS, Drummond MJ, Dickinson JM, Timmerman KL, Gundermann DM, Jennings K, Volpi E, and Rasmussen BB. (2012) Pax7+ satellite cells in young and older adults following resistance exercise. Muscle Nerve, In Press.

142. Thalacker-Mercer AE, Fleet JC, Craig BA, et al. (2007) Inadequate protein intake affects skeletal muscle transcript profiles in older humans. Am J Clin Nutr. 85: 1344–1352.

143. Houston DK, Nicklas BJ, Ding J, et al. (2008) Dietary protein intake is associated with lean mass change in older, community-dwelling adults: the Health, Aging, and Body Composition (Health ABC) Study. Am J Clin Nutr. 87: 150–155.

144. Symons TB, Schutzler SE, Cocke TL, et al. (2007) Aging does not impair the anabolic response to a protein-rich meal. Am J Clin Nutr. 86: 451–456.

145. Campbell WW, Trappe TA, Wolfe RR, et al. (2001) The recommended dietary allowance for protein may not be adequate for older people to maintain skeletal muscle. J Gerontol A Biol Sci Med Sci. 56: M373–80.

146. Wolfe RR and Miller SL. (2008) The recommended dietary allowance of protein: a misunderstood concept. JAMA. 299: 2891–2893.

147. Dreyer HC, Drummond MJ, Pennings B, et al. (2008) Leucine-enriched essential amino acid and carbohydrate ingestion following resistance exercise enhances mTOR signaling and protein synthesis in human muscle. Am J Physiol Endocrinol Metab. 294: E392–400.

148. Louard RJ, Barrett EJ, and Gelfand RA. (1995) Overnight branched-chain amino acid infusion causes sustained suppression of muscle proteolysis. Metabolism. 44: 424–429.

149. Verhoeven S, Vanschoonbeek K, Verdijk LB, et al. (2009) Long-term leucine supplementation does not increase muscle mass or strength in healthy elderly men. Am J Clin Nutr. 89: 1468–1475.

150. Walrand S, Short KR, Bigelow ML, et al. (2008) Functional impact of high protein intake on healthy elderly people. Am J Physiol Endocrinol Metab. 295: E921–8.

151. Phillips SM, Tipton KD, Ferrando AA, et al. (1999) Resistance training reduces the acute exercise-induced increase in muscle protein turnover. Am J Physiol. 276: E118–24.

152. MacDougall JD, Gibala MJ, Tarnopolsky MA, et al. (1995) The time course for elevated muscle protein synthesis following heavy resistance exercise. Can J Appl Physiol. 20: 480–486.

153. Phillips SM, Tipton KD, Aarsland A, et al. (1997) Mixed muscle protein synthesis and breakdown after resistance exercise in humans. Am J Physiol. 273: E99–107.

154. Biolo G, Maggi SP, Williams BD, et al. (1995) Increased rates of muscle protein turnover and amino acid transport after resistance exercise in humans. Am J Physiol. 268: E514–20.

155. Borsheim E, Aarsland A, and Wolfe RR. (2004) Effect of an amino acid, protein, and carbohydrate mixture on net muscle protein balance after resistance exercise. Int J Sport Nutr Exerc Metab. 14: 255–271.

156. Biolo G, Tipton KD, Klein S, et al. (1997) An abundant supply of amino acids enhances the metabolic effect of exercise on muscle protein. Am J Physiol. 273, E122–9.

157. Tipton KD, Ferrando AA, Phillips SM, et al. (1999) Postexercise net protein synthesis in human muscle from orally administered amino acids. Am J Physiol. 276: E628–34.

158. Rasmussen BB, Tipton KD, Miller SL, et al. (2000) An oral essential amino acid-carbohydrate supplement enhances muscle protein anabolism after resistance exercise. J Appl Physiol. 88: 386–392.

159. Andersen LL, Tufekovic G, Zebis MK, et al. (2005) The effect of resistance training combined with timed ingestion of protein on muscle fiber size and muscle strength. Metabolism. 54: 151–156.

160. Bird SP, Tarpenning KM, and Marino FE. (2006) Independent and combined effects of liquid carbohydrate/essential amino acid ingestion on hormonal and muscular adaptations following resistance training in untrained men. Eur J Appl Physiol. 97: 225–238.

161. Rankin JW, Goldman LP, Puglisi MJ, et al. (2004) Effect of post-exercise supplement consumption on adaptations to resistance training. J Am Coll Nutr. 23: 322–330.

162. Ballard TL, Clapper JA, Specker BL, et al. (2005) Effect of protein supplementation during a 6-mo strength and conditioning program on insulin-like growth factor I and markers of bone turnover in young adults. Am J Clin Nutr. 81: 1442–1448.

163. Hulmi JJ, Tannerstedt J, Selanne H, et al. (2009) Resistance exercise with whey protein ingestion affects mTOR signaling pathway and myostatin in men. J Appl Physiol. 106: 1720–1729.

164. Willoughby DS, Stout JR, and Wilborn CD. (2007) Effects of resistance training and protein plus amino acid supplementation on muscle anabolism, mass, and strength. Amino Acids. 32: 467–477.

165. Campbell WW and Leidy HJ. (2007) Dietary protein and resistance training effects on muscle and body composition in older persons. J Am Coll Nutr. 26: 696S–703S.

166. Verdijk LB, Jonkers RA, Gleeson BG, et al. (2009) Protein supplementation before and after exercise does not further augment skeletal muscle hypertrophy after resistance training in elderly men. Am J Clin Nutr. 89: 608–616.

167. Fujita S, Dreyer HC, Drummond MJ, et al. (2009) Essential amino acid and carbohydrate ingestion before resistance exercise does not enhance postexercise muscle protein synthesis. J Appl Physiol. 106: 1730–1739.

168. Kraemer WJ, Adams K, Cafarelli E, et al. (2002) American College of Sports Medicine position stand. Progression models in resistance training for healthy adults. Med Sci Sports Exerc. 34: 364–380.

169. Holm L, Reitelseder S, Pedersen TG, et al. (2008) Changes in muscle size and MHC composition in response to resistance exercise with heavy and light loading intensity. J Appl Physiol. 105: 1454–1461.

170. Abe T, Kearns CF, and Sato Y. (2006) Muscle size and strength are increased following walk training with restricted venous blood flow from the leg muscle, Kaatsu-walk training. J Appl Physiol. 100: 1460–1466.

171. Shinohara M, Kouzaki M, Yoshihisa T, et al. (1998) Efficacy of tourniquet ischemia for strength training with low resistance. Eur J Appl Physiol Occup Physiol. 77: 189–191.

172. Takarada Y, Sato Y, and Ishii N. (2002) Effects of resistance exercise combined with vascular occlusion on muscle function in athletes. Eur J Appl Physiol. 86: 308–314.

173. Takarada Y, Takazawa H, Sato Y, et al. (2000) Effects of resistance exercise combined with moderate vascular occlusion on muscular function in humans. J Appl Physiol. 88: 2097–2106.

174. Takarada Y, Tsuruta T, and Ishii N. (2004) Cooperative effects of exercise and occlusive stimuli on muscular function in low-intensity resistance exercise with moderate vascular occlusion. Jpn J Physiol. 54: 585–592.

175. Abe T, Yasuda T, Midorikawa T, et al. (2005) Skeletal muscle size and circulating IGF-1 are increased after two weeks of twice daily KAATSU resistance training. Int J Kaatsu Training Res. 1: 6–12.

176. Manini TM and Clark BC. (2009) Blood flow restricted exercise and skeletal muscle health. Exerc Sport Sci Rev. 37: 78–85.

177. Fujita S, Abe T, Drummond MJ, et al. (2007) Blood flow restriction during low-intensity resistance exercise increases S6K1 phosphorylation and muscle protein synthesis. J Appl Physiol. 103: 903–910.

178. Drummond MJ, Fujita S, Takashi A, et al. (2008) Human Muscle Gene Expression following Resistance Exercise and Blood Flow Restriction. Med Sci Sports Exerc. 40: 691–698.

179. Fry CS, Glynn EL, Drummond MJ, Timmerman KL, Fujita S, Abe T, Dhanani S, Volpi E, and Rasmussen BB. (2010) Blood flow restriction exercise stimulates mTORC1 signaling and muscle protein synthesis in older men. J Appl Physiol 108: 1199–1209.

CHAPTER 4

The Role of the Nervous System in Muscle Atrophy

Minal Bhanushali and Robin Conwit
National Institute of Neurological Disorders and Stroke and National Institute of Health, Rockville, MD, USA

Jeffrey Metter and Luigi Ferrucci
National Institute of Aging, Clinical Research Branch, Harbor Hospital, Baltimore, MD, USA

INTRODUCTION

Understanding the mechanisms of loss of mobility and physical performance that occur in many older individuals has been the main focus of geriatric and gerontological research over the last three decades. Based on the findings of many epidemiological and clinical studies, it has been suggested that physical performance is the most robust biomarker of the aging process, and accelerated decline in physical performance, mostly lower extremity performance, tracks accelerated aging. In fact, poor lower extremity performance is an independent risk factor for multiple negative health outcomes including disability, nursing home admission, health care resources utilization and death, independent of and stronger than other biomedical measures of health status [1–3].

Many researchers have launched projects aimed at understanding the causes of physical function decline with aging and to better understand why physical function is such a strong prognostic marker. When talking about changes of mobility and physical performance with aging it is logical to immediately think of muscle. In the absence of muscle, mobility is impossible, and it is well known that aging is associated with decline in lean body mass, which is a good proxy of skeletal muscle mass. A number of studies have measured muscle mass in clinical and epidemiological populations using a range of different techniques to test the hypothesis that decline in muscle mass was the main cause of mobility and physical function decline in late life [3–7]. The results of these studies were somewhat surprising and have generated more questions than answers. It is useful to summarize briefly the findings of these studies: a) Muscle mass was a very poor predictor of physical function and mobility, and was only weakly related to mortality; b) Muscle mass and muscle strength were highly

Sarcopenia, First Edition. Edited by Alfonso J. Cruz-Jentoft and John E. Morley.

related but the relationship was less than expected, especially in very old individuals; c) Aging was characterized by a decline of both muscle strength and muscle mass, but the decline in strength substantially exceeded the decline in mass d) the relationship between muscle strength and physical performance, especially lower extremity performance was statistically significant but far from being exhaustive. For example, the variance in walking speed explained by lower extremity muscle strength was less than 15%, and after adjusting for lower extremity strength, the effect of chronological age on walking speed was still highly significant.

These findings suggest that: a) The decline in muscle strength with aging is caused by a combination of decline in skeletal mass and an even more important decline in muscle quality (strength per unit of mass; b) Even strength (and power), which is the most direct measure of the contribution of muscle to movement, explains only in small part physical performance and decline of physical performance with aging. Considering these studies, it is not surprising that interventions that have attempted to improve physical function in older persons by increasing muscle mass (i.e. testosterone, Insulin growth factor or IGF-1/Growth hormone) have been only minimally successful in improving muscle strength [8,9]. We are left with a conundrum: if muscle strength explains only a small percentage of physical function what important components are we missing?

One of the possible solutions is the old concept that 'force is useless without control'. Adequate control and graduation of muscle contraction in different muscle groups in a volitional movement is a very complex process, which requires the participation of different organ systems. It is almost naive to believe that by just studying muscle, the ultimate effector of movement, we can understand the effect of aging on physical function. The neurological control of movement is the 'white elephant' that only very recently has received some attention as a possible cause of age-associated mobility disability, and even as a direct cause of sarcopenia.

Before we continue, one important corollary should be established right away. This book focuses on sarcopenia, and there is no doubt that anatomical and functional changes in the central and peripheral nervous system participate in sarcopenia through multiple mechanisms, for example by removing trophic signals and facilitating the transaction of myocells to senescence and apoptosis. However, the organization of optimally coordinated contraction is by far the most essential prerequisite to the maintenance of muscle mass and muscle strength. When the importance of physical activity to sarcopenia is considered, the role of the nervous system spans well beyond the simple effect on muscle tissue and involves the area of movement control and its changes with aging. To better explain this concept it is useful to make an example. Let's focus on a very simple task such as a simple 'knee extension', we know that in young individuals we can obtain the same strength by supra maximal electrical stimulation of the quadriceps muscle and volitional maximal contraction [10–12].

However, in old individuals, the electrical stimulation generates significantly more strength than maximal volitional contraction [13,14]. Thus, the global neurological strategy to obtain maximal contraction becomes less effective with aging or, in other words, the nervous system component of contraction becomes impaired with aging. Although few studies have attempted to expand this model to more complex tasks, it is logical to hypothesize that the more complex is the motor task, the stronger is the role played by the neurological control system in controlling spatial and temporal patterns of contraction among myofibers, single muscles and muscle groups to optimize force generation. In this view, the boundaries

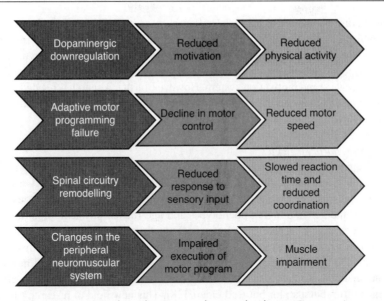

Figure 4.1   Neural mechanisms and events leading to Sarcopenia.

between the role of neurological control on force generation (neurological component of muscle impairment) and the role of 'sarcopenia' in the genesis of disability are blurred.

To start exploring the 'neurological component of muscle impairment' we will start by describing the chain of events that leads to the generation of a volitional task. Then we will summarize the literature concerning the effect of aging on the functionality of each ring in the chain, and attempt to estimate their relative importance. Then, we will describe the mechanism by which a neurological dysfunction can lead to muscle atrophy and changes in muscle quality. Finally, using the limited data available in the literature, we will try to hypothesize a time course narrative of role played by different neurological dysfunction on muscle impairment and mobility disability with aging in a life-course perspective.

In our view, and with a great deal of simplification, the rings in the chain are as follows (See Figure 4.1):

1. *Motivation*

   Historically older subjects were thought to lack a biological imperative to reproduce or 'hunt and gather.' When individuals are followed longitudinally over many years from early adult life, they report a progressive decline in the amount of leisure time physical activity particularly for high intensity activity [15] and show a progressive decline in aerobic fitness [16]. As noted by Ingram [17], similar changes in activity levels are observed across a number of species of animals. Age related changes in brain function also play important roles. Various studies have demonstrated changes in the dopaminergic system with aging that lead to reduced levels of dopamine [18], reduction in the postsynaptic dopamine receptors [19,20] and presynaptic dopamine transporters [21] which collectively result in altered reward processing [22]. Moreover, apart from rewards, the brain's reward system tracks energetic and other costs of effort during selection of action [23–25]. The down-regulation of dopamine signaling with aging results in diminished reward signals and/or increased cost signals and altered dynamics upon which decision making is based [26]. With aging, the effort required for movement may out-weigh expected rewards resulting in decreased motivation for movement. It has been postulated that such changes result in the down regulation of the dopamine mediated reward and motivation system. However, further research is needed to delineate the exact mechanism and the extent of the role of the reward and motivational pathways in motor slowing [27].

2. *Generation of the motor program*

   (a) *Motor control strategies*

   The analysis of the age-related modifications of motor control strategies is a topic of extreme interest with important theoretical and practical implications. Understanding the mechanisms by which the brain develops motor programs continuously adapted to the emergence of aging phenotypes and age-related physical impairments opens a window in the mechanism of neuronal plasticity. Failure of adaptive mechanisms probably plays an important role in the development of physical disability with aging. On the other hand, a better comprehension of the principles of motor control may help develop advanced technological solutions not only for seniors affected by disabilities but also for but frail elders [28]. This new field of research (often called 'gerontechnology' which is the combination of 'gerontology' – the scientific study of aging – and 'technology') cannot be successful without a thorough analysis of the age-related modifications of motor control strategies.

   It is well known that older persons rely on more widespread CNS engagement for motor control [27], and it has been suggested that a wider engagement of neurological structures reflects increased reliance on cognitive control mechanisms as a compensatory strategy to offset age-related sensorimotor decline. The basal ganglia and prefrontal cortex play a predominant role in motor planning and execution. Strong feedback loops exist between the two structures, with the basal ganglia (along with the cerebellum) being directly involved in the motor programming of movement, and the prefrontal regions dealing more directly with the direction and the extent of movement. According to a diffuse theory, basal ganglia 'age functionally' faster than the rest of the brain, and therefore the prefrontal regions must assume a greater role in the generation of movement programs, such as during movement preparation [29] and execution [30] or when switching between complex coordinated movements [31]. Frontal networks also mediate automaticity for certain movements that, once automated, can be performed with lesser cortical activation [32,33]. However, studies have also observed substantial declines in size and connectivity of prefrontal structures, which may contribute to further compromise in motor control [27]. MRI based volumetric studies and Diffusion tensor imaging (DTI) studies have shown that grey and white matter in the prefrontal and frontal areas show the most severe decline in volume and hence are most vulnerable to aging [34–36] whereas aging selectively impairs the efficiency of the function of frontal networks [37]. Finally, aging impairs basic mechanisms of cortical plasticity [38], which may impair new motor learning [39].

   (b) Movement speed

   Reduced velocity of movement has been reported by a myriad of studies on aging. Slowness is one of the most robust effects of aging on movement performance. Decreases in movement speed for 30%–70% of older adults compared with young adults have been demonstrated on a variety of motor tasks [40,41]. The slowing of movement with aging is attributable to changes in structural elements. For example, age-related slowing of maximum running speed was characterized by a decline in stride length and an increase in contact time along with a lower magnitude of ground reaction forces. The sprint-trained athletes demonstrated an age-related selective muscular atrophy and reduced force capacity that contributed to the deterioration in sprint running ability with age [42].

It has been hypothesized that degradation of the white matter systems in normal aging may contribute greatly to slow performance. Sullivan et al. assessed quantitative fiber tracking using DTI imaging and performance of functional measures using unilateral and bilateral fine finger movement test, digit symbol test and measures of ataxia in 120 men and women between ages 20-81 years. They found that fine finger movement speed was related to the integrity of fibers of the internal and external capsules, which are the systems interconnecting striatal and motor cortical regions sub-serving motor control. Also, changes in the cerebellar hemispheric fiber bundles contributed to slower finger movements. In addition, age-related balance impairment and ataxia was found with degradation of supratentorial white matter, rather than changes in cerebellum [43]. Finally, aging-related white matter hyperintensities result in reduced velocity, irrespective of their exact anatomical location [44].

At a biochemical level, decline in the dopamine transporters after the fifth decade of life, contributes to slow motor performance, deficits in response selection and motor adjustments [45]. The dopamine transporter has been noted to decline starting early in adult life [46]. Studies have found that lower striatal dopamine transporter levels are associated with reductions in speed, cadence, single and double support durations, thereby contributing to impaired gait [47]. Van Dyke et al. reported that loss of striatal dopamine transporter may contribute to slowing of motor reaction speed with advancing age [48]. Motor deficits due to decline in dopamine signaling cannot be separated from deficits in reward processing, given that the motor cortex receives dopaminergic reward signals similarly to prefrontal cortex [49,50].

(c) Quality of motor programs:

There is some evidence that movement programs are less redundant and precise and require more corrections in older compared to younger individuals. Balance becomes impaired, there is increased sway while walking a straight line and stepping to avoid falling becomes slower and less effective [51,52] and as a consequence the risk for falls substantially increases [53,54]. To better understand the genesis of these functional impairments, it is useful to consider a simple movement such as reaching to grab something. Such movement can be divided into a primary movement and secondary compensatory sub-movements. The primary movement, which consists in getting the hand to the target, is performed with smooth, bell-shaped velocity profile (increasing velocity to get the hand close and then deceleration as the hand approaches the target) and is generally considered a pre-programmed ballistic movement. Inaccuracy of the initial control plan affects the precision of the movement and may cause slowing and deviations of the primary movement from the target. The secondary sub-movements during the final approach to the target are corrective adjustments aimed at improving movement accuracy [55,56]. Since neuromuscular noise increases with aging, older adults tend to shorten the primary movement and increase the role of corrective sub-movements to improve precision [57]. Analogously, it can be assumed that wider corrective movements may be required during static and dynamic balance adjustments.

3. *Verification and scaling of the motor program and on line correction based on sensory inputs*

(a) Decline in sensory feedback:

Proprioceptive feedback is important for postural control and motor coordination. Toe position matching test and tandem stance stability test assessing lower limb proprioceptive acuity showed age related decline and positive correlation with falls in previous 12 months [58–60]. As a result of the sensory decline, there is increased reliability on visual feedback for motor performance [61]. There is increased vulnerability of the motor and somatosensory region of the brain to age-related atrophy [27,62]. This could be secondary to prominent cortical atrophy in frontal cortex near primary motor cortex, calcarine cortex near primary visual cortex which occurs by middle age and later spans widespread cortical regions that include primary and association sensory cortex [63]. Impaired cortical integration of available sensory signals may explain why gait, posture and postural stability are preferentially affected by parietal white matter hyperintensities [44].

In addition, age associated striatal dopaminergic denervation is a contributing factor for recurrent falls in the elderly [64]. The central ability to inhibit balance destabilizing vision-related postural control processes and ability to tune muscle tone on standing depends at least partially on striatal dopaminergic pathways in older individuals. The level of presynaptic dopaminergic denervation in the anteroventral striatum contributed 20-25% of the variability in antero-posterior body sway magnitude, which is a measure of impaired balance [65].

In the peripheral nervous system, changes occur with age at the level of the individual proprioceptors. Aged muscle spindles show reduced density with fewer intrafusal fibers and morphological changes like decreased spindle diameter, axonal swelling and expanded motor endplates that may be a result of denervation [58,66]. Similarly cutaneous and joint mechanoreceptors show reduced number and mean density of receptors with aging [67,68]. These changes could potentially contribute to decline in proprioceptive acuity.

(b) Reaction time

Simple reaction time shortens from infancy into the late 20s, then increases slowly until the 50s and 60s, and then lengthens faster as the person gets into his 70s and beyond [69–72]. This effect is more marked for complex reaction time tasks [69,70]. Reaction time also becomes more variable with age and cognitive impairment as in Alzheimer's disease [73,74]. MacDonald *et al*. found that reaction time variability in older adults was usually associated with slower reaction times and worse recognition of stimuli, and suggested that variability might be a useful measure of general neural integrity [75]. Welford speculates that slowing reaction time with age is not merely the consequence of slower nervous conduction times but also results from increased tendency of older people to be more careful and monitor their responses more thoroughly [76,77]. When troubled by a distraction, older people also tend to devote their exclusive attention to one stimulus, and ignore another stimulus, more completely than younger people [78]. Lajoie and Gallagher found that old people who tend to fall in nursing homes had a significantly slower reaction time than those who did not tend to fall [79]. Furthermore, performing dual tasks such as walking while incrementally counting backwards is also associated with increased risk of falling, particularly in older adults. There is greater relative reduction in gait velocity and the increased variability in stride velocity in older adults in comparison to younger subjects, when performing dual tasks [80]. Similarly, decreased attentional resources may also contribute to the diminished proprioceptive abilities of elderly individuals [58]. Doumas et al., 2008 M. Doumas, C. Smolders and R. Krampe, Task prioritization in aging: effects of sensory information on concurrent posture and memory performance. *Exp. Brain Res.*, (2008). Doumas *et al.* tested upright stance in older adults (mean age = 71.0 years) during a concurrent 'n-back' working memory task. With vision, and a fixed support surface, postural sway increased when attention was divided [81].

(c) Motor coordination and changes in the brain:

Subcortical structures important for motor performance and coordination including cerebellum and the caudate nucleus exhibit accelerated decrease in volume with age [82]. Better performance on an eye-hand coordinated task was related to greater callosal integrity, with greatest contribution to performance from the genu, parietal and temporal sectors of corpus callosum [83]. Other studies using fMRI and bimanual tasks assessing the strength of activation in the motor cortex in relation to cross-sectional surface area of the corpus callosum showed that the size of the corpus callosum modulated activity of the supplementary motor area and cingulate cortex in a manner that was dependent upon task complexity [84]. The age-related bimanual coordination deficits may be differentially higher for more complex tasks and callosal decline may lead to these deficits[27].

4. *Execution of the motor program through the spinal cord and nerves.*

The corticospinal tracks transform volitional motor programs into action by inducing activation of spinal motoneurons. The excitatory postsynaptic potentials (EPSP) in spinal motoneurons induced by fast-conducting descending volleys show a linear decline with age [85], although many other measures of corticospinal communication appear unaffected by aging [86]. Moreover, qualitative changes in corticospinal communication may occur, such as anticipatory modulation of corticospinal excitability to speed up response generation seen in simple reaction time tasks [87]. Data on change in spinal cord and spinal cord neurons with aging is scant. Animal studies mostly performed in rats found signs of spinal cord degeneration, including de-myelination of individual axons starting in the ventral roots and later developing in the dorsal roots followed by fibrosis. Autopsy studies in humans have shown that the number and diameter of anterior horn motor neurons decline with increasing age [88] [89–91]. Studies have estimated a 25 to 50% decline in the number of spinal motor neurons between the age of 20 and 90, with most of the loss coming in later years. Both in animal models and in human studies, the loss of motor neurons is associated with an increase in the number of astrocytes and with an apparent alteration in the dendritic networks of the neurons [92]. Associated with these changes, there is a slowing of conduction latencies in the spinal cord. Transcranial Magnetic Stimulation studies have shown reduced excitability of efferent corticospinal pathways in elderly [93].

These changes may cause reduction of muscle strength, mass and performance with aging, although direct evidence of this association is lacking. The exact nature of the mechanism that cause such a decline in motor neurons is not understand but hypothesized mechanisms include a reduction in endocrine and paracrine production of IGF-1, a

pro-inflammatory with chronically elevated levels of IL-6 and TNF-alpha but also modification of signaling input from the upstream neurological structure that act as trophic
stimulus.

(a) Changes in the motor units:

Younger subjects, 20 to 40 years of age, have approximately twice as many motor
units in comparison to older subjects between 63 and 81 years of age [94]. This
reduction of motor neurons is partially compensated by increased sprouting that
results in progressively less and larger motor units [95]. Moreover, reorganization
occurs in the motor units with an increase in their size due to increased number
of fibers per motor unit, which in turn increases the force generated by that unit
[94,96,97].

In addition, the pattern of motor unit activation changes with aging. The pattern
of motor unit activation observed in the youngest age group, with recruitment of
progressively larger units and increases in firing rate at higher force levels, is consistent with the Henneman's size principle [98]. As more motor units are recruited
and/or as motor unit firing rates increase, the force of contraction increases. In contrast, in older adults, motor unit size and firing rate are already higher at low force
levels with a progressive recruitment of larger units as force increases [96]. In spite
of this compensatory reorganization, the ability to produce intended force declines
with age. A study assessing the force and discharge characteristics of motor units
in the hand muscle of young and old adults demonstrated that the difference in
force between the recruitment of successive motor units does not differ between age
groups, but that motor unit recruitment may be more transient in older persons and
contribute to the greater variability in force observed in old adults during graded
ramp contractions [99].

Variable rate of motor unit discharges contributes to greater muscle force fluctuations during sub-maximal contraction in older adults [100,101]. These fluctuations
in the muscle force impair the ability to move the limb accurately to a desired target. This is demonstrated by experiments assessing abduction of the index finger
i.e. contractions of the first dorsal interosseous muscle with a submaximal load at
different movement velocities [102,103].

(b) Changes in the peripheral nerves:

It is known that peripheral nerves and conduction velocities change with age.
Conwit and Metter reported slow linear decline in peripheral nerve conduction
velocity beginning after 30 to 40 years of age [104]. The values normally change
by less than 10 m/s by the age of 60 to 80 years [105]. Similarly, there is a gradual
decline of the amplitude of compound muscle action potentials and sensory nerve
action potentials (SNAPs) [104]. At least in part, the reduction in axonal conduction
speed is due to drop outs of the largest axonal fibers and reduced myelination. There
is some evidence that sensory afferent axons are more affected than effect motor
axons [106]. These changes in the conduction velocities with age are related to
loss of muscle strength. Metter et al. studied the relation of age-related changes in
the median nerve function to grip strength in the Baltimore longitudinal study of
aging. They found that median nerve conduction velocity declined linearly with age
and had a relatively small but significant independent predictive role in loss of grip
strength. The level of independent effect was about one third of the effect attributed
to forearm muscle mass or age [107].

(c) Changes at the neuromuscular junction:

Due to neuroaxonal degeneration as described above, there is loss of synaptic input at the neuromuscular junction (NMJ). In addition, substantial age-related changes occur at the level of the NMJ. As a response to this partial denervation of myofibers within a motor unit, the intact axons sprout to reinnervate surrounding denervated muscle end plates [108,109]. The perisynaptic Schwaan cells at the NMJ guide axonal sprouts to denervated endplates [110]. However, animal studies have suggested that the capacity for axonal and motor endplate sprouting is relatively limited with aging. Reduced neuromuscular inactivity inhibits axonal sprouting due to failure of perisynpatic Schwaan cells and/or reduced calcium influx into the nerve terminals to support sprout growth [110]. The motor neuron reinnervation of the regenerating muscle fibers is critical for the final differentiation into mature myofibers. This may contribute to slowed myofiber regeneration in the sarcopenic muscle and further adds to neuromuscular impairment [109].

Widening of synaptic clefts and degeneration of junctional folds at the post synaptic region have been reported in a study assessing external intercostal muscles in subjects between 4 to 77 years of age [111]. The distribution and morphology of acetylcholine receptors changes with age. An increase in the number of perijunctional acetylcholine receptors and a greater number of smaller conglomerates of acetylcholine receptors are seen in older persons compared to younger persons [112]. This anatomical remodeling is coupled with age-related neurophysiological alterations including increased quantal content, with a more rapid rundown of endplate potential strength during continuous stimulation of the pre-synaptic neuron. The direct functional impact of these changes remains unknown.

5. *The Excito-Contraction (EC) coupling in muscle fibers.*

EC coupling is a physiological process of converting the neural signal for muscle activation i.e. the sarcolemmal action potential into muscle contraction and force generation [113]. Aging results in reduced number of dihydropyridine receptors and expression of a junctional face membrane protein of the sarcoplasmic reticulum (JP 45) resulting in altered protein-protein interaction and deficits in calcium supply to contractile proteins. This ultimately leads to a reduced contractile force of the skeletal muscle [114–116]. In addition, structural changes of myosin lead to changes in the kinetics of the cross-bridge cycle, which further contributes to reduced contractile force [117].

Many studies performed in different muscle groups have shown definite age-related changes in the functional properties of contractile muscle fibers. A significant increase in time to peak tension and the time to relaxation following evoked twitches have been demonstrated in triceps surae as well as plantar and dorsiflexors of the ankle in elderly persons [118,119]. Vandervoot and McComas found a linear increase of twitch times with age from 20 to 100 years although changes in muscle strength did not become evident until the seventh decade of life [119]. Such changes in muscle fiber type may contribute to enhanced muscle fatigue resistance with maximal stimulation in the elderly. However, reports have suggested that muscle fatigue in older individuals is greater [120–122], less than [123,124], or similar [125] to young individuals.

It is important to underline that slowing of the muscle contraction also reduces capacity for rapid force production in protective reflexes and amplifies the impact of muscle weakness on mobility [126,127]. In addition, slowing of the peripheral nerve conduction velocity and rate of torque development of a muscle contraction further contributes to this effect [104,126]. A study by Klass et al. showed that maximal rate of torque development and integrated intramuscular electromyogram (EMGs) at peak rate of torque development during fast contractions were lower in elderly (48%) in comparison to young adults (16.5%; P value <0.05). These age-related changes during fast voluntary contraction of tibialis anterior were accompanied by a decline in motor unit discharge frequency. This suggests that the age-related decline in maximal motor unit discharge frequency limit the performance of fast voluntary contractions in addition to the slowing of muscle contractile properties [128].

6. *The role of nervous system in muscle skeletal development and sarcopenia*:
Aging results in a substantial impairment of the supraspinal or central nervous system drive due to anatomical and functional changes in the frontal cortex, white matter tracts, dopaminergic system and all the systems that contribute to motor neuron excitation. These changes are accompanied by slowing of peripheral nerves, degradation of the neuromuscular junction and changes in the contractile properties of the muscle including the excitation-contraction uncoupling, and all ultimately contributes to a dysfunction of the muscle and possibly also contributes to the progressive muscle atrophy that characterizes the aging process. There is little doubt that the neurological contribution to sarcopenia contributes to physical disability and morbidity, either as a primary cause or because of interference with compensatory strategies. Because most of these changes occur late in life, the reason why muscle mass and muscle strength start to decline with aging relatively early in life remains an open question. Studies that use a life-course perspective are now in the field, hopefully, they will provide some answers to this specific question. However, based on the current literature, we would like to propose a hypothetical model that may help to organize the next set of studies in humans and, if confirmed, may shed light on new effective strategies for prevention. In particular, we propose that the life-course process of sarcopenia could be divided six critical phases: 1) Development. The program for the development of the motor system is inscribed in our genes, but its execution is certainly driven by the nervous system. There is very strong evidence that a number of environmental conditions can affect the final realization of the muscle phenotype, including early nutrition and physical activity [129]. During this phase there is an almost perfect proportionality between increments in muscle mass and increments in muscle strength; 2) Early adulthood: (20-35 years): In this phase the musculoskeletal system attains maximal physical potential and performance, which is strongly affected by the level of physical activity and exercise, which may substantially affect the genetic programs of muscle development and affect peak mass; 3) Late early adulthood (30-45 years): During this period functional capability starts changing with slight losses in muscle strength and slowing of reaction and movement times, although the age of onset varies widely between individuals. Muscle quality also starts changing, especially in obese and sedentary individuals, because of muscle fat infiltration and because the force generated by muscle fibers per unit of cross-sectional area is reduced. Note that up to this phase, performance is mostly affected by muscle mass and by the neurological drive to contraction. In fact, the number of motor neurons, nerve conduction velocity, and functional anatomy of motor units are substantially intact. During this period, what is most striking is a marked decline in most individuals in the level of physical activity in which they participate. While not well studied, we speculate that this loss in physical activity appears to be based on an innate loss of motivation resulting in gradual muscle atrophy from decreasing muscle

use, and likely represents a form of disuse atrophy. The motivational changes may relate to changes that are observed beginning in the third decade of life in brain regional volumes, including caudate, cerebellum and prefrontal regions, and lower numbers of striatal dopamine transporters. The feedback relationship between the frontal lobe, basal ganglia and dopaminergic system are strongly related to motor control and movement motivation, as well as the drive/reward systems. Roth and Joseph noted that dopamine receptor content which declines with increasing age in the brains of aging rats could be slowed by alternate day fasting and temporarily altered by prolactin with improvement in motor performance [130]. 4) Middle age (40-65 years): The decline in muscle mass, and especially muscle strength become more evident although they are still compensated by a great deal of reserve capacity and they have little impact on habitual physical function, but maximal performance levels in athletic activities clearly decline. In most individuals there is clear decline in muscle quality, which again is particularly evident in those who are obese and sedentary. In this period, women go through the menopause which is associated with changes in hormonal patterns with associated changes in body fat mass, and men are showing declines in testosterone levels that are associated with losses of lean mass. 5) Older age (65+ years) large losses of muscle mass and strength challenge the ability of individuals in strenuous activities and in some cases even in daily life activities. Ability to compensate for other co-impairment is also reduced. This is the end-stage of the process and results in significant motor disability, postural instability and falls in elderly.

CONCLUSION

Sarcopenia is a lifelong process in adults. The causes are partially understood but underlying changes in the brain are likely critical to the cascade that leads to this progressive course. A striking myriad of changes in the central nervous and neuromuscular systems occurring throughout the lifespan cumulates and are associated with progressive decline in physical activity levels. This occurs in humans and other species. It is plausible that there is a central pacemaker orchestrating the various central processes contributing to sarcopenia, such as aging-related changes in the dopaminergic system. Additional mechanisms like hormonal loss, inflammation, disease and physical inactivity contribute to the early phases. However a critical question is what factors cause these declines and how can this process be altered or slowed down. The answer to this question will help us not only understand and hopefully slow down the normal aging process, but also give us insights and open new frontiers in treatment of various disorders with accelerated neurodegeneration like Alzheimer's or Parkinson's disease.

ACKNOWLEDGMENT

We thank Dimitros Kapogiannis, MD for his input and review of the manuscript. Disclaimer: This report does not represent the official view of the National Institute of Neurological disorders and Stroke (NINDS), the National Institute of Aging (NIA), the National Institutes of Health (NIH), or any part of the US Federal Government. No official support or endorsement of this article by the NINDS, NIA or NIH is intended or should be inferred.

REFERENCES

1. Hairi, N.N., et al., Loss of muscle strength, mass (sarcopenia), and quality (specific force) and its relationship with functional limitation and physical disability: the Concord Health and Ageing in Men Project. J Am Geriatr Soc, 2010. 58(11): p. 2055–2062.

2. Janssen, I., et al., The healthcare costs of sarcopenia in the United States. J Am Geriatr Soc, 2004. 52(1): p. 80–85.

3. Reid, K.F., et al., Lower extremity muscle mass predicts functional performance in mobility-limited elders. J Nutr Health Aging, 2008. 12(7): p. 493–498.

4. Goodpaster, B.H., et al., Attenuation of skeletal muscle and strength in the elderly: The Health ABC Study. J Appl Physiol, 2001. 90(6): p. 2157–2165.

5. Iannuzzi-Sucich, M., K.M. Prestwood, and A.M. Kenny, Prevalence of sarcopenia and predictors of skeletal muscle mass in healthy, older men and women. J Gerontol A Biol Sci Med Sci, 2002. 57(12): p. M772–7.

6. Janssen, I., S.B. Heymsfield, and R. Ross, Low relative skeletal muscle mass (sarcopenia) in older persons is associated with functional impairment and physical disability. J Am Geriatr Soc, 2002. 50(5): p. 889–896.

7. Lexell, J., C.C. Taylor, and M. Sjostrom, What is the cause of the ageing atrophy? Total number, size and proportion of different fiber types studied in whole vastus lateralis muscle from 15- to 83-year-old men. J Neurol Sci, 1988. 84(2–3): p. 275–294.

8. Bhasin, S., Testosterone supplementation for aging-associated sarcopenia. J Gerontol A Biol Sci Med Sci, 2003. 58(11): p. 1002–1008.

9. Giovannini, S., et al., Modulation of GH/IGF-1 axis: potential strategies to counteract sarcopenia in older adults. Mech Ageing Dev, 2008. 129(10): p. 593–601.

10. Miller, M., D. Downham, and J. Lexell, Effects of superimposed electrical stimulation on perceived discomfort and torque increment size and variability. Muscle Nerve, 2003. 27(1): p. 90–98.

11. Mohr, T., et al., The effect of high volt galvanic stimulation on quadriceps femoris muscle torque. J Orthop Sports Phys Ther, 1986. 7(6): p. 314–318.

12. Westing, S.H., J.Y. Seger, and A. Thorstensson, Effects of electrical stimulation on eccentric and concentric torque-velocity relationships during knee extension in man. Acta Physiol Scand, 1990. 140(1): p. 17–22.

13. Hakkinen, K., et al., Neuromuscular performance in voluntary bilateral and unilateral contraction and during electrical stimulation in men at different ages. Eur J Appl Physiol Occup Physiol, 1995. 70(6): p. 518–527.

14. Yue, G.H., et al., Older adults exhibit a reduced ability to fully activate their biceps brachii muscle. J Gerontol A Biol Sci Med Sci, 1999. 54(5): p. M249–53.

15. Talbot, L.A., et al., Changes in leisure time physical activity and risk of all-cause mortality in men and women: the Baltimore Longitudinal Study of Aging. Prev Med, 2007. 45(2–3): p. 169–176.

16. Fleg, J.L., et al., Accelerated longitudinal decline of aerobic capacity in healthy older adults. Circulation, 2005. 112(5): p. 674–682.

17. Ingram, D.K., Age-related decline in physical activity: generalization to nonhumans. Med Sci Sports Exerc, 2000. 32(9): p. 1623–1629.

18. Garnett, E.S., G. Firnau, and C. Nahmias, Dopamine visualized in the basal ganglia of living man. Nature, 1983. 305(5930): p. 137–138.

19. Kaasinen, V., et al., Age-related dopamine D2/D3 receptor loss in extrastriatal regions of the human brain. Neurobiol Aging, 2000. 21(5): p. 683–688.

20. Suhara, T., et al., Age-related changes in human D1 dopamine receptors measured by positron emission tomography. Psychopharmacology (Berl), 1991. 103(1): p. 41–45.

21. Volkow, N.D., et al., Decreased dopamine transporters with age in health human subjects. Ann Neurol, 1994. 36(2): p. 237–239.

22. Dreher, J.C., et al., Variation in dopamine genes influences responsivity of the human reward system. Proc Natl Acad Sci U S A, 2009. 106(2): p. 617–622.

23. Day, J.J., J.L. Jones, and R.M. Carelli, Nucleus accumbens neurons encode predicted and ongoing reward costs in rats. Eur J Neurosci, 2011. 33(2): p. 308–321.

24. Hauber, W. and S. Sommer, Prefrontostriatal circuitry regulates effort-related decision making. Cereb Cortex, 2009. 19(10): p. 2240–2247.

25. Phillips, P.E., M.E. Walton, and T.C. Jhou, Calculating utility: preclinical evidence for cost-benefit analysis by mesolimbic dopamine. Psychopharmacology (Berl), 2007. 191(3): p. 483–495.

26. Eppinger, B., D. Hammerer, and S.C. Li, Neuromodulation of reward-based learning and decision making in human aging. Ann N Y Acad Sci, 2011. 1235(1): p. 1–17.

27. Seidler, R.D., et al., Motor control and aging: links to age-related brain structural, functional, and biochemical effects. Neurosci Biobehav Rev, 2010. 34(5): p. 721–733.

28. Micera, S., P. Bonato, and T. Tamura, Gerontechnology. IEEE Eng Med Biol Mag, 2008. 27(4): p. 10–14.

29. Sterr, A. and P. Dean, Neural correlates of movement preparation in healthy ageing. Eur J Neurosci, 2008. 27(1): p. 254–260.

30. Marchand, W.R., et al., Age-related changes of the functional architecture of the cortico-basal ganglia circuitry during motor task execution. Neuroimage, 2011. 55(1): p. 194–203.

31. Coxon, J.P., et al., Reduced basal ganglia function when elderly switch between coordinated movement patterns. Cereb Cortex, 2010. 20(10): p. 2368–2379.

32. Floyer-Lea, A. and P.M. Matthews, Changing brain networks for visuomotor control with increased movement automaticity. J Neurophysiol, 2004. 92(4): p. 2405–2412.

33. Poldrack, R.A., et al., The neural correlates of motor skill automaticity. J Neurosci, 2005. 25(22): p. 5356–5364.

34. Courchesne, E., et al., Normal brain development and aging: quantitative analysis at in vivo MR imaging in healthy volunteers. Radiology, 2000. 216(3): p. 672–682.

35. Malykhin, N., et al., Structural organization of the prefrontal white matter pathways in the adult and aging brain measured by diffusion tensor imaging. Brain Struct Funct, 2011. 216(4): p. 417–431.

36. Westlye, L.T., et al., Life-span changes of the human brain white matter: diffusion tensor imaging (DTI) and volumetry. Cereb Cortex, 2010. 20(9): p. 2055–2068.

37. Achard, S. and E. Bullmore, Efficiency and cost of economical brain functional networks. PLoS Comput Biol, 2007. 3(2): p. e17.

38. Freitas, C., et al., Changes in cortical plasticity across the lifespan. Front Aging Neurosci, 2011. 3: p. 5.

39. Rogasch, N.C., et al., Corticomotor plasticity and learning of a ballistic thumb training task are diminished in older adults. J Appl Physiol, 2009. 107(6): p. 1874–1883.

40. Cooke, J.D., S.H. Brown, and D.A. Cunningham, Kinematics of arm movements in elderly humans. Neurobiol Aging, 1989. 10(2): p. 159–165.

41. Pohl, P.S., C.J. Winstein, and B.E. Fisher, The locus of age-related movement slowing: sensory processing in continuous goal-directed aiming. J Gerontol B Psychol Sci Soc Sci, 1996. 51(2): p. P94–102.

42. Korhonen, M.T., et al., Biomechanical and skeletal muscle determinants of maximum running speed with aging. Med Sci Sports Exerc, 2009. 41(4): p. 844–856.

43. Sullivan, E.V., T. Rohlfing, and A. Pfefferbaum, Quantitative fiber tracking of lateral and inter-hemispheric white matter systems in normal aging: relations to timed performance. Neurobiol Aging, 2010. 31(3): p. 464–481.

44. Murray, M.E., et al., Functional impact of white matter hyperintensities in cognitively normal elderly subjects. Arch Neurol, 2010. 67(11): p. 1379–1385.

45. Troiano, A.R., et al., Dopamine transporter PET in normal aging: dopamine transporter decline and its possible role in preservation of motor function. Synapse, 2010. 64(2): p. 146–151.

46. van Dyck, C.H., et al., Age-related decline in dopamine transporters: analysis of striatal subre-gions, nonlinear effects, and hemispheric asymmetries. Am J Geriatr Psychiatry, 2002. 10(1): p. 36–43.

47. Cham, R., et al., Striatal dopaminergic denervation and gait in healthy adults. Exp Brain Res, 2008. 185(3): p. 391–398.

48. van Dyck, C.H., et al., Striatal dopamine transporters correlate with simple reaction time in elderly subjects. Neurobiol Aging, 2008. 29(8): p. 1237–1246.

49. Kapogiannis, D., et al., Reward-related activity in the human motor cortex. Eur J Neurosci, 2008. 27(7): p. 1836–1842.

50. Kapogiannis, D., et al., Reward processing abnormalities in Parkinson's disease. Mov Disord, 2011. 26(8): p. 1451–1457.

51. McIlroy, W.E. and B.E. Maki, Age-related changes in compensatory stepping in response to unpredictable perturbations. J Gerontol A Biol Sci Med Sci, 1996. 51(6): p. M289–96.

52. Woollacott, M.H. and P.F. Tang, Balance control during walking in the older adult: research and its implications. Phys Ther, 1997. 77(6): p. 646–660.

53. Englander, F., T.J. Hodson, and R.A. Terregrossa, Economic dimensions of slip and fall injuries. J Forensic Sci, 1996. 41(5): p. 733–746.

54. Speechley, M. and M. Tinetti, Falls and injuries in frail and vigorous community elderly persons. J Am Geriatr Soc, 1991. 39(1): p. 46–52.

55. Abrams, R.A. and J. Pratt, Rapid aimed limb movements: differential effects of practice on component submovements. J Mot Behav, 1993. 25(4): p. 288–298.

56. Chua, R. and D. Elliott, Visual regulation of manual aiming. Human Movement Science, 1993. 12(4): p. 365–401.

57. Walker, N., D.A. Philbin, and A.D. Fisk, Age-related differences in movement control: adjusting submovement structure to optimize performance. J Gerontol B Psychol Sci Soc Sci, 1997. 52(1): p. P40–52.

58. Goble, D.J., et al., Proprioceptive sensibility in the elderly: degeneration, functional conse-quences and plastic-adaptive processes. Neurosci Biobehav Rev, 2009. 33(3): p. 271–278.

59. Lord, S.R., R.D. Clark, and I.W. Webster, Physiological factors associated with falls in an elderly population. J Am Geriatr Soc, 1991. 39(12): p. 1194–1200.

60. Lord, S.R., et al., Lateral stability, sensorimotor function and falls in older people. J Am Geriatr Soc, 1999. 47(9): p. 1077–1081.

61. Lord, S.R. and I.W. Webster, Visual field dependence in elderly fallers and non-fallers. Int J Aging Hum Dev, 1990. 31(4): p. 267–277.

62. Good, C.D., et al., A voxel-based morphometric study of ageing in 465 normal adult human brains. Neuroimage, 2001. 14(1 Pt 1): p. 21–36.

63. Salat, D.H., et al., Thinning of the cerebral cortex in aging. Cereb Cortex, 2004. 14(7): p. 721–730.

64. Bohnen, N.I., et al., Age-associated striatal dopaminergic denervation and falls in community-dwelling subjects. J Rehabil Res Dev, 2009. 46(8): p. 1045–1052.

65. Cham, R., et al., Striatal dopamine denervation and sensory integration for balance in middle-aged and older adults. Gait Posture, 2007. 26(4): p. 516–525.

66. Liu, J.X., et al., Fiber content and myosin heavy chain composition of muscle spindles in aged human biceps brachii. J Histochem Cytochem, 2005. 53(4): p. 445–454.

67. Aydog, S.T., et al., Decrease in the numbers of mechanoreceptors in rabbit ACL: the effects of ageing. Knee Surg Sports Traumatol Arthrosc, 2006. 14(4): p. 325–329.

68. Iwasaki, T., et al., The aging of human Meissner's corpuscles as evidenced by parallel sectioning. Okajimas Folia Anat Jpn, 2003. 79(6): p. 185–189.

69. Der, G. and I.J. Deary, Age and sex differences in reaction time in adulthood: results from the United Kingdom Health and Lifestyle Survey. Psychol Aging, 2006. 21(1): p. 62–73.

70. Luchies, C.W., et al., Effects of age, step direction, and reaction condition on the ability to step quickly. J Gerontol A Biol Sci Med Sci, 2002. 57(4): p. M246–9.

71. Welford, A.T., Motor Performance, in Handbook for the Psychology of Aging, J.E. Birren, Schaie, K.W., Editor 1977, Van Nostrand Reinhold: New York.

72. Yan, J.H., et al., Developmental features of rapid aiming arm movements across the lifespan. J Mot Behav, 2000. 32(2): p. 121–140.

73. Gorus, E., et al., Reaction times and performance variability in normal aging, mild cognitive impairment, and Alzheimer's disease. J Geriatr Psychiatry Neurol, 2008. 21(3): p. 204–218.

74. Hultsch, D.F., S.W. MacDonald, and R.A. Dixon, Variability in reaction time performance of younger and older adults. J Gerontol B Psychol Sci Soc Sci, 2002. 57(2): p. P101–15.

75. MacDonald, S.W., et al., Increased response-time variability is associated with reduced inferior parietal activation during episodic recognition in aging. J Cogn Neurosci, 2008. 20(5): p. 779–786.

76. Botwinick, J., Cautiousness in advanced age. J Gerontol, 1966. 21(3): p. 347–353.

77. Welford, A.T., Between bodily changes and performance: some possible reasons for slowing with age. Exp Aging Res, 1984. 10(2): p. 73–88.

78. Redfern, M.S., et al., Attentional dynamics in postural control during perturbations in young and older adults. J Gerontol A Biol Sci Med Sci, 2002. 57(8): p. B298–303.

79. Lajoie, Y. and S.P. Gallagher, Predicting falls within the elderly community: comparison of postural sway, reaction time, the Berg balance scale and the Activities-specific Balance Confidence (ABC) scale for comparing fallers and non-fallers. Arch Gerontol Geriatr, 2004. 38(1): p. 11–26.

80. Hollman, J.H., et al., Age-related differences in spatiotemporal markers of gait stability during dual task walking. Gait Posture, 2007. 26(1): p. 113–119.

81. Doumas, M., C. Smolders, and R.T. Krampe, Task prioritization in aging: effects of sensory information on concurrent posture and memory performance. Exp Brain Res, 2008. 187(2): p. 275–281.

82. Raz, N., et al., Regional brain changes in aging healthy adults: general trends, individual differences and modifiers. Cereb Cortex, 2005. 15(11): p. 1676–1689.

83. Sullivan, E.V., T. Rohlfing, and A. Pfefferbaum, Longitudinal study of callosal microstructure in the normal adult aging brain using quantitative DTI fiber tracking. Dev Neuropsychol, 2010. 35(3): p. 233–256.

84. Stancak, A., et al., The size of corpus callosum correlates with functional activation of medial motor cortical areas in bimanual and unimanual movements. Cereb Cortex, 2003. 13(5): p. 475–485.

85. Eisen, A., M. Entezari-Taher, and H. Stewart, Cortical projections to spinal motoneurons: changes with aging and amyotrophic lateral sclerosis. Neurology, 1996. 46(5): p. 1396–1404.

86. Smith, A.E., et al., Male human motor cortex stimulus-response characteristics are not altered by aging. J Appl Physiol, 2011. 110(1): p. 206–212.

87. Levin, O., et al., Age-related differences in human corticospinal excitability during simple reaction time. Neurosci Lett, 2011. 487(1): p. 53–57.

88. Zhang, C., et al., Age-related reductions in number and size of anterior horn cells at C6 level of the human spinal cord. Okajimas Folia Anat Jpn, 1996. 73(4): p. 171–177.

89. Cruz-Sanchez, F.F., et al., Evaluation of neuronal loss, astrocytosis and abnormalities of cytoskeletal components of large motor neurons in the human anterior horn in aging. J Neural Transm, 1998. 105(6–7): p. 689–701.

90. Mittal, K.R. and F.H. Logmani, Age-related reduction in 8th cervical ventral nerve root myelinated fiber diameters and numbers in man. J Gerontol, 1987. 42(1): p. 8–10.

91. Tomlinson, B.E. and D. Irving, The numbers of limb motor neurons in the human lumbosacral cord throughout life. J Neurol Sci, 1977. 34(2): p. 213–219.

92. Cruz-Sanchez, F.F., et al., Synaptophysin in spinal anterior horn in aging and ALS: an immunohistological study. J Neural Transm, 1996. 103(11): p. 1317–1329.

93. Sale, M.V. and J.G. Semmler, Age-related differences in corticospinal control during functional isometric contractions in left and right hands. J Appl Physiol, 2005. 99(4): p. 1483–1493.

94. Doherty, T.J. and W.F. Brown, The estimated numbers and relative sizes of thenar motor units as selected by multiple point stimulation in young and older adults. Muscle Nerve, 1993. 16(4): p. 355–366.

95. Wang, F.C., V. de Pasqua, and P.J. Delwaide, Age-related changes in fastest and slowest conducting axons of thenar motor units. Muscle Nerve, 1999. 22(8): p. 1022–109.

96. Ling, S.M., et al., Age-associated changes in motor unit physiology: observations from the Baltimore Longitudinal Study of Aging. Arch Phys Med Rehabil, 2009. 90(7): p. 1237–1240.

97. Thomas, C.K., et al., Twitch properties of human thenar motor units measured in response to intraneural motor-axon stimulation. J Neurophysiol, 1990. 64(4): p. 1339–1346.

98. Henneman, E. and C.B. Olson, Relations between Structure and Function in the Design of Skeletal Muscles. J Neurophysiol, 1965. 28: p. 581–598.

99. Jesunathadas, M., et al., Recruitment and derecruitment characteristics of motor units in a hand muscle of young and old adults. J Appl Physiol, 2010. 108(6): p. 1659–1667.

100. Laidlaw, D.H., M. Bilodeau, and R.M. Enoka, Steadiness is reduced and motor unit discharge is more variable in old adults. Muscle Nerve, 2000. 23(4): p. 600–612.

101. Tracy, B.L., et al., Variability of motor unit discharge and force fluctuations across a range of muscle forces in older adults. Muscle Nerve, 2005. 32(4): p. 533–540.

102. Christou, E.A., M. Shinohara, and R.M. Enoka, Fluctuations in acceleration during voluntary contractions lead to greater impairment of movement accuracy in old adults. J Appl Physiol, 2003. 95(1): p. 373–384.

103. Kornatz, K.W., E.A. Christou, and R.M. Enoka, Practice reduces motor unit discharge variability in a hand muscle and improves manual dexterity in old adults. J Appl Physiol, 2005. 98(6): p. 2072–2080.

104. Conwit RA, M.E., Age related changes in peripheral and central conduction. *Clinical Neurophysiology and neuromuscular diseases2001*, Philadelphia: WB Saunders.

105. Norris, A.H., N.W. Shock, and I.H. Wagman, Age changes in the maximum conduction velocity of motor fibers of human ulnar nerves. J Appl Physiol, 1953. 5(10): p. 589–593.

106. Scaglioni, G., et al., Plantar flexor activation capacity and H reflex in older adults: adaptations to strength training. J Appl Physiol, 2002. 92(6): p. 2292–2302.

107. Metter, E.J., et al., The relationship of peripheral motor nerve conduction velocity to age-associated loss of grip strength. Aging (Milano), 1998. 10(6): p. 471–478.

108. Aagaard, P., et al., Role of the nervous system in sarcopenia and muscle atrophy with aging: strength training as a countermeasure. Scand J Med Sci Sports, 2010. 20(1): p. 49–64.

109. Edstrom, E., et al., Factors contributing to neuromuscular impairment and sarcopenia during aging. Physiol Behav, 2007. 92(1–2): p. 129–135.

110. Tam, S.L. and T. Gordon, Mechanisms controlling axonal sprouting at the neuromuscular junction. J Neurocytol, 2003. 32(5–8): p. 961–974.

111. Wokke, J.H., et al., Morphological changes in the human end plate with age. J Neurol Sci, 1990. 95(3): p. 291–310.

112. Oda, K., Age changes of motor innervation and acetylcholine receptor distribution on human skeletal muscle fibres. J Neurol Sci, 1984. 66(2–3): p. 327–338.

113. MacIntosh BR, G.P., McComas AJ, Skeletal muscle form and function. 2nd ed. Human kinetics 2006, Champaign IL.

114. Delbono, O., et al., Loss of skeletal muscle strength by ablation of the sarcoplasmic reticulum protein JP45. Proc Natl Acad Sci U S A, 2007. 104(50): p. 20108–13.

115. Jimenez-Moreno, R., et al., Sarcoplasmic reticulum Ca2+ release declines in muscle fibers from aging mice. Biophys J, 2008. 94(8): p. 3178–3188.

116. Russ, D.W. and J.S. Grandy, Increased desmin expression in hindlimb muscles of aging rats. J Cachexia Sarcopenia Muscle, 2011. 2(3): p. 175–180.

117. Lowe, D.A., D.D. Thomas, and L.V. Thompson, Force generation, but not myosin ATPase activity, declines with age in rat muscle fibers. Am J Physiol Cell Physiol, 2002. 283(1): p. C187–92.

118. Davies, C.T., D.O. Thomas, and M.J. White, Mechanical properties of young and elderly human muscle. Acta Med Scand Suppl, 1986. 711: p. 219–226.

119. Vandervoort, A.A. and A.J. McComas, Contractile changes in opposing muscles of the human ankle joint with aging. J Appl Physiol, 1986. 61(1): p. 361–367.

120. Cupido, C.M., A.L. Hicks, and J. Martin, Neuromuscular fatigue during repetitive stimulation in elderly and young adults. Eur J Appl Physiol Occup Physiol, 1992. 65(6): p. 567–572.

121. Lennmarken, C., et al., Skeletal muscle function in man: force, relaxation rate, endurance and contraction time-dependence on sex and age. Clin Physiol, 1985. 5(3): p. 243–255.

122. Petrella, J.K., et al., Age differences in knee extension power, contractile velocity, and fatigability. J Appl Physiol, 2005. 98(1): p. 211–220.

123. Ditor, D.S. and A.L. Hicks, The effect of age and gender on the relative fatigability of the human adductor pollicis muscle. Can J Physiol Pharmacol, 2000. 78(10): p. 781–790.

124. Kent-Braun, J.A., R.G. Miller, and M.W. Weiner, Phases of metabolism during progressive exercise to fatigue in human skeletal muscle. J Appl Physiol, 1993. 75(2): p. 573–580.

125. Lindstrom, B., et al., Skeletal muscle fatigue and endurance in young and old men and women. J Gerontol A Biol Sci Med Sci, 1997. 52(1): p. B59–66.

126. Vandervoort, A.A. and K.C. Hayes, Plantarflexor muscle function in young and elderly women. Eur J Appl Physiol Occup Physiol, 1989. 58(4): p. 389–394.

127. Whipple, R.H., L.I. Wolfson, and P.M. Amerman, The relationship of knee and ankle weakness to falls in nursing home residents: an isokinetic study. J Am Geriatr Soc, 1987. 35(1): p. 13–20.

128. Klass, M., S. Baudry, and J. Duchateau, Age-related decline in rate of torque development is accompanied by lower maximal motor unit discharge frequency during fast contractions. J Appl Physiol, 2008. 104(3): p. 739–746.

129. Marcell, T.J., Sarcopenia: causes, consequences, and preventions. J Gerontol A Biol Sci Med Sci, 2003. 58(10): p. M911–6.

130. Roth, G.S. and J.A. Joseph, Peculiarities of the effect of hormones and transmitters during aging: modulation of changes in dopaminergic action. Gerontology, 1988. 34(1–2): p. 22–28.

CHAPTER 5

Nutrition, Protein Turnover and Muscle Mass

Stéphane Walrand and Christelle Guillet

Clermont Université, Université d'Auvergne, Unité de Nutrition Humaine, Clermont-Ferrand, France; and INRA, UMR 1019, Unite de Nutrition Humaine, Clermont-Ferrand, France

Yves Boirie

Clermont Université, Université d'Auvergne, Unité de Nutrition Humaine, Clermont-Ferrand, France; INRA, UMR 1019, Unite de Nutrition Humaine, Clermont-Ferrand, France; and CHU Clermont-Ferrand, Service de Nutrition Clinique, Clermont-Ferrand, France

INTRODUCTION

Muscle erosion, which begins after the age of 55 years, is one of the most important factors of disability in elderly people. The cumulative decline in muscle mass reaches 40% from 20 to 80 years. The magnitude of this phenomenon as a public health problem is not well established as there are few epidemiological and longitudinal studies focusing on the decrements of strength and muscle mass with advancing age [1]. However, it is known that sarcopenia becomes more prevalent as individuals age and it has to be differentiated from cachexia [2,3]. The reduction in muscle mass and strength provokes an impaired mobility and increased risk for falls and fall-related fractures. In addition, muscle loss is associated with a decrease in overall physical activity levels with subsequent metabolic alterations such as obesity, insulin resistance and a reduction in bone density in the elderly. Sedentary individuals, subjects with poor protein intakes, low vitamin D, low testosterone levels and those suffering from debilitating diseases are at greater risks of sarcopenia. As the elderly population increases around the world, the involuntary loss of muscle mass with aging may become a major health problem in years to come.

Sarcopenia is believed to be due predominantly to atrophy of skeletal muscle fibers, mainly type II fibers. This results in a relative elevation in type I fibers density related to a supposed preservation of muscle endurance and a reduction in muscle strength. On a metabolic point of view, muscle size, function and composition are closely regulated by

Sarcopenia, First Edition. Edited by Alfonso J. Cruz-Jentoft and John E. Morley.
© 2012 John Wiley & Sons, Ltd. Published 2012 by John Wiley & Sons, Ltd.

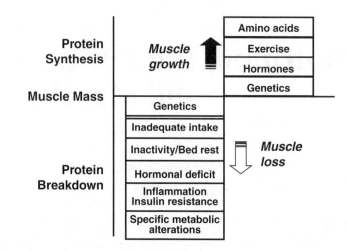

Figure 5.1 Regulation of muscle protein mass.

muscle protein turnover rate. Consequently, the age-related loss of muscle proteins is a consequence of an imbalance between protein synthesis and degradation rates (Figure 1). Until now, most reports have indicated that muscle protein synthesis declines with age [4,5]. These studies have demonstrated that synthesis rates of various muscle fractions, such as myofibrillar and mitochondrial fractions, decline in elderly or even by middle age. Reduced protein turnover adversely affects muscle function by inducing protein loss and damaged protein accumulation. Data suggest that sarcopenia is not only due to failure of muscle protein synthesis in the postabsorptive, but also to a lack of response of muscle protein metabolism in the fed state [6]. Other factors such as neurodegenerative processes with loss of alpha motor neurons in the spinal column, dysregulation of anabolic hormone (insulin, growth and sex hormones) and cytokine productions, modifications in the response to inflammatory events, inadequate nutritional intakes and sedentarity also participate in muscle loss during aging.

The determinants of sarcopenia include likely both genetic and environmental factors, with a complex series of poorly understood interactions. Likewise it is possible that epigenetic events may influence muscle fiber types evolution [7]. In fact, it is still unknown whether muscle loss of aged people is an inevitable condition of aging *per se*, or if illnesses, inappropriate nutrition, sedentarity and other lifestyle habits are major causes of sarcopenia. Currently, as the pathophysiology of sarcopenia is poorly understood, interventions to either prevent, retard or reverse this condition are extremely limited [8,9].

EVIDENCES FOR A ROLE FOR NUTRITION IN SARCOPENIA

'Anabolic resistance' of skeletal muscle to nutrition in elderly subjects

Some authors have argued that muscle loss in elderly subjects partly depends upon inadequate nutritional intake and/or an impaired response of skeletal muscle to nutrients, e.g. amino acids [8]. By using femoral arterio-venous balance and biopsies of vastus lateralis, muscle protein synthesis and breakdown have been measured in response to oral or intravenous infusions of amino acid mixture in young and elderly subjects [10,11]. When amino acids are infused intravenously, a significant increase of amino acid delivery to the leg, of amino acid transport, and muscle protein synthesis is reported irrespective of age [10]. So, although protein breakdown was not modified during amino acid infusion, a positive net balance of amino acids across the muscle was achieved. These data suggest that despite an age-related decline in muscle mass, muscle protein anabolism can be stimulated by high amino acid availability in the elderly [10]. Muscle protein turnover and amino acid transport in healthy young and elderly people were also determined during an oral administration of an amino acid mixture. As already shown by Boirie et al. for leucine [12], amino acid first-pass splanchnic extraction of phenylalanine was significantly higher in the elderly during ingestion of amino acids, but the delivery to the leg increased to the same extent in both groups. In addition, amino acid transport into muscle cells, muscle protein synthesis, and net balance increased similarly in both the young and the elderly [11]. Thus, despite an increased splanchnic extraction, muscle protein anabolism can be stimulated by oral amino acids in elderly as well as in young subjects as far as the dietary protein intakes or the amount of amino acid mixture administered is high enough to induce a great amino acid availability for muscle. Interestingly, muscle protein synthesis increased to the same extent after an oral intake of either balanced amino acids or essential amino acids only in healthy elderly [13], suggesting that non-essential amino acids may not be required to stimulate muscle protein anabolism in older adults, but specific studies on which and how much of these essential amino acids has to be performed. From these studies it seems that the amount of amino acids/protein intakes is crucial for triggering protein synthesis. Indeed, it was demonstrated that a smaller amount of protein during meal intake was not able to stimulate muscle protein synthesis as efficiently as higher doses [14]. This concept of a limited response to feeding was already demonstrated in animal studies involving old rodents [15,16]. When amino acids and glucose are administered either orally or intra-venously during an euglycemic hyperinsulinemic clamp [17,18] an increased amino acid delivery and transport into the muscle and a decreased muscle protein breakdown occurs in both groups. However, the stimulation of muscle protein synthesis in the young subjects was not depicted in the elderly despite the elevation in plasma amino acids and an even higher insulinemia [17,18]. Interestingly the response of whole body protein breakdown was lower in the elderly in response to insulin or to the meal [19–21]. The adaptation of muscle protein anabolism to hyperaminoacidemia and hyperinsulinemia seems to be due to an impaired response to insulin as demonstrated by direct infusion into the arterial side of the muscle area [22]. When muscle protein fractions within the muscle were separated, it was shown that the mitochondrial proteins were particularly affected by the age-related insulin resistance [17,23]. More recent studies from Volpi's group have indicated that the blunted response of protein synthesis in healthy elderly was the result of a decreased adaptation of leg blood flow to insulin [24]. Indeed blood flow is a crucial determinant of amino acid delivery and of the protein synthesis process through amino acids transport [25]. When blood flow was restored by using nitroprussiate in the elderly, muscle protein synthesis was also normalized [26]. These studies lead us to open the question of muscle sensitivity to hormones like insulin or to substrates like amino acids suggesting that a threshold needs to be reached to induce muscle protein synthesis and that this threshold may be higher in the case of inflammation (Figure 2). Recent studies have shown that reducing inflammation by using anti-inflammatory agents is able to restore muscle protein synthesis in old rats [27]. It also demonstrates that substrates delivery has to be controlled by acting on the plasma availability or the blood flow. In addition, it is known that lipid intakes modulate insulin sensitivity and inflammation. In a recent study, an oleate-enriched diet decreased

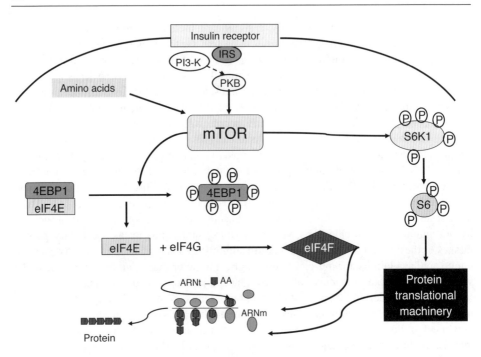

Figure 5.2   Activation of insulin signaling pathway by amino acids.

inflammation markers in the plasma and in the adipose tissue of old rats [28]. However, the major effect of feeding old rats a high-oleate diet was to restore muscle protein synthesis in response to amino acid and insulin.

So the lack of anabolic response to a complete meal in the muscles is likely to contribute to the development, over the long term, of sarcopenia in the elderly. The consecutive issue is whether nutrition, i.e. an adapted protein intake, could reverse the phenomenon.

What is the basis of protein requirement during aging?

Protein requirement is defined as the lowest dietary protein intake able to compensate for the obligatory losses of nitrogen from the body and to preserve bodily functions [29]. The current mean dietary requirement for healthy adult men and women of all ages, was set by the 1985 joint FAO/WHO/UNU expert consultation, and estimated to be 0.6 g protein/kg/d, with a suggested safe level of intake set at 0.75 g protein/kg/d [30]. However, because of many changes in body organs functions and metabolism with age, such as body composition, insulin resistance, altered protein metabolism especially in skeletal muscle, some authors [31–34] have suggested that the utilization of dietary proteins and amino acids may differ between the young and the older adults. Consequently, the same authors, using various methodologies, i.e. nitrogen balance and tracer procedures, have tried to define the modifications of protein requirement with advancing age [31–34]. Taken together, studies based on nitrogen balance using the same formula, showed that protein requirement increases in elderly people, especially in aged individuals during compulsory inactivity such as bed rest [35]. When the recalculated data from all studies were combined by weighted mean averages, a mean protein requirement of 0.89 g protein/kg/d was estimated [31,32]. Nevertheless, other works based on tracer methodology reported that the rate of whole body protein turnover, a commonly assumed determinant of protein requirement, exhibited no significant modifications with age when expressed per kg of fat free mass [33,34]. These studies also demonstrated that because metabolic demands for protein are reduced by one third, with no impairment in efficiency of protein utilization, apparent protein requirements seemed not to be increased in the elderly population [33,34]. However, there are still a lot of discussions ongoing arguing for or against an increasing requirement of protein for elderly populations [36,37]. It is generally difficult to establish firm recommendations for protein intake for this population, but it is safe to consider that protein requirement can be slightly increased in elderly people to limit loss of lean body mass and preserve a better response to any critical stress like sepsis or trauma. This comment is reflected by recent data from the Health ABC study showing that despite adequate intakes of protein, appendicular muscle mass (reflecting whole body muscle mass) was lost during a three-year follow up and that the less protein that is eaten the more muscle is lost [38]. Thus, it is possible that nitrogen balance may not exactly reflect the small changes in protein metabolism that happen everyday at a low scale, but cumulating for months can result in a significant decline in muscle protein mass. In this case, it is hypothesized that adaptation of elderly subjects to protein restriction may be inadequate as already reported by Castaneda et al. [39] . This is the reason why most of the research should also focus on the incomplete recovery of muscle mass following stress also called 'the catabolic crisis model' [40]. For instance in hospitalized elderly subjects, nitrogen balance studies indicate that 1.3 to 1.6g/kg/d should be applied [41].

How to improve protein retention in elderly subjects: beyond protein quantity?

What is the response to increasing protein intakes?

Surprisingly, only a few experiments were designed to study the effect of increased protein intake in an elderly population. When the protein amount in the diet increases from 12% to 21% of total energy, whole body protein turnover was enhanced in elderly men and women [42]. Following a low protein intake (50% of usual intake), no modification of whole body protein synthesis and breakdown was noticed in a group of aged women [43]. However, whole body protein oxidation, nitrogen balance, muscle mass and function and immune response were significantly affected in the group fed a low protein diet [39]. Collectively, these observations highlight the importance of maintaining adequate protein intakes in elderly people to counteract the negative effect of aging on protein metabolism. These previous observations were repeated recently indicating some adaptations using muscle specific transcript profiles [44]. Of course the other important question is about the upper limit of protein intakes in the elderly subjects, knowing that a reduced glomerular filtration capacity is occurring. To address this issue, we recently demonstrated [45] that a high protein ingestion, i.e. 3 g/kg fat free mass/d for 10 days, was inefficient to enhance protein synthesis at whole body as well as the skeletal muscle levels of healthy elderly subjects in the postabsorptive state. Interestingly, although a high protein diet normally enhanced glomerular filtration rate in young adults, it reduced renal function in the aged group [45]. Other data have shown long ago that the maximal adaptive capacity of ureagenesis in adults (for a mean weight of 70 kg) was about 22 mg of urea nitrogen/kg body weight/h [46]. These data correspond to a maximal protein consumption of ~3.3g/kg/d, so that the safe upper limit for protein intake has been fixed to less than 2.2 g/kg/d by the French group on protein recommendation for elderly subjects [47].

Is there an effect of the protein source?

The consumption of different protein sources and its effect on protein metabolism have been assessed in elderly women [48]. One diet was composed half of animal proteins and half of vegetable proteins, whereas one-third of the proteins consumed in a second diet were from vegetable and two-thirds from animals, and inversely in a third diet. Nitrogen balance was not modified in this study, but whole body protein breakdown was not inhibited to the same extent by the meal when the protein source was from vegetables in comparison with meat [48]. This study showed that intake of high quality proteins may be an important issue in elderly people, suggesting also that aging may be associated with more specific amino acid requirements especially for the essential amino acids. The quality of dietary proteins and its impact on muscle protein synthesis may be less important when protein intake is sufficient. In a recent study, we compared milk and soy proteins for their potential impact on muscle protein synthesis using a classical steady state approach [49]. No differences could be found between the different sources of dietary proteins despite changes in leg amino acid uptakes. However, there is not enough data in the field of aging regarding the issue of essential amino acids especially at low protein intakes.

Optimizing protein digestion rate to improve AA availability?

By analogy with carbohydrates, the concept of 'fast' and 'slow' proteins was established according to the speed at which protein are digested and absorbed from the gut [50]. The two main milk proteins, i.e. casein and whey protein, have different metabolic fates in the intestinal tract. Whey protein, a soluble protein, is considered as a 'fast' protein since the plasma appearance of its constituting amino acids after its digestion and absorption is high, fast, but transient. On the contrary, casein clots in the stomach, which delays its gastric emptying and therefore results in a slower, lower but prolonged release and absorption of amino acids. This concept was applied to study the response of postprandial protein metabolism during aging [51]. In this population, the duration and magnitude of elevated plasma amino acids are key factors to counteract the decrease in muscle sensitivity to amino acids. Accordingly, whole body protein gain was higher after a meal containing 'fast' protein, i.e. whey protein, than 'slow' protein, i.e. casein, in the elderly, when considering either isonitrogenous or isoleucine (as leucine is a well-known anabolic factor) meals. In addition, post-prandial protein utilization by the body was significantly higher with the fast protein than with the slow one [51]. A report from Paddon-Jones et al. [52] showed that whey proteins were able to stimulate muscle protein synthesis rate in a group of healthy elderly individuals as well as the free amino acid mixture but the essential amino acids content of the two diets was not similar. More recently, we measured the postprandial muscle protein synthesis in response to a bolus of either whey protein, casein or casein hydrolysate in healthy elderly subjects [53]. It was clearly demonstrated that not only the speed of protein absorption, but also the leucine content were key factors for the stimulation of muscle protein anabolism. These data clearly suggest that a dietary protein mixture which can be quickly digested and absorbed might be more efficient to limit protein loss during aging than a mixture yielding slower kinetics. This data illustrates that age-related anabolic resistance could be overcome by a better availability of dietary amino acids especially essential amino acids. For instance, muscle function is improved in the elderly during bed rest after essential amino acids supplementation [35]. Another way to optimize amino acid availability from solid foods is to improve chewing capacity since it may influence postprandial amino acid kinetics. Indeed, it has been demonstrated that chewing alterations induced by dental prosthesis could modulate postprandial AA kinetics following meat ingestion [54].

Is there a specific daily protein feeding pattern?

A 'pulse' protein feeding pattern that combines meals rich and low in proteins during the day may improve protein retention in elderly persons [19,55]. A 'spread' diet composed of four meals, spreading daily protein intake over 12 hours was compared to a pulse diet providing 80% of daily protein intake concentrated at midday. The pulse protein pattern was more efficient at improving nitrogen balances and whole body protein retention in aged people after 15 days. Concerning the potential explanation, it can be argued that the pulse protein diet possesses a couple of advantages: a) the midday protein pulse meal may stimulate whole body synthesis by highly increasing amino acid concentration, b) high carbohydrate and low protein meals are known to limit protein loss by reducing protein breakdown rate via postprandial hyperinsulinemia, c) it is combined with the daily physical activity associated with everyday life. Interestingly, the beneficial effect of the pulse protein pattern on protein accretion still persisted several days after the end of the diet [55]. The pulse protein diet also restored a significant anabolic response of skeletal muscle protein synthesis to feeding without affecting protein breakdown in old rats [56]. These studies suggest that the use of a 'pulse' protein pattern increases body protein retention, in particular in skeletal muscle. This concept represents an attractive and safe approach rather than simply increased protein intake in the elderly subjects since it may be difficult to achieve a high amount of dietary protein in this population.

Improvement of protein retention by amino acids?

Animal and human studies have focused on the potential mechanism of the decreased skeletal muscle sensitivity to amino acids in elderly individuals. A defect in branched chain amino acid (BCAA) pathway activation may be responsible for this alteration [17]. Consequently, the alteration of muscle protein synthesis response to anabolic signals may be counteracted by nutritional strategies aiming at improving BCAA availability. For example, in vitro or in vivo high leucine administration is able to stimulate muscle protein synthesis rate in aged rodents [15,57,58]. In these models, leucine acts as an actual mediator able to modulate specific intracellular pathway linked with the stimulation of protein translation

[59]. Interestingly, when given to old rats for 10 days, the beneficial effect of leucine supplementation persisted, indicating that a long-term utilization of leucine-enriched diets may limit muscle wasting in aged individuals [60]. In addition, these data suggest that nutritional manipulations increasing the availability of leucine into skeletal muscle, such as the utilization of a leucine-rich fast protein, i.e. whey protein, could be beneficial to improve protein retention during aging. The beneficial effect of such a diet on muscle protein synthesis in aged humans has been determined in several studies [52,61–63]. It is concluded that leucine is able to stimulate muscle protein synthesis in the short term but may not on a longer term [64].

More recently, special attention has been focused on the impact of citrulline on muscle protein synthesis. Indeed this AA not incorporated in the protein matrix during protein synthesis may play a role since it may stimulate muscle protein synthesis in malnourished animals [65]. Other amino acids, like glutamine, may be helpful to preserve skeletal muscle in elderly subjects, especially in stressed conditions [66].

ANABOLIC RESPONSE TO PHYSICAL EXERCISE IN THE ELDERLY

The anabolic effect of resistance exercise should be used to amplify the anabolic action of dietary proteins on muscle protein synthesis. Yarasheski et al. determined the rate of *vastus lateralis* muscle protein synthesis by using the *in vivo* incorporation of intravenously infused ^{13}C-leucine into mixed muscle protein in both young and elderly men before and at the end of two weeks of resistance exercise training [67]. Although the muscle fractional synthesis rate was lower in the elderly before training, it increased to reach a comparable rate irrespective of the age of the subjects after two weeks of exercise. In contrast to these results, Welle et al. found no improvement in myofibrillar protein synthesis rate in either young or old men who completed 12 weeks of resistance training [68]. The discrepancy of these observations could be explained by the different experimental designs used in these studies. The training stimulus may not have been powerful enough to affect protein turnover in the investigation by Welle et al. [68]. In addition, the timings of measurements relative to the last bout of exercise were also different in these investigations. Further, other measurements of synthesis rate of individual muscle proteins showed that a 2-week weight-lifting program increased MHC synthesis rate in 23-32 and 78-84-year-old subjects [69]. However, the protein synthesis rate of actin was increased after exercise only in the younger group, showing that the anabolic effect of resistance exercise in elderly subjects is protein-dependent. Age-related lowering of the transcript levels of MHC IIa and IIx is not reversed by 3 months of resistance exercise training [70], whereas exercise resulted in a higher synthesis rate of MHC in association with an increase in MHC I isoform transcript levels [71]. Other results showed that the stimulation of MHC synthesis rate by resistance exercise is mediated by more efficient translation of mRNA [72]. Furthermore, the effect of 16 weeks of endurance exercise on MHC isoform protein composition and mRNA abundance was tested in a recent study [73]. The regulation of MHC isoform transcripts remained robust in older muscle after endurance exercise, but this did not result in corresponding changes in MHC protein expression [73].

Few data are currently available concerning the rate of muscle protein breakdown after exercise in elderly subjects. A session of 45 minutes of eccentric exercise produced a similar increase in whole body protein breakdown irrespective of the age of the volunteers [74].

However, myofibrillar proteolysis, based on 3-methylhistidine (3-MH)/creatinine measurements, did not increase until 10 days' post-exercise in the young group but remained high through the same period in the older men [74]. In addition, the urinary 3-MH-to-creatinine ratio was not affected at the end of 2 weeks of resistance exercise in either the younger or older volunteers [69].

From this section, it may be concluded that ageing muscle still responds to physical activity but there are no clear-cut recommendations for any specific type of physical activity.

COMBINATION OF NUTRITIONAL AND TRAINING STRATEGIES

Most of the studies failed to show any beneficial effect of nutritional supplementations on muscle anabolic properties in exercising elderly subjects. For example, Welle et al. reported that high protein meals (0.6-2.4 g protein/kg per day) did not enhance the myofibrillar protein synthesis rate in *vastus lateralis* muscle following three sessions of resistance exercise in 62-75-year-old men and women [75]. In frail very old people (87 years old), high-intensity resistance exercise training with or without concomitant multinutrient supplementation had the same efficiency on muscle weakness reversibility [75]. Of note, reports showed that ingestion of oral pre or post-exercise amino acid supplements can improve net muscle protein balance in young volunteers [76,77]. The response to amino acid intake with concomitant exercise is dependent upon the composition and amount, as well as the pattern and timing of ingestion in relation to the performance of exercise [78]. The response of net muscle protein synthesis to consumption of an essential amino acid-carbohydrate supplement solution immediately before resistance exercise is greater than when the solution is consumed after exercise, primarily because of an increase in muscle protein synthesis as a result of increased delivery of amino acids to the leg [79]. Whether amino acid and carbohydrate intakes immediately before or after resistance exercise can enhance the anabolic effect of training in older individuals as shown in the younger group is still controversial. In a recent study, it was shown that dietary protein digestion and absorption kinetics were not impaired after exercise at an older age. Moreover, exercising before protein intake allows for a greater use of dietary protein-derived amino acids for de novo muscle protein synthesis in both young and elderly men [80].

CONCLUDING REMARKS AND FUTURE DIRECTION

Loss of muscle mass involves a number of underlying mechanisms including intrinsic changes in the muscle and central nervous system, humoral and lifestyle factors. However, nutrition is the key regulator of muscle maintenance through its numerous biological actions on protein synthesis machinery. Many data demonstrate that nutritional means to counter sarcopenia exist. These strategies aim at improving amino acid availability since postprandial elevation of plasma AA is the main determinant of muscle anabolism. Other metabolic aspects can modulate sensitivity of skeletal muscle to nutrients, like the quality and the pattern of daily protein intakes rather than simply increasing the amount of proteins which should be cautiously used in an aged population with a potentially reduced kidney function. Inactivity also induces anabolic resistance and regular exercise could reverse this phenomenon. The combination of specific nutritional and physical activity programs may have a significant effect on muscle protein balance in young subjects. This strategy has to be tested in a large trial of elderly people. Furthermore, the possibility of therapeutical approach to enhance protein synthesis and to limit sarcopenia has been emphasized by studies in the care management of heart failure [81] or hypertension [82,83] or COPD [84]. Other approaches using angiotensin-converting enzyme inhibitors have resulted in a reduction of strength and walking speed decline in comparison with other antihypertensive agents [85]. This evidence of pharmacological approaches is able to help age-related weakness and dependence. So, interventional strategies using nutritional advices, drugs and/or exercise in large epidemiological studies are required before being applied to the general public. The ultimate objective of such investigations is to restore mobility and to limit physical dependence of elderly people in order to improve their quality of life.

REFERENCES

1. Cruz-Jentoft, A. J., Baeyens, J. P., Bauer, J. M., Boirie, Y., Cederholm, T., Landi, F., Martin, F. C., Michel, J. P., Rolland, Y., Schneider, S. M., Topinkova, E., Vandewoude, M. & Zamboni, M. (2010) Sarcopenia: European consensus on definition and diagnosis: Report of the European Working Group on Sarcopenia in Older People. Age Ageing 39:412–423.

2. Muscaritoli, M., Anker, S. D., Argiles, J., Aversa, Z., Bauer, J. M., Biolo, G., Boirie, Y., Bosaeus, I., Cederholm, T., Costelli, P., Fearon, K. C., Laviano, A., Maggio, M., Rossi Fanelli, F., Schneider, S. M., Schols, A. & Sieber, C. C. (2010) Consensus definition of sarcopenia, cachexia and pre-cachexia: joint document elaborated by Special Interest Groups (SIG) 'cachexia-anorexia in chronic wasting diseases' and 'nutrition in geriatrics'. Clin Nutr 29:154–159.

3. Argiles, J. M., Anker, S. D., Evans, W. J., Morley, J. E., Fearon, K. C., Strasser, F., Muscaritoli, M. & Baracos, V. E. (2010) Consensus on cachexia definitions. J Am Med Dir Assoc 11: 229–230.

4. Nair, K. S. (2005) Aging muscle. Am J Clin Nutr 81:953–963.

5. Walrand, S. & Boirie, Y. (2003) Muscle protein and amino acid metabolism with respect to age-related sarcopenia. Boca Raton: CRC Press.

6. Walrand, S., Guillet, C., Salles, J., Cano, N. & Boirie, Y. (2011) Physiopathological Mechanism of Sarcopenia. Saunders.

7. Baar, K. (2010) Epigenetic control of skeletal muscle fibre type. Acta Physiol (Oxf) 199:477–487.

8. Short, K. R. & Nair, K. S. (2000) The effect of age on protein metabolism. Curr Opin Clin Nutr Metab Care 3:39–44.

9. Walrand, S. & Boirie, Y. (2005) Optimizing protein intake in aging. Curr Opin Clin Nutr Metab Care 8:89–94.

10. Volpi, E., Ferrando, A. A., Yeckel, C. W., Tipton, K. D. & Wolfe, R. R. (1998) Exogenous amino acids stimulate net muscle protein synthesis in the elderly. J Clin Invest 101:2000–2007.

11. Volpi, E., Mittendorfer, B., Wolf, S. E. & Wolfe, R. R. (1999) Oral amino acids stimulate muscle protein anabolism in the elderly despite higher first-pass splanchnic extraction. Am J Physiol 277:E513–520.

12. Boirie, Y., Gachon, P. & Beaufrere, B. (1997) Splanchnic and whole-body leucine kinetics in young and elderly men. Am J Clin Nutr 65:489–495.

13. Volpi, E., Kobayashi, H., Sheffield-Moore, M., Mittendorfer, B. & Wolfe, R. R. (2003) Essential amino acids are primarily responsible for the amino acid stimulation of muscle protein anabolism in healthy elderly adults. Am J Clin Nutr 78:250–258.

14. Katsanos, C. S., Kobayashi, H., Sheffield-Moore, M., Aarsland, A. & Wolfe, R. R. (2005) Aging is associated with diminished accretion of muscle proteins after the ingestion of a small bolus of essential amino acids. Am J Clin Nutr 82:1065–1073.

15. Dardevet, D., Sornet, C., Bayle, G., Prugnaud, J., Pouyet, C. & Grizard, J. (2002) Postprandial stimulation of muscle protein synthesis in old rats can be restored by a leucine-supplemented meal. J Nutr 132:95–100.

16. Mosoni, L., Valluy, M. C., Serrurier, B., Prugnaud, J., Obled, C., Guezennec, C. Y. & Mirand, P. P. (1995) Altered response of protein synthesis to nutritional state and endurance training in old rats. Am J Physiol 268:E328–335.

17. Guillet, C., Prod'homme, M., Balage, M., Gachon, P., Giraudet, C., Morin, L., Grizard, J. & Boirie, Y. (2004) Impaired anabolic response of muscle protein synthesis is associated with S6K1 dysregulation in elderly humans. FASEB J 18:1586–1587.

18. Volpi, E., Mittendorfer, B., Rasmussen, B. B. & Wolfe, R. R. (2000) The response of muscle protein anabolism to combined hyperaminoacidemia and glucose-induced hyperinsulinemia is impaired in the elderly. J Clin Endocrinol Metab 85:4481–4490.

19. Arnal, M. A., Mosoni, L., Boirie, Y., Houlier, M. L., Morin, L., Verdier, E., Ritz, P., Antoine, J. M., Prugnaud, J., Beaufrere, B. & Mirand, P. P. (1999) Protein pulse feeding improves protein retention in elderly women. Am J Clin Nutr 69:1202–1208.

20. Boirie, Y., Gachon, P., Cordat, N., Ritz, P. & Beaufrere, B. (2001) Differential insulin sensitivities of glucose, amino acid, and albumin metabolism in elderly men and women. J Clin Endocrinol Metab 86:638–644.

21. Guillet, C., Zangarelli, A., Gachon, P., Morio, B., Giraudet, C., Rousset, P. & Boirie, Y. (2004) Whole body protein breakdown is less inhibited by insulin, but still responsive to amino acid, in nondiabetic elderly subjects. J Clin Endocrinol Metab 89:6017–6024.

22. Rasmussen, B. B., Fujita, S., Wolfe, R. R., Mittendorfer, B., Roy, M., Rowe, V. L. & Volpi, E. (2006) Insulin resistance of muscle protein metabolism in aging. FASEB J 20:768–769.

23. Boirie, Y., Short, K. R., Ahlman, B., Charlton, M. & Nair, K. S. (2001) Tissue-specific regulation of mitochondrial and cytoplasmic protein synthesis rates by insulin. Diabetes 50:2652–2658.

24. Fujita, S., Rasmussen, B. B., Cadenas, J. G., Grady, J. J. & Volpi, E. (2006) Effect of insulin on human skeletal muscle protein synthesis is modulated by insulin-induced changes in muscle blood flow and amino acid availability. Am J Physiol Endocrinol Metab 291:E745–754.

25. Biolo, G., Declan Fleming, R. Y. & Wolfe, R. R. (1995) Physiologic hyperinsulinemia stimulates protein synthesis and enhances transport of selected amino acids in human skeletal muscle. J Clin Invest 95:811–819.

26. Timmerman, K. L., Lee, J. L., Fujita, S., Dhanani, S., Dreyer, H. C., Fry, C. S., Drummond, M. J., Sheffield-Moore, M., Rasmussen, B. B. & Volpi, E. (2010) Pharmacological vasodilation improves insulin-stimulated muscle protein anabolism but not glucose utilization in older adults. Diabetes 59:2764–2771.

27. Rieu, I., Magne, H., Savary-Auzeloux, I., Averous, J., Bos, C., Peyron, M. A., Combaret, L. & Dardevet, D. (2009) Reduction of low grade inflammation restores blunting of postprandial muscle anabolism and limits sarcopenia in old rats. J Physiol 587:5483–5492.

28. Tardif, N., Salles, J., Landrier, J. F., Mothe-Satney, I., Guillet, C., Boue-Vaysse, C., Combaret, L., Giraudet, C., Patrac, V., Bertrand-Michel, J., Migne, C., Chardigny, J. M., Boirie, Y. & Walrand, S. (2011) Oleate-enriched diet improves insulin sensitivity and restores muscle protein synthesis in old rats. Clin Nutr 30:799–806.

29. Clugston, G., Dewey, K. G., Fjeld, C., Millward, J., Reeds, P., Scrimshaw, N. S., Tontisirin, K., Waterlow, J. C. & Young, V. R. (1996) Report of the working group on protein and amino acid requirements. Eur J Clin Nutr 50 Suppl 1: S193–195.

30. FAO, WHO & UNU (1985) Energy and protein requirements. Report of a joint expert consultation, p. 724.

31. Campbell, W. W., Crim, M. C., Dallal, G. E., Young, V. R. & Evans, W. J. (1994) Increased protein requirements in elderly people: new data and retrospective reassessments. Am J Clin Nutr 60:501–509.

32. Campbell, W. W. & Evans, W. J. (1996) Protein requirements of elderly people. Eur J Clin Nutr 50 Suppl 1: S180–183; discussion S183–185.

33. Millward, D. J. (1999) Optimal intakes of protein in the human diet. Proc Nutr Soc 58:403–413.

34. Millward, D. J., Fereday, A., Gibson, N. & Pacy, P. J. (1997) Aging, protein requirements, and protein turnover. Am J Clin Nutr 66:774–786.

35. Ferrando, A. A., Paddon-Jones, D., Hays, N. P., Kortebein, P., Ronsen, O., Williams, R. H., McComb, A., Symons, T. B., Wolfe, R. R. & Evans, W. (2010) EAA supplementation to increase nitrogen intake improves muscle function during bed rest in the elderly. Clin Nutr 29:18–23.

36. Briefel, R. R. & Johnson, C. L. (2004) Secular trends in dietary intake in the United States. Annu Rev Nutr 24:401–431.

37. Millward, D. J., Layman, D. K., Tome, D. & Schaafsma, G. (2008) Protein quality assessment: impact of expanding understanding of protein and amino acid needs for optimal health. Am J Clin Nutr 87:1576S–1581S.

38. Houston, D. K., Nicklas, B. J., Ding, J., Harris, T. B., Tylavsky, F. A., Newman, A. B., Lee, J. S., Sahyoun, N. R., Visser, M. & Kritchevsky, S. B. (2008) Dietary protein intake is associated with lean mass change in older, community-dwelling adults: the Health, Aging, and Body Composition (Health ABC) Study. Am J Clin Nutr 87:150–155.

39. Castaneda, C., Charnley, J. M., Evans, W. J. & Crim, M. C. (1995) Elderly women accommodate to a low-protein diet with losses of body cell mass, muscle function, and immune response. Am J Clin Nutr 62:30–39.

40. English, K. L. & Paddon-Jones, D. (2010) Protecting muscle mass and function in older adults during bed rest. Curr Opin Clin Nutr Metab Care 13:34–39.

41. Gaillard, C., Alix, E., Boirie, Y., Berrut, G. & Ritz, P. (2008) Are elderly hospitalized patients getting enough protein? J Am Geriatr Soc 56:1045–1049.

42. Pannemans, D. L., Halliday, D. & Westerterp, K. R. (1995) Whole-body protein turnover in elderly men and women: responses to two protein intakes. Am J Clin Nutr 61:33–38.

43. Castaneda, C., Dolnikowski, G. G., Dallal, G. E., Evans, W. J. & Crim, M. C. (1995) Protein turnover and energy metabolism of elderly women fed a low-protein diet. Am J Clin Nutr 62:40–48.

44. Thalacker-Mercer, A. E., Fleet, J. C., Craig, B. A., Carnell, N. S. & Campbell, W. W. (2007) Inadequate protein intake affects skeletal muscle transcript profiles in older humans. Am J Clin Nutr 85:1344–1352.

45. Walrand, S., Short, K. R., Bigelow, M. L., Sweatt, A. J., Hutson, S. M. & Nair, K. S. (2008) Functional impact of high protein intake on healthy elderly people. Am J Physiol Endocrinol Metab 295:E921–928.

46. Rudman, D., DiFulco, T. J., Galambos, J. T., Smith, R. B., Salam, A. A. & Warren, W. D. (1973) Maximal rates of excretion and synthesis of urea in normal and cirrhotic subjects. J Clin Invest 52:2241–2249.

47. Groupe & travail, d. (2007) Apport en protéines : consommation, qualité, besoin et recommandations.

48. Pannemans, D. L., Wagenmakers, A. J., Westerterp, K. R., Schaafsma, G. & Halliday, D. (1998) Effect of protein source and quantity on protein metabolism in elderly women. Am J Clin Nutr 68:1228–1235.

49. Luiking, Y. C., Engelen, M. P., Soeters, P. B., Boirie, Y. & Deutz, N. E. (2011) Differential metabolic effects of casein and soy protein meals on skeletal muscle in healthy volunteers. Clin Nutr 30:65–72.

50. Boirie, Y., Dangin, M., Gachon, P., Vasson, M. P., Maubois, J. L. & Beaufrere, B. (1997) Slow and fast dietary proteins differently modulate postprandial protein accretion. Proc Natl Acad Sci U S A 94:14930–14935.

51. Dangin, M., Guillet, C., Garcia-Rodenas, C., Gachon, P., Bouteloup-Demange, C., Reiffers-Magnani, K., Fauquant, J., Ballevre, O. & Beaufrere, B. (2003) The rate of protein digestion affects protein gain differently during aging in humans. J Physiol 549:635–644.

52. Paddon-Jones, D., Sheffield-Moore, M., Katsanos, C. S., Zhang, X. J. & Wolfe, R. R. (2006) Differential stimulation of muscle protein synthesis in elderly humans following isocaloric ingestion of amino acids or whey protein. Exp Gerontol 41:215–219.

53. Pennings, B., Boirie, Y., Senden, J. M., Gijsen, A. P., Kuipers, H. & van Loon, L. J. (2011) Whey protein stimulates postprandial muscle protein accretion more effectively than do casein and casein hydrolysate in older men. Am J Clin Nutr 93:997–1005.

54. Remond, D., Machebeuf, M., Yven, C., Buffiere, C., Mioche, L., Mosoni, L. & Patureau Mirand, P. (2007) Postprandial whole-body protein metabolism after a meat meal is influenced by chewing efficiency in elderly subjects. Am J Clin Nutr 85:1286–1292.

55. Arnal, M. A., Mosoni, L., Boirie, Y., Gachon, P., Genest, M., Bayle, G., Grizard, J., Arnal, M., Antoine, J. M., Beaufrere, B. & Mirand, P. P. (2000) Protein turnover modifications induced by the protein feeding pattern still persist after the end of the diets. Am J Physiol Endocrinol Metab 278:E902–909.

56. Arnal, M. A., Mosoni, L., Dardevet, D., Ribeyre, M. C., Bayle, G., Prugnaud, J. & Patureau Mirand, P. (2002) Pulse protein feeding pattern restores stimulation of muscle protein synthesis during the feeding period in old rats. J Nutr 132:1002–1008.

57. Dardevet, D., Sornet, C., Balage, M. & Grizard, J. (2000) Stimulation of in vitro rat muscle protein synthesis by leucine decreases with age. J Nutr 130:2630–2635.

58. Guillet, C., Zangarelli, A., Mishellany, A., Rousset, P., Sornet, C., Dardevet, D. & Boirie, Y. (2004) Mitochondrial and sarcoplasmic proteins, but not myosin heavy chain, are sensitive to leucine supplementation in old rat skeletal muscle. Exp Gerontol 39:745–751.

59. Anthony, J. C., Anthony, T. G., Kimball, S. R. & Jefferson, L. S. (2001) Signaling pathways involved in translational control of protein synthesis in skeletal muscle by leucine. J Nutr 131:856S–860S.

60. Rieu, I., Sornet, C., Bayle, G., Prugnaud, J., Pouyet, C., Balage, M., Papet, I., Grizard, J. & Dardevet, D. (2003) Leucine-supplemented meal feeding for ten days beneficially affects postprandial muscle protein synthesis in old rats. J Nutr 133:1198–1205.

61. Katsanos, C. S., Chinkes, D. L., Paddon-Jones, D., Zhang, X. J., Aarsland, A. & Wolfe, R. R. (2008) Whey protein ingestion in elderly persons results in greater muscle protein accrual than ingestion of its constituent essential amino acid content. Nutr Res 28:651–658.

62. Rieu, I., Balage, M., Sornet, C., Debras, E., Ripes, S., Rochon-Bonhomme, C., Pouyet, C., Grizard, J. & Dardevet, D. (2007) Increased availability of leucine with leucine-rich whey proteins improves postprandial muscle protein synthesis in aging rats. Nutrition 23:323–331.

63. Rieu, I., Balage, M., Sornet, C., Giraudet, C., Pujos, E., Grizard, J., Mosoni, L. & Dardevet, D. (2006) Leucine supplementation improves muscle protein synthesis in elderly men independently of hyperaminoacidaemia. J Physiol 575:305–315.

64. Verhoeven, S., Vanschoonbeek, K., Verdijk, L. B., Koopman, R., Wodzig, W. K., Dendale, P. & van Loon, L. J. (2009) Long-term leucine supplementation does not increase muscle mass or strength in healthy elderly men. Am J Clin Nutr 89:1468–1475.

65. Osowska, S., Duchemann, T., Walrand, S., Paillard, A., Boirie, Y., Cynober, L. & Moinard, C. (2006) Citrulline modulates muscle protein metabolism in old malnourished rats. Am J Physiol Endocrinol Metab 291:E582–586.

66. Coeffier, M. & Dechelotte, P. (2005) The role of glutamine in intensive care unit patients: mechanisms of action and clinical outcome. Nutr Rev 63:65–69.

67. Yarasheski, K. E., Zachwieja, J. J. & Bier, D. M. (1993) Acute effects of resistance exercise on muscle protein synthesis rate in young and elderly men and women. Am J Physiol 265:E210–214.

68. Welle, S., Thornton, C. & Statt, M. (1995) Myofibrillar protein synthesis in young and old human subjects after three months of resistance training. Am J Physiol 268:E422–427.

69. Hasten, D. L., Pak-Loduca, J., Obert, K. A. & Yarasheski, K. E. (2000) Resistance exercise acutely increases MHC and mixed muscle protein synthesis rates in 78–84 and 23–32 yr olds. Am J Physiol Endocrinol Metab 278:E620–626.

70. Balagopal, P., Schimke, J. C., Ades, P., Adey, D. & Nair, K. S. (2001) Age effect on transcript levels and synthesis rate of muscle MHC and response to resistance exercise. Am J Physiol Endocrinol Metab 280:E203–208.

71. Williamson, D. L., Godard, M. P., Porter, D. A., Costill, D. L. & Trappe, S. W. (2000) Progressive resistance training reduces myosin heavy chain coexpression in single muscle fibers from older men. J Appl Physiol 88:627–633.

72. Welle, S., Bhatt, K. & Thornton, C. A. (1999) Stimulation of myofibrillar synthesis by exercise is mediated by more efficient translation of mRNA. J Appl Physiol 86:1220–1225.

73. Short, K. R., Vittone, J. L., Bigelow, M. L., Proctor, D. N., Coenen-Schimke, J. M., Rys, P. & Nair, K. S. (2005) Changes in myosin heavy chain mRNA and protein expression in human skeletal muscle with age and endurance exercise training. J Appl Physiol 99:95–102.

74. Fielding, R. A., Meredith, C. N., O'Reilly, K. P., Frontera, W. R., Cannon, J. G. & Evans, W. J. (1991) Enhanced protein breakdown after eccentric exercise in young and older men. J Appl Physiol 71:674–679.

75. Welle, S. & Thornton, C. A. (1998) High-protein meals do not enhance myofibrillar synthesis after resistance exercise in 62- to 75-yr-old men and women. Am J Physiol 274:E677–683.

76. Tipton, K. D., Borsheim, E., Wolf, S. E., Sanford, A. P. & Wolfe, R. R. (2003) Acute response of net muscle protein balance reflects 24-h balance after exercise and amino acid ingestion. Am J Physiol Endocrinol Metab 284:E76–89.

77. Tipton, K. D., Ferrando, A. A., Phillips, S. M., Doyle, D., Jr. & Wolfe, R. R. (1999) Postexercise net protein synthesis in human muscle from orally administered amino acids. Am J Physiol 276:E628–634.

78. Wolfe, R. R. (2002) Regulation of muscle protein by amino acids. J Nutr 132:3219S–3224S.

79. Tipton, K. D., Rasmussen, B. B., Miller, S. L., Wolf, S. E., Owens-Stovall, S. K., Petrini, B. E. & Wolfe, R. R. (2001) Timing of amino acid-carbohydrate ingestion alters anabolic response of muscle to resistance exercise. Am J Physiol Endocrinol Metab 281:E197–206.

80. Pennings, B., Koopman, R., Beelen, M., Senden, J. M., Saris, W. H. & van Loon, L. J. (2011) Exercising before protein intake allows for greater use of dietary protein-derived amino acids for de novo muscle protein synthesis in both young and elderly men. Am J Clin Nutr 93: 322–331.

81. Parmley, W. W. (1998) Evolution of angiotensin-converting enzyme inhibition in hypertension, heart failure, and vascular protection. Am J Med 105:27S–31S.

82. Schaufelberger, M., Andersson, G., Eriksson, B. O., Grimby, G., Held, P. & Swedberg, K. (1996) Skeletal muscle changes in patients with chronic heart failure before and after treatment with enalapril. Eur Heart J 17:1678–1685.

83. Vescovo, G., Dalla Libera, L., Serafini, F., Leprotti, C., Facchin, L., Volterrani, M., Ceconi, C. & Ambrosio, G. B. (1998) Improved exercise tolerance after losartan and enalapril in heart failure: correlation with changes in skeletal muscle myosin heavy chain composition. Circulation 98:1742–1749.

84. Guzun, R., Aguilaniu, B., Wuyam, B., Mezin, P., Koechlin-Ramonatxo, C., Auffray, C., Saks, V. & Pison, C. (2011) Effects of Training at Mild Exercise Intensities on Quadriceps Muscle Energy Metabolism in Patients with Chronic Obstructive Pulmonary Disease. Acta Physiol (Oxf).

85. Onder, G., Penninx, B. W., Balkrishnan, R., Fried, L. P., Chaves, P. H., Williamson, J., Carter, C., Di Bari, M., Guralnik, J. M. & Pahor, M. (2002) Relation between use of angiotensin-converting enzyme inhibitors and muscle strength and physical function in older women: an observational study. Lancet 359:926–930.

CHAPTER 6

The Complex Relation between Muscle Mass and Muscle Strength

Todd M. Manini

*Institute on Aging & The Department of Aging and Geriatric Research,
University of Florida, Gainesville, FL, USA*

David W. Russ

*Ohio Musculoskeletal and Neurological Institute (OMNI); and
School of Rehabilitation and Communication Sciences, Ohio University,
Athens, OH, USA*

Brian C. Clark

*Ohio Musculoskeletal and Neurological Institute (OMNI); and
Department of Biomedical Sciences, Ohio University, Athens, OH, USA*

INTRODUCTION

Over the past several decades the scientific and medical communities have recognized that skeletal muscle dysfunction (e.g., muscle weakness, muscle atrophy, poor muscle coordination, etc.) is a debilitating and life threatening condition in older persons. The age-associated loss of muscle strength is highly associated with both mortality and physical disability [1–5], and maintenance of muscle mass with advancing age is critical because it serves as a metabolic reservoir that is needed to effectively withstand disease [6]. However, while it is clearly understood that muscle strength and mass are inter-correlated (larger-sized muscle produces greater force), the decline in muscle strength that occurs with aging does not follow the same trajectory as the loss in muscle mass. These overt differences have prompted scientists to encourage the community to consider these phenomena – loss in mass strength and mass – as separate entities with their own respective etiology [7].

This chapter will discuss the complex relationship between muscle strength and mass by evaluating the epidemiological, randomized trial and physiological literature. With regard to the former, recent epidemiological evidence has provided a better understanding of the

Sarcopenia, First Edition. Edited by Alfonso J. Cruz-Jentoft and John E. Morley.
© 2012 John Wiley & Sons, Ltd. Published 2012 by John Wiley & Sons, Ltd.

degree to which the loss in muscle mass is associated with the loss in muscle strength with aging. Next, discussion of randomized trials will provide unbiased evidence that changes in muscle strength and mass are dissociated. Finally, the muscular and neural control of muscle strength will be described.

DISSOCIATION OF MUSCLE STRENGTH AND MASS IN POPULATION-BASED EPIDEMIOLOGICAL STUDIES

It was originally thought that the loss of skeletal muscle mass largely explained muscle weakness observed in older adults [8]. In fact, cross-sectional design studies indicated that muscle size explained approximately 50% of the variance in force capability of that same muscle [9]. Therefore, it was a logical deduction that the visible decrease in muscle size that occurs with aging was in large part responsible for the loss in muscle strength and increased rates of physical limitations seen in old age. Throughout the 1990s and even today, basic science research was largely focused on factors that dictate muscle catabolic and anabolic processes. At that same time, longitudinal studies in humans were initiated to precisely estimate the loss in muscle size that occurs in late-life and how this loss impacts muscle strength. One of the first studies by Hughes and colleagues found that after 10 years of follow-up in a small subset of individuals between 46–78 years old the decline of strength was 60% greater than estimates from cross-sectional comparisons and that the age-associated changes in muscle mass only explained 4% of the change in muscle strength [10]. More data from maturing longitudinal studies with larger samples like the Health, Aging and Body Composition study arrived to the literature and supported this same notion [11,12]. They showed that changes in muscle mass explained only a small proportion of the change in muscle strength. These findings certainly contradicted the initially postulated role of muscle mass in dictating the age-related loss in muscle strength. In summary, the longitudinal data indicate that the decline in muscle strength is significantly more rapid than the concomitant loss of muscle mass, and that the change in quadriceps muscle area explains <10% of the between-subject variability in the change in knee extensor muscle strength [11]. Moreover, maintaining or gaining muscle mass does not prevent aging-related declines in muscle strength [11]. These data – also originating from the Health ABC study and depicted in Figure 6.1 – demonstrate that older adults who gained ≥3% body weight did not lose leg muscle mass, but they exhibited a similar degree of muscle strength loss (2–4% per year) as older adults who lost ≥3% of their body weight (and also demonstrated substantial muscle wasting) [11]. This study clearly showed that changes in leg strength followed over six years showed little, if any, resemblance to changes in leg muscle mass. Accordingly, these findings indicate that the loss of muscle strength in older adults is weakly associated with the loss of lean body mass and that the preservation of the muscle mass does not prevent muscle strength loss per se. Despite the evidence on the disconnection between muscle strength and mass, basic science research continues to focus effort on factors that control muscle tissue size [13].

The dissociation of muscle strength and mass is also revealed by their relative association with physical limitations (e.g., mobility limitation, poor physical performance and physical disability). Manini and Clark conducted a systematic literature search of MEDLINE articles that yielded 2,666 hits [7]. After evaluating these articles, it was concluded that the literature was not appropriate to conduct a meta-analysis of findings because of the following issues: 1) the outcomes were not uniform across studies, 2) there were limited prospective cohorts

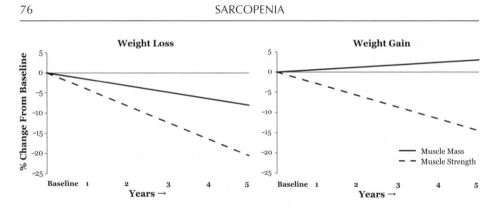

Figure 6.1   The age-related loss of muscle strength is weakly associated with the loss of muscle mass. These figures were adapted from published data obtained from the Health ABC Study to examine the relationship between changes in knee extensor strength and quadriceps femoris cross-sectional area muscle (measured *via* computed tomography) in a five-year longitudinal study of older adults [11]. These data represent the annualized rate of loss over five years in older adults that lost body weight (left panel; n=309 men) and gained body weight (right panel; n=143 men). Note that 1) muscle strength is lost at a substantially faster rate than muscle mass, and 2) that gaining muscle mass does not prevent the aging-related loss of muscle strength (right panel). Adapted from Delmonico MJ, Harris TB, Visser M, Park SW, Conroy MB, Velasquez-Mieyer P, Boudreau R, Manini TM, Nevitt M, Newman AB, and Goodpaster BH. Longitudinal study of muscle strength, quality, and adipose tissue infiltration. Am J Clin Nutr. 1579–1585, 2009. Created figure approved by the corresponding author (Personal Communication with MJ Delmonico). Reprinted with permission from Manini and Clark 2011 [7].

available, 3) there was excessive variability in the measurement of muscle mass and strength, and 4) biases noted in many cross-sectional observational studies were not considered in the analyses. Despite these limitations in the literature, data from seven studies for muscle strength [2,14–19], and nine studies for muscle mass [16,17,19–26] that met pre-determined quality criteria are illustrated in Figure 6.2. Studies examining the association between low muscle strength and poor physical performance or disability were significant 90% of the time (18 out of 20 associations), whereas those examining the same association with low muscle mass were significant 35% of the time (10 out of 28 associations). Furthermore, the unweighted average of the relative risks for low muscle strength was 2.20 (95% CI: 1.5–3.1), while low muscle mass exhibited a relative risk of 1.37 (0.87–2.0). These findings suggest that the number and magnitude of associations for low physical performance or disability are greater for low muscle strength than low muscle mass.

DISSOCIATION OF MUSCLE STRENGTH AND MASS FOUND AMONG INTERVENTION STUDIES (RANDOMIZED TRIALS)

An even greater understanding of the disassociation between muscle mass and strength can be garnered from the examination of the changes in strength associated with increased (i.e. resistance exercise training) and decreased physical activity levels. It is clear that resistance exercise is a potent stimulus to increase muscle strength, but it is well recognized that these adaptations are mediated by a combination of neural and muscular factors. In fact, there are several excellent review papers dedicated to this discussion [27,28].

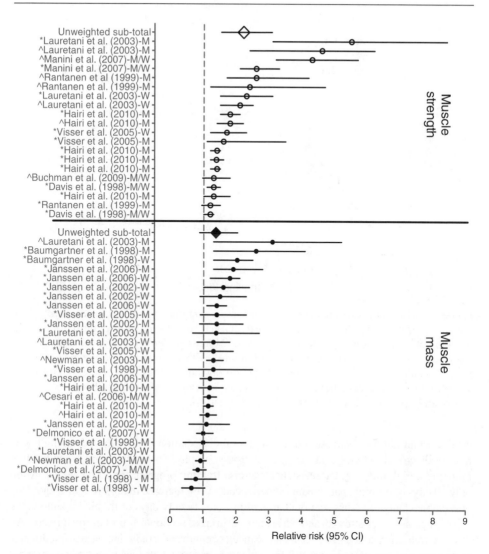

Figure 6.2 Relative risk of poor physical performance, functional limitation or physical disability in older adults with dynapenia (low muscle strength) or sarcopenia (low muscle mass). The counterfactuals are older adults with normal muscle strength or mass. Studies investigating multiple outcomes or expressing findings by sex are repeated. The author of each study is followed with whether the relative risk was estimated in Males (M), Females (F), or both (M/F). Symbols indicate whether outcome was self-report physical function/disability (*) or observed physical performance (^). Reprinted with permission from Manini and Clark 2011 [7].

There are generally two pieces of evidence that support the notion that muscle strength and mass disassociate with resistance exercise. *First*, increased strength observed during the early phases of resistance training occurs before the exercise stimulus is actually capable of eliciting gross morphological increases in a cross sectional area of muscle fibers. For example, training increases strength prior to any measurable difference in muscle properties as demonstrated by an increase in maximal *voluntary* force without a change in maximal force observed when the muscle is electrically stimulated [29]. Seynnes and colleagues

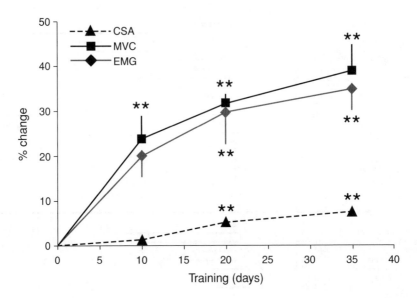

Figure 6.3 Time course of changes in proximal cross-sectional area (CSA), maximal voluntary contraction (MVC), and electromyographical (EMG) activity of the quadriceps muscle following initiation of high intensity leg extension resistance exercise performed 3 days per week. Values are means (SE). **$p < 0.01$ vs. baseline. Reprinted with permission from Seynnes OR, de Boer M, Narici MV. Early skeletal muscle hypertrophy and architectural changes in response to high-intensity resistance training. *Journal of Applied Physiology* 2007;102:368–73. © The American Physiological Society (APS). All rights reserved.

conducted a thorough evaluation of the temporal dissociation in muscle size, strength and muscle electrical activity (via surface electromyography) in healthy young adults after initiating a high intensity leg resistance exercise training program for 35 days [30]. After only 10 days of training, participants experienced ∼20% increase in leg strength without an observable change in cross sectional area of muscle. Twenty days of training resulted in a ∼30% increase in leg strength and ∼5% increase in cross sectional area of the quadriceps. At 35 days, training resulted in a 38% increase in leg strength and a 6.5% increase in quadriceps cross-sectional area (See Figure 6.3 for temporal changes). Changes in electromyography closely followed the temporal pattern of muscle strength. These results suggest that short-term gains in strength are primarily related to a complex interaction between changes in activation and discharge properties of motor units as well as the adaptation in the central command for learning. In summary, muscle strength adaptations during the early phases of resistance exercise are minimally related to factors associated with the size of the muscle.

Second, the increase in strength as a result of resistance training can spread to a contralateral limb not being trained [31]. When muscles of one limb undergo chronic training the contralateral limb increases strength to about half of the level observed from the limb that was actually trained [32]. Additionally, there is no adaptation in muscle morphology in the contralateral limb [33]. A recent study by Fimland and colleagues demonstrated that four weeks of unilateral leg resistance exercise enhanced neural drive (efferent neural drive) to the contralateral agonist muscles, but not sensory afferent drive [34]. Additional measures found that enhanced neural drive was due to either higher descending motor drive to the contralateral limb from supraspinal areas or changes in presynaptic inhibition that would mediate recruitment and discharge rate of motor units. The cross-transfer effect to non-trained muscle groups provides additional evidence that adaptations to the intrinsic muscle tissue are not necessary to modulate muscle strength.

Interventions that use imagined or intended muscle contractions strongly support a clear disconnection between muscle mass and strength. We often imagine ourselves conducting various movements, a process called motor imagery [35]. Archers, for example, might imagine themselves pulling a bow and aiming at a target. Mentally rehearsing these actions can improve performance of the actual movements [36]. Research on mental practice of motor tasks clearly demonstrates that it improves motor skills [37,38], and even increases muscle strength [39]. Ranganathan and colleagues demonstrated that 12 weeks of motor imagery training of both the little finger abductor and the elbow flexors increased muscle strength ~35% and 14%, respectively [40]. This improvement in muscle strength was accompanied by increases in electroencephalogram-derived cortical potential leading the authors to suggest that the strength increase was due to 'enhancement in the central command to muscle' [40]. Neuroimaging studies demonstrate that motor imagery and actual movements share, at least in part, common neural pathways as imagery has been shown to activate several cortical areas, including the primary motor cortex [41]. Accordingly, interventional studies using imagined or intended muscle actions strongly support a clear disconnection between muscle mass and strength.

A similar phenomenon of the muscle strength and mass dissociation associated with resistance training is found with the opposite paradigm of prolonged disuse of muscle. Here, excessive loss of strength is often found with minor to modest reductions in muscle mass following prolonged unweighting (disuse atrophy). For example, we have previously reported that young adults who underwent four weeks of leg muscle unloading experienced a marked loss in muscle strength (~15%) and muscle mass (~9%) [42,43]. However, close inspection of this data utilizing multiple regression analytical techniques indicated that 'neurological factors' explained nearly 50% of the between-subject loss of strength while 'muscular factors' explained around 40%. While the loss of muscle mass (atrophy) was significantly associated with the between-subject loss of strength, its individual contribution (<10%) was less than the contribution from alterations in central neural deficits and indices of excitation-contraction uncoupling.

Another example of the dissociation of strength from muscle mass is demonstrated by studies investigating the exogenous supplementation of androgens or growth factors in order to ameliorate sarcopenia/dynapenia and improve physical function. While these experiments largely rescue the age-related declines in both testosterone and insulin-like growth factor-1 yielding increased muscle mass, the effect on muscle performance is marginally altered [44]. For example, Snyder et al. showed that three years of testosterone replacement in hypogonadal men resulted in a 3.1 kg average increase in lean body mass without a significant change in either maximal knee extension or flexion strength [45]. Additionally, Papadakis et al. found that six months of growth hormone supplementation increased lean body mass 4.4% without significant changes in knee extension or hand grip strength [44]. These studies suggest that clinically significant increases in muscle mass don't carry forward to adaptation in muscle strength.

More recent work on testosterone therapy to increase lean mass has shown more favorable adaptations that transfer to clinically significant increases in muscle strength. Schroeder and colleagues found that men randomized to physiological doses of transdermal testosterone or recombinant human growth hormone+testosterone had increases in both strength and muscle size [46]. However, after eight weeks, men in both groups actually had a reduction in their muscle strength when expressed as a function of muscle mass. Interestingly, after 17 weeks, muscle strength increased above what was expected from the increase in mass, but only in the group randomized to testosterone. These data suggest that the early effects of anabolic hormones might be a result of fluid accumulation in muscle and any muscle strength adaptations might require a long duration supplementation. In a more recent study, Travison and coworkers found in a large sample of 165 men aged >65 years that six months of testosterone supplementation increased appendicular muscle mass by 1 kg (a ~4% increase) compared to a placebo group [47]. The increase in muscle mass was associated with an ~8% increase in leg strength and the group receiving testosterone was more likely to achieve clinically meaningful increases in upper and lower body muscle strength. Lastly, Bhasin and colleagues showed that supraphysiologic doses of testosterone increased leg strength between 11–19% [48]. These more recent studies argue that interventions targeted to increase muscle mass might be effective at increasing muscle strength. However, it is unclear the degree to which and length of anabolic hormone therapy required to increase muscle strength.

In summary, based on a synthesis of the literature we believe the commonly assumed equivalence between muscle mass and strength is not the case because (i) longitudinal aging studies indicate a disassociation between the loss of muscle mass and strength, and (ii) the changes in muscle mass and the changes in strength resulting from alterations in physical activity levels (i.e., exercise training or disuse) do not follow the same time course. Thus, adaptations in other properties in the human neuromuscular system must be involved in the regulation of strength, suggesting that muscle mass should not be used as an intermediate endpoint in interventions designed to improve functional or physical capacity. Unfortunately, these other modulating mechanisms have received far less attention than those associated with muscle growth. Below we will briefly review some of the physiological sites and properties that alter strength with special reference to age-associated losses.

FACTORS THAT DICTATE THE DISSOCIATION BETWEEN MUSCLE STRENGTH AND MUSCLE MASS: MUSCULAR AND NEURAL FACTORS

The mechanisms accounting for an increase or decrease in strength can arise from two broad categories: (i) neural and (ii) skeletal muscle factors, as it is well known that the output from these sources control force production (see Figure 6.4 for a schematic). As such, "muscle strength" is probably a misnomer and "neuromuscular strength" a more apt alternative. The neuromuscular system contains several potential sites that can affect maximal voluntary force output, such as excitatory drive from supraspinal centers, a-motoneuron excitability, motor unit recruitment and rate coding, neuromuscular transmission, muscle mass, E-C coupling processes, and muscle morphology (fat infiltration). In the next sections we will discuss age-related changes in neural and muscular factors that potentially explain the dissociation between muscle mass and strength.

Central (voluntary) activation

As stated earlier, aging is commonly associated with muscle weakness. This loss of muscle strength is likely due to a wide variety of physiologic reasons, including reductions in

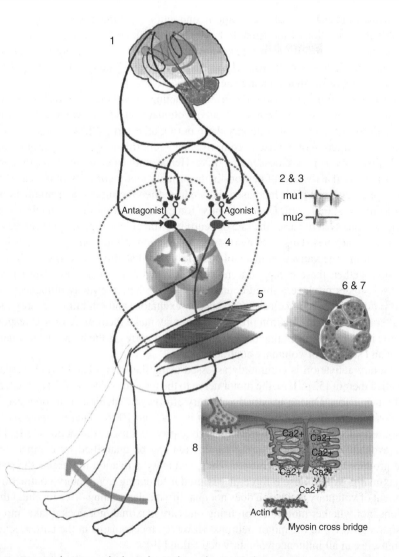

Figure 6.4 Potential sites and physiological mechanisms that regulate strength. The neuro-muscular system contains several potential sites that can affect voluntary force or power production, such as excitatory drive from supraspinal centers, α-motoneuron excitability, antagonistic muscle activity, motor unit recruitment and rate coding, neuromuscular transmission, muscle mass, excitation-contraction (E-C) coupling processes, and muscle morphology and architecture. There is evidence of aging-induced alterations at nearly every denoted site within the system such as, but not limited to, the following: 1. Decreased cortical excitability [78]; 2. Decreased spinal excitability [161]; 3. Decreased maximal motor unit discharge rate [162]; 4. Slowed nerve conduction [163]; 5. Alterations in muscle architecture (reduced fascicle length, pennation angle and tendon stiffness) [164]; 6. Decreased muscle mass (sarcopenia) [12]; 7. Increased myocellular lipid content [106]; 8. Excitation-Contraction Uncoupling (i.e. decreased number of dihydropyridine receptors) [165]. Figure reprinted with permission from Clark and Manini 2008 [166].

muscle mass and changes in the excitation-contraction coupling process. However, it is also probable that a portion of the strength loss is attributable to the nervous system's ability – or lack thereof – to fully activate skeletal muscle. Thus, it is imperative that scientists and clinicians understand the role of the central nervous system in mediating the muscle weakness observed with advancing age.

Prior to more fully discussing the effects of aging on voluntary activation we will first provide a brief overview of the assessment of voluntary activation. Voluntary activation has been defined as the level of voluntary drive during an effort [49]. A voluntary effort, or a voluntary contraction of a muscle, comprises the recruitment of motor neurons, and hence muscle fibers, by increased descending drive. Hence, with an increased force of contraction there is increased activation of neurons in the primary motor cortex with increased firing of corticospinal neurons [50]. Increased descending drive recruits greater numbers of motor neurons in the spinal cord. Concomitantly, force summates more effectively because the central nervous system varies the rate of neuronal firing, thereby generating increased force at higher frequencies. This is known as rate modulation or rate coding. Nevertheless, each motor neuron innervates a number of muscle fibers that fire one-to-one with the motor neuron. Together, these comprise a motor unit. When a motor unit fires sufficiently fast, its muscle fibers produce a fused contraction. While there are many influences on motor neurons during voluntary contractions, such as excitatory and inhibitory sensory feedback, and alterations in motor neuron properties that may make them more or less responsive to synaptic input [51], descending drive from the motor cortex is the major determinant of the timing and strength of voluntary contractions.

Voluntary activation is commonly assessed using the interpolated twitch method, or a derivative thereof [52]. Here, the motor nerve to the muscle is electrically stimulated during a voluntary effort. During maximal voluntary efforts, any increment in force evoked by a stimulus indicates that voluntary activation is less than 100%. That is, some motor units are not recruited or are not firing fast enough to produce fused contractions [53]. The extra force evoked by stimulation during contraction can be quantified by comparison to the force produced by the whole muscle. Thus, voluntary activation represents the proportion of maximal possible muscle force that is produced during a voluntary contraction. Measurement of voluntary activation does not quantify the descending drive reaching the motor neurons, nor whether motor neuron firing rates are maximal, nor does it take into account the source of drive to the motor neurons. However, mechanisms in the cortex, spinal cord and muscle can all influence voluntary activation [49].

Evidence for the role of central activation in modulating muscle strength loss can be garnered from studies of disuse and aging. Regarding the former, young adults undergoing prolonged muscle disuse through unweighting or immobilization experience up to a 70% loss in muscle strength that is not explained by muscle atrophy [42,43]. The correlation between change in muscle strength and voluntary activation of muscle following prolonged disuse is illustrated in Figure 6.5. These data, which represent a compilation of numerous studies from the Clark Lab over the past decade, demonstrate strength loss is highly associated with the nervous system's inability to voluntarily activate muscle in both the upper and lower extremities [42,54,55]. Note that the amount of strength loss experienced during disuse in young adults is greater than that seen with aging and thus the relationship is unlikely to explain strength loss with increased age. Nevertheless, there is evidence to suggest that aging results in impaired voluntary activation of agonist muscles [56]; however,

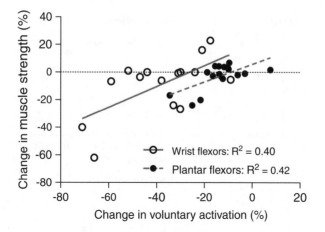

Figure 6.5 Muscle weakness as a result of prolonged disuse is associated with the nervous system's ability to voluntarily activate muscle. Data are from young adults who underwent four weeks of cast immobilization of the wrist flexor or unweighting of the plantar-flexors. Maximal voluntary contraction (MVC) and voluntary activation was measured by evaluating the added force following a supramaximal electrical stimulus (100 Hz doublet) to the peripheral nerve during the MVC. Data represent a compilation of numerous studies from the Clark Lab, including unpublished and published data. Data from published studies include Clark et al. 2006 and Clark et al. 2008 and Clark et al. 2010 [43,54,55].

the effects are not universal across muscle groups (for review see Brooke and colleagues [57]).

A synthesis of the literature does provide some insight into potential explanations of these equivocal reports. Specifically, several studies examining the effect of age on voluntary isometric activation of the knee extensors (Figure 6.6A) and the elbow flexors (Figure 6.6B) suggest that older adults, particularly those greater than 70–75 years of age, exhibit a decrease in voluntary activation; whereas investigations on the age-related changes in voluntary activation of the dorsiflexors yield null findings (Figure 6.6C). Due to the functional differences between these muscles, as well as differences in their physiologic profiles (e.g. motor unit innervations and fiber type characteristics) these muscle-group specific effects are not overly surprising. Differences in activation of different muscle groups are reported in young subjects [58]. The knee extensors are generally reported at a lower activation level whereas the ankle dorsiflexors are reported as being fully activated [59]. Aging may amplify these intermuscle differences in activation. For example, slowing of muscle contraction and relaxation with age is greater for the ankle dorsiflexors than the knee extensors [60]. Consistent with this difference, motor unit firing rates recorded during contractions of different forces show similar rates in young and old men for the knee extensor, vastus lateralis, but slower rates for old men than young men for the ankle dorsiflexor, tibialis anterior [60]. This suggests that for the ankle dorsiflexors, old adults may be able to achieve high levels of voluntary activation with levels of output from the nervous system that are lower than those in young adults, whereas similar output in young and old is required for the knee extensors. Muscle slowing in upper limb muscles, including the elbow flexors, is also reported as minor (∼10%) [61]. We should note that three studies indicating a dramatic

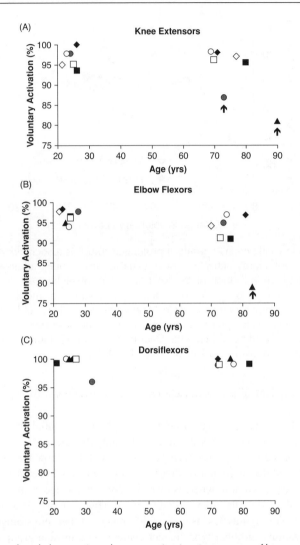

Figure 6.6 Age-related changes in voluntary activation (a measure of how much of a muscle's possible force is produced by a voluntary contraction) is muscle group specific. Studies quantifying age-related differences in voluntary activation of the knee extensors (A), elbow flexors (B), and ankle dorsiflexors (C) during isometric contractions. Selected studies have been highlighted with an arrow pointing to them (see main text for further discussion on these specific papers). Data points in A correspond to the following articles: Filled circles: Stevens et al. 2003, Filled squares: Roos et al. 1999, Filled diamonds: Callahan et al. 2009, Filled triangle: Harridge et al. 1999 [167], Open circles: Wilder and Cannon 2009 [168], Open Squares: Cannon et al. 2007 [169], Open diamonds: Knight and Kamen 2001 [170], Data points in B correspond to the following articles: Filled circles: DeSerres and Enoka 1998 [171], Filled squares: Bilodeau et al. 2001 [172], Filled diamonds: Klein et al. 2001 [173], Filled triangle: Jakobi and Rice 2002 [63], Open circles: Yue et al. 1999 [174], Open Squares: Hunter et al. 2008 [175], Open diamonds: Yoon et al. 2008 [176]. Data points in C correspond to the following articles: Filled circles: Kent-Braun and Ng 1999 [177], Filled squares: Connelly et al. 1999 [178], Filled diamonds: Lanza et al. 2004 [179], Filled triangle: Klass et al. 2005 [180], Open circles: Simoneau et al. 2005 [181], Open Squares: Chung et al. 2007 [182]. Reprinted with permission from Clark, B.C. and Taylor, J.L. Age-related changes in motor cortical properties and voluntary activation of skeletal muscle. *Current Aging Science*. 4(3): 193–200, 2011.

impairment in voluntary activation are highlighted with an arrow in Figure 6.6. Two of these (Figure 6.6A) relate to the knee extensor muscles and one relates to the elbow flexors (Figure 6.6B). With regard to the knee extensors, a number of reports show no differences between old and young adults, but two reports stand out as showing a deficit in voluntary activation with aging (Figure 6.6A, vertical arrows) [62–64]. One of these represents data from the oldest known cohort of individuals that has been examined to date (n=11, age range: 85–97 years) [62], and this observation suggests that deficits in the neural drive can contribute to much of the muscle weakness observed in the very elderly – at least in the knee extensor muscles. The second of the highlighted studies deserves particular attention because it is the largest to date (young adults: n=46, 18–32 years, older adults: n=46, 64–84 years) [64]. Here, when a novel curvilinear relationship between measured voluntary activation and the percentage of maximal voluntary force was considered, the voluntary activation of older adults was calculated to produce 87% of maximal muscle force in comparison to 98% maximal force produced by younger subjects. Together, these studies provide proof of principle that losses in muscle strength are associated with the nervous system's ability to activate muscle with older adults exhibiting impairments in this ability.

Age-related change in supraspinal properties

The neurons in the premotor and primary motor cortex form a complex network of glutamatergic interneurons, afferent projections, and pyramidal neurons that project to the striatum and spinal cord, among other areas of the central nervous system. Although it is often widely assumed that there are neuropathic processes that decay the primary motor cortex (M1) neurons in normal aging, it does not appear that an actual decrease in cortical neurons occurs [65]. However, there are substantial morphometric changes in the motor cortex that do occur with normal aging. For example, cadaveric dissections from humans who died without neurological signs suggest that individuals over 65 years of age exhibit a 43% volumetric reduction in the premotor cortex neuron cell body size in comparison to adults younger than 45 years, which have more recently been corroborated in living humans using high-resolution magnetic resonance imaging (MRI) [66]. In the MRI work, Salat and colleagues calculated the thicknesses of several different areas of the cortex to examine the atrophy in specific cortical regions and observed that cortical thinning occurs by middle age. Moreover, areas near the precentral gyrus, show marked atrophy [66]. Furthermore, there is also evidence to suggest that age-related differences exist in mass of white matter and of myelinated nerve fiber length with individuals losing ~45% of the total length of the myelinated fibers, mostly in the smallest white matter nerve fibers [67]. Also, cross-sectional studies further suggest that aging disrupts the integrity of white matter [68]. Functionally, it appears that these changes due to aging would affect the connectivity of the cortex with itself as well as the rest of the central nervous system.

In addition to morphometric changes, there has long been interest regarding the neurochemical changes within the basal ganglia that can be attributed to aging. This interest was largely driven by the hypothesis that changes in neurotransmitters and their receptors may be attributed to decreases in cognitive as well as motor functions. Certainly, it has been shown that impaired neurotransmission is responsible for at least some age-related behavioral abnormalities [69], including the serotonergic [70,71], cholinergic [72], adrenergic [71], dopaminergic, GABAergic, and glutamatergic systems [73,74]. Reductions in neurotrophic factors have been shown within the motor cortex as well [75]. Age-related changes in the dopaminergic system are perhaps best understood from work on different neurological conditions such as Parkinson's disease. Older adults exhibit reduced dopamine transporter availability [76], and animal findings show that older rodents have decreased dopamine (D_2) receptors [77].

Aging also affects motor cortical properties at the systems level. Specifically, aging is associated with a decrease in cortical excitability [78], increased activation in areas of sensorimotor processing and integration [79–81], and reduced cortical plasticity [82,83]. The effect of aging on cortical excitability is most commonly examined using transcranial magnetic stimulation (TMS), which also allows for the assessment of intracortical excitability [84]. A recent investigation on age-related changes in intracortical facilitatory and inhibitory properties using paired-pulse TMS suggests that middle-aged adults exhibit reduced cortical excitability in comparison to younger adults, as it has been observed that individuals in their late 50s and early 60s exhibit more intracortical inhibition and less intracortical facilitation than adults in their 20s [85]. More recent findings in the elders (mean age of 71 years) support these previous data, which show substantially more intracortical inhibition and less intracortical facilitation in comparison to young adults [86].

In addition to age-related changes in excitability and activation, the human motor cortex also displays an age-dependent decrease in cortical plasticity [82]. For example, Fathi et al. reported that paired-associative electrical stimulation of the median nerve at the wrist resulted in an increased amplitude of the motor evoked potential elicited using TMS in young (21–39 years) and middle-aged (40–59 years); however, this increase did not occur in older adults (60+ years) [82].

Collectively, these findings suggest that aging results in numerous changes in supraspinal properties, such as cortical atrophy, altered neurochemistry, and reduced motor cortical excitability. All of these factors could be mechanistically linked to impairments in voluntary activation capacity and contribute to age-related reductions in motor weakness.

Age related change in spinal properties and the neuromuscular junction

The neuromuscular system is comprised of individual motor units, each of which features a single motor neuron and all the muscle fibers it innervates. The neuromuscular junction serves as the communication bridge between the nerve terminal and the muscle fibers it innervates. While the motor neuron and its behavior (recruitment and firing rate characteristics) are the 'final common pathway' for all motor commands, each motor neuron typically has 50,000 synapses to convey these commands [87], and can thus be influenced by numerous factors such as physical size and dendritic synaptic input current. It is well-known that motor unit recruitment is primarily regulated on a biophysical basis with smaller diameter neurons being recruited first due to having a reduced surface area with fewer parallel ion channels and therefore a higher overall resistance resulting in a greater change in membrane potential based on Ohm's Law [88]. However, in addition to the size principle of recruitment, discharge patterns of motor neurons are influenced by both the characteristics of their presynaptic input and their intrinsic properties. The regularity of the discharge of motor neurons is thought to reflect their prominent post-spike after hyperpolarization [89]. Additionally, motor neurons exhibit a 'bistable' behavior that is characterized by neurons with greater excitability (depolarized closer to threshold) exhibiting a firing rate with a much higher frequency than one that is hyperpolarized [90]. This phenomenon is thought to be explained by dendrite properties known as the persistent inward current which is only expressed when sufficient levels of monoamine (i.e. norepinephrine) neuromodulatory input is present [90]. In essence, the persistent inward currents action is to amplify synaptic input, with it being estimated to enhance ionotropic inputs by fivefold or more thus allowing the firing rates required for maximal activation of muscle fibers to be generated by surprisingly small inputs.

Motor units demonstrate numerous age-related adaptations, including changes in morphology, behavior, and electrophysiology. With regards to changes in morphology, advancing age is thought to result in a reduced motor unit number as well as an increased number of fibers per motor unit (increased innervation ratio) due to the compensatory collateral sprouting by surviving neurons [91]. Aging also elicits remodeling of the neuromuscular junctions endplate [92]. Specifically, aged neuromuscular junctions exhibit elevations in pre-synaptic nerve terminal branching, and in the post-synaptic distribution of receptor sites for neurotransmitter [92]. Interestingly, recent evidence indicates that disuse further compounds these age-associated changes as muscle unloading was observed to result in significant remodeling (expanded area and circumference length both in pre- and post-synaptic regions stained for acetylcholine vesicles/receptors and increase in neural cell adhesion molecule expression) of aged rats neuromuscular junction, but not in those of young, healthy rats [92]. Accordingly, these findings may indicate that the combination of aging and disuse, at least among aged rats, results in partial denervation leading to morphological remodeling of the neuromuscular junction.

Aging has also been shown to result in changes in spinal excitability. For example, Kido and colleagues reported that both the maximum soleus H-reflex (H-max, a measure of global spinal excitability) and the maximum soleus M-wave (M-max, also known as the compound muscle action potential or CMAP) decrease gradually with age, with the decrease in the H-max being more pronounced (reduced H-max to M-ma ratio; Figure 6.7). The H-reflex only provides a global measure of spinal excitability, as it can be modulated by a number of

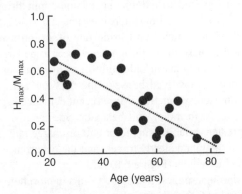

Figure 6.7 Age-related decline in the human soleus muscles H-max to M-max ratio suggesting that advancing age results in a decrease in global spinal excitability. Data were obtained during standing while the muscle was activated at an intensity equal to 15% of its maximum voluntary contraction. Reprinted with permission from Kido, A., Tanaka, N., and Stein, R.B. Spinal excitation and inhibition decrease as humans age. *Can J Physiol Pharmacol.* 82: 238–248, 2004.

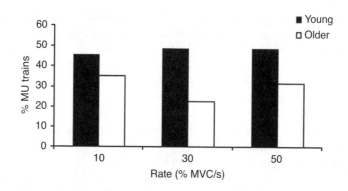

Figure 6.8   Percentage of motor unit trains in which doublets were observed in young (black) and older (white) individuals at three rates of force production. There were no significant differences among rates of force production, but significant differences between groups were found, indicating that the young subjects tended to display more doublet discharges. Reprinted with permission from Christie, A., and Kamen, G. Doublet discharges in motorneurons of young and older adults. *J Neurophysiol.* 95(5): 2787–2795, 2006

potential factors (e.g., presynaptic inhibition, variation in the amount of neurotransmitter released by the Ia terminal, fluctuations in the membrane potential arising, alterations in the intrinsic properties in the motorneurons, etc.). As such, the aforementioned findings suggest that overall spinal excitability is depressed in older adults. However, others have observed that heteronymous facilitation [93] and oligosynaptic reflexes [57] also decrease with age, which provides collective evidence that there is a general decrease in the excitability of spinal reflexes with age.

The end result of the morphological and physiological adaptations in motor units with aging is alterations in the behavioral discharge properties of motor units. For instance, older adults have been reported to exhibit mean motor unit firing rates of the tibialis anterior across a variety of contraction intensities that are ~30–35% lower than young adults [94], and the maximum motor unit firing rate of an intrinsic hand muscle is also comparably reduced [94]. These lower firing rates appear to be largely inter-related to the longer twitch contraction durations in older muscle, which further illustrates the critical integrative control processes involved between the nervous and muscular systems as it relates to overall neuromuscular function. More recent evidence suggests that more subtle age-related differences exist in motor unit behavior. Specifically, older adults have been reported to exhibit a greater variability in motor unit discharge rates that appears to largely influence their ability to maintain steady forces, and the occurrence of motor unit doublet discharges is lower in older adults (Figure 6.8) [95].

Collectively, these findings suggest that aging results in morphological changes in motor units, including an actual reduction in functional motor units. A change of this nature (i.e., loss of motor units resulting in some muscle fibers not undergoing re-innervation) would theoretically result in a reduction in muscle weakness. Additionally, age-related changes in spinal properties and the neuromuscular junction, such as decreased spinal excitability and a reduction in maximal motor unit discharge rates, may contribute to impairments in voluntary activation capacity (and thus muscle weakness).

MUSCULAR CONTRIBUTORS TO FORCE GENERATION

In this section we will discuss age-related changes in muscular properties as they relates to muscle size and composition, excitation-contraction coupling, and cross-bridge function and energetics.

Age-related changes in muscle size and composition

Much atrophy undoubtedly occurs with advancing age. In fact, data from the Health, Aging, and Body Composition (Health ABC) Study —which followed 1,678 older adults between 70–79 years of age longitudinally over a five-year period – indicates that, on average, older men lose approximately 1% of their thigh muscle area per year and older women lose approximately 0.65% of their thigh muscle area per year [11]. With this stated it should be noted that there is a large between-subject variability in the degree of atrophy observed with aging, and some older adults appear to exhibit no or nominal losses in muscle mass. To study the effects of increasing age on human skeletal muscle size and composition, Lexell et al. examined 15-micron cross-sections of autopsied whole vastus lateralis muscle from 43 previously physically healthy men between 15 and 83 years of age [96]. They reported that age-related muscle atrophy begins during the third decade of life and accelerates thereafter. The observed atrophy appeared to be primarily caused by a loss of fibers, with no predominant effect on any fiber type, and to a lesser extent by a reduction in fiber size – predominantly type II fibers. This finding was later corroborated by Lee and colleagues who reported that aging resulted in a decreased fiber area percentage, fiber number percentage, and mean fiber area of type IIA and IIB muscle fibers, but that type I fibers increased in area and number but not in size [97]. Moreover, the type II fibers appeared morphologically smaller and flatter, which is consistent with other reports suggesting pathological abnormalities in aged human muscle fibers such as central nuclei, ring fibers, fiber splitting, scattered highly atrophic fibers, moth-eaten fibers and even vacuoles [98]. Hence, deterioration of the size and structure of a muscle reduces force-generating capacity.

There are many interacting factors leading to muscle wasting in older adults, and they often present themselves concurrently. Changes in muscle protein metabolism have been proposed as an explanatory factor in muscle wasting in older adults, as the balance between protein synthesis and degradation is largely responsible for the maintenance of lean mass [99]. However, recent findings suggest that basal muscle protein synthesis rates do not differ between young and old adults [100,101], and today it is generally accepted that the difference in fasted rates of muscle protein synthesis or breakdown are not altered at resting among healthy older adults [99]. Current hypotheses related to causative factors affecting muscle protein turnover surround the concept of older adults being resistant to anabolic stimuli, such as those associated with feeding, insulin, or physical activity. For example, while the ingestion or infusion of large quantities of amino acids/protein ($\sim$30–40 g) yield similar increases in muscle protein synthesis in both young and older individuals [102], recent studies indicate that older adults exhibit a diminished accretion of muscle proteins after the ingestion of smaller amounts of essential amino acids (6–15 g) [101,103]. Similarly, several recent studies have reported a blunted muscle protein synthesis response following an acute bout of resistance exercise in older subjects [104]. These effects are likely due to deficits in the mammalian target of rapamycin (mTOR) signaling pathway [100], extracellular-related kinase (ERK) 1/2 signaling pathway, and/or upregulation of the ubiquitin proteasome pathway in the elderly [105].

In addition to muscle size and anatomical structure, aged muscle also appears to differ in other compositional manners. For instance, over the past decade numerous studies have reported that aging increases the adipocyte content between muscle groups (intermuscular adipose tissue) and between muscle fascicles (intramuscular adipose tissue) [11,106]. The earliest of these studies suggested that greater muscle fat content was associated with reduced muscle strength [107] suggesting a potential mechanistic link between increases in fat infiltration in muscle and muscle weakness. Indeed, cytokine production from adipose tissue has been linked to depressed muscle force production [92,108], thus providing a theoretical basis to this assertion. However, more recent longitudinal data has failed to observe a direct relationship between increased levels of intermuscular adipose tissue and strength loss with age [11].

Age-related changes in contractile filaments

As noted, age-related declines in muscular force production were considered to be solely a function of reduced muscle mass for some time. It is no surprise then that substantial attention has been devoted to age-related changes in the contractile proteins actin and myosin, which make up the majority of the volume of a skeletal muscle cell. Although sarcomeric actin seems to be quite uniform across muscle cells, myosin, in particular the myosin heavy chain (MHC), is not. In fact, muscle cells (fibers) are frequently differentiated by which isoform(s) of myosin they express. These different myosin isoforms are associated with different levels of ATP consumption – Type I (i.e., slow) consume less ATP than Type II (i.e., fast) isoforms at maximum levels of contractile activation [109–111]. Studies suggest that metabolic cost of Type I < Type IIa < Type IIx < Type IIb fibers. While humans do not express Type IIb myosin, this pattern appears to hold for the three principal isoforms expressed in human muscle. Aging is associated with a loss of skeletal muscle mass (sarcopenia), and since actin and myosin are the predominant proteins in skeletal muscle, an overall loss in these proteins is observed with aging [112]. Some investigators have reported an age-related decline in the myosin:actin ratio in rat muscles [113], which might be expected to alter force production, as has been suggested in studies of disuse and microgravity [114]. Of note, this change occurred in the semimembranosus, but not the soleus muscle, and was observed only in very old, but not old animals [113].

In addition to loss of muscle mass, aging is also generally associated with a shift in fiber type. Although not universal, most studies of aging muscle reflect a shift in overall muscle phenotype from faster to slower MHC, such that a larger proportion of the remaining contractile mass is composed of slower MHC isoforms [115]. Consistent with a slower overall muscle phenotype are observations of reduced potentiation in aged skeletal muscle [116]. This shift is believed to be the result of both greater atrophy of Type II fibers as well as a relatively small loss of fast, Type II fibers [96]. Such a shift may inherently alter muscle quality, as the specific tension of Type II fibers is greater than that of Type I fibers [117]. Although the underlying mechanisms are not entirely clear, apoptotic loss of the α-motor neurons has been implicated [118]. A decline in overall habitual physical activity has been shown to occur with increasing age, but MHC changes due to disuse and detraining are typically observed to be the opposite of those seen with aging (i.e., from slower to faster isoforms).

In addition to the absolute amount of contractile protein, some investigators have reported age-related functional impairments of these proteins within single fibers [119] and even at the level of isolated myosin molecules [120]. Lowe and colleagues demonstrated a reduction in the number of strongly bound crossbridges in maximally-activated fibers of aged vs. young rats using electron paramagnetic resonance [121]. These functional deficits may be the result of a reduced mixed muscle protein and MHC turnover [122], which could in turn contribute to the accumulation of post-translational modifications that impair crossbridge function.

Finally, the thin filaments also contain tropomyosin and the troponin isoforms. Although these regulatory proteins are not part of the actin-myosin crossbridge, they are critical in opening up the myosin binding site on actin, which makes crossbridge formation possible. If either tropomyosin or troponin are not functioning properly, it is possible that fewer crossbridges will form (in effect reducing the calcium sensitivity of the muscle), generating less force which would result in reduced muscle quality [123]. Recent proteomics studies have suggested that increased age is associated with reduced expression of these proteins and increased post-translational modifications (e.g. nitration) [124], either of which could impair protein function. These proteins have received much less attention in the aging literature than the contractile proteins, and this area clearly needs more study in the future.

Age-related changes in muscular force transmission

Although actin and myosin are proteins responsible for the generation of muscular force (*via* the crossbridge cycle), functional force needs to be effectively transmitted to produce optimal function. Much force transmission in skeletal muscle takes place through a complex array of cytoskeletal proteins, and it is possible that deficiencies in these cytoskeletal proteins could reduce muscle quality by impairing force transmission. This topic has been largely unexplored, despite evidence from knockout animals that loss of at least one cytoskeletal protein, desmin, is associated with reduced muscle quality [125]. However, the few existing studies indicate that, if anything, desmin is increased with aging [126,127]. Interestingly, one group [128] has reported increased specific force in muscles from desmin knockout mice, speculating desmin acts a 'viscous element that dissipates mechanical energy'. If this is the case, then an age-associated increase in desmin could indeed contribute to impaired muscle quality with aging. Clearly, further work needs to be done to explore the potential role of cytoskeletal changes in aging muscle function.

AGE-RELATED CHANGES IN EXCITATION-CONTRACTION COUPLING

Excitation-contraction coupling converts the neural signal for muscle activation (muscle action potential) into muscle contraction and force development through a series of bio-physical steps (Figure 6.9). Briefly, the action potential spreads throughout the muscle *via*

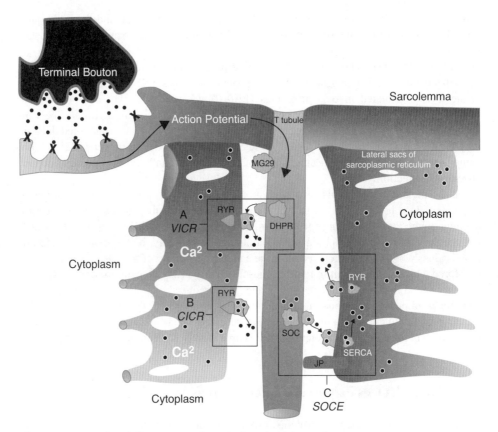

Figure 6.9 Graphical illustration voltage-induced calcium release.
VICR = voltage-induced calcium release; CICR = calcium-induced calcium release; SOCE = store-operated calcium entry; RYR = Ryanodine receptor; DHPR = Dihydropyridine receptor; SERCA = Sarcoplasmic/endoplasmic reticulum calcium ATPase; JP = juntophilin.

the t-tubular system, activating the voltage-sensitive dihydropyridine receptors (DHPRs), which subsequently open the ryanodine receptors (RYRs; Ca^{2+} release channels). This releases Ca^{2+} from its membranous storage area known (the sarcoplasmic reticulum (SR)). The newly-released Ca^{2+} binds to Troponin C which promotes crossbridge formation and force production. The Ca^{2+} is then returned to the SR by the sarcoplasmic reticulum Ca^{2+} pump (SR-ATPase) [129]. Although the process of Ca^{2+} re-uptake is important to force-relaxation and age-related changes may play a significant role in phenomena such as task performance (i.e. motor coordination) and muscle fatigue, the process of Ca^{2+} release is much more directly related to force production. Thus, the rest of the review on E-CC will focus on age-related changes in Ca^{2+} release.

The description of E-CC above outlines the predominant mechanism of Ca^{2+} release in skeletal muscle, also referred to as voltage induced calcium release (VICR) and does not require transmembrane movement of extracellular calcium [130]. However, Ca^{2+} induced calcium release (CICR), which predominates in cardiac muscle, has also been shown to occur in skeletal muscle [131,132]. In this process, direct entry of extra cellular Ca^{2+} into the myoplasm *via* activation of DHPRs that are not associated with RyRs occurs, and triggers further mobilization of intracellular Ca^{2+} stores by activating RyRs. It has been suggested that this CICR may amplify the effects of VICR [133]. Finally, store operated calcium entry (SOCE) is thought to serve to renew depleted Ca^{2+} in the SR via the opening of plasma membrane-located store-operated Ca^{2+} channels (SOCC) [134]. This allows extracellular Ca^{2+} to accumulate in the cytoplasm in order to replenish SR Ca^{2+} [135]. Theoretically, disruption at any point in the E-CC process can prevent optimal activation of muscle mass and thus reduce muscle quality, which would result in muscle weakness.

Impairments in SR Ca^{2+} release have been suggested to explain deficits of muscle quality in aged muscle [136–138]. Arguably, the idea that changes in E-CC were contributing to age-related weakness began with reports of 'excitation-calcium release uncoupling' in single fibers from aged human muscles [139]. Perhaps the most obvious mechanism for 'uncoupling' of E-CC to account for loss of force production would be a reduction in the expression of the principal proteins in VICR. Although some early work indicated that RYR expression might be reduced with age, at least in fast muscles [136], a number of studies have not supported this hypothesis [140]. There is more support for the age-related loss of DHPR (particularly the α-1s subunit), such that a greater number of RYRs are not associated with DHPR, causing the uncoupling and disrupting the VICR process [141,142]. More recently, attention has been focused on the β-1a subunit of the DHPR. This subunit has roles in chaperoning the α-1s subunit to the t-tubule membrane and regulating Ca^{2+} current [142,143]. It also interacts directly with RyR [144], and may impair E-CC by binding to charged residues on RyR [145]. Taylor et al., 2009 determined that DHPR-β1a increases significantly with age in fast, slow and mixed murine muscle fibers, and that overexpression of the subunit results in a decrease in α-1s subunits and a decline in specific force [146]. Finally, Payne et al. (2009) found that RNA inhibition of DHPR-β1a expression in FDB muscles of young and old mice caused a significant reduction of charge movement in young mice, but restored charge movement to young control levels in old mice [147].

Although the case for alterations of DHPR contributing to the age-related decline in muscle quality is compelling, other processes may be impaired as well. Others suggest that aging may impair SR calcium release, independent of DHPR function [149]. In these experiments, the RYR was stimulated directly through pharmacological means in an SR vesicle preparation. Thus, SR function was compromised. Interestingly, this study found that the older muscles also exhibited a reduced RYR-FKBP binding [149]. FKBP is a small immunophilin known to associate with the RYR, and reduced RYR-FKBP interaction has been linked to reduced muscle quality and impaired calcium release in models of aging, heart failure and exhaustion [150]. While the cause of the reduced protein-protein interaction has not been definitively identified, data suggest that an age-related increase in RYR oxidation may be at work [150]. Such a modification may be the result of reduced protein turnover with increasing age, allowing for greater accumulation of post-translational modifications such as oxidation [151].

Investigators have also begun examining a potential role for SR-related proteins that are not directly involved in SR Ca^{2+} release, with much attention given to junctophilin and mitsugumin 29 (MG29). These proteins are both associated with the triadic junctions between the t-tubules and terminal cisternae, and both appear necessary for normal triad organization and optimal E-CC [152]. Interestingly, MG29 has been linked to SOCE and has been shown to decline with aging [153], and may contribute to the fragmentation of the SR, resulting in fragments of Ca^{2+}-containing SR disconnected from the t-tubule membranes [154]. It has been hypothesized that this fragmentation occurs in a subpopulation of fibers that became at least partially dependent on extracellular Ca^{2+} for SR Ca^{2+}. This phenomenon essentially shifts the E-CC mechanism from VICR to CICR [155]. Muscles containing higher percentages of such fibers dependent on SOCE would be at a force-generating disadvantage compared to normal skeletal muscle fibers that are not dependent upon the influx of Ca^{2+} from the t-tubule, particularly if the SR were depleted of Ca^{2+}. The role for an age-associated decline in SOCE in impaired muscle quality remains unclear, however, as others have not found that age adversely affects either SOCE or calcium stores [147], and the conditions under which impairments in SOCE may affect force (i.e., prolonged, high-rate stimulation with long-duration pulses) may not occur during normal muscle function [156].

Because of the role of E-CC in linking neural signals to muscular responses, it is not surprising that a direct biochemical interaction between muscle and nerve may influence E-CC. There is evidence to suggest that muscle-specific IGF-1 may act in a paracrine, retrograde manner to preserve motor neuron function [157]. This in turn is thought to lead to the preservation of E-CC and muscle quality [158], possibly through the regulation of DHPR expression. However, questions regarding the exact mechanisms and outcomes of IGF-1 over expression remain.

Finally, it is worth noting that age-related changes in membrane composition of the SR itself may occur. While much attention has been focused on the age-related alterations of the proteins associated with the SR, it is well known that the function of integral membrane proteins is affected by the composition of the membranes in which they are situated [159]. Investigation along these lines has been quite limited. However, age related changes in the SR phospholipid and fatty acid composition have been demonstrated [160]. The contribution of such alterations in membrane composition to age-related changes in muscle function have not been characterized, but at least one group has observed an increased susceptibility to heat inactivation of SERCA function in the SR of aging rats [160].

CONCLUSION

The age-related loss of muscle mass only partially explains the reduction in muscle strength, and as such – to a large extent – these two issues are seemingly independent of one another. Salient points for consideration are that: 1) recent data from longitudinal studies on aging indicate that maintaining or gaining muscle mass does not prevent aging-related declines in muscle strength; and 2) muscle weakness is independently associated with physical disability and mortality. The physiologic mechanisms of muscle weakness with aging are multifactorial and arise from deficits in neural activation, reductions in the intrinsic force-generating capacity of muscle, as well as muscle wasting. Research continues to determine the relative contribution of the various segmental components of the neuromuscular system associated with muscle strength loss that is not related to the size of muscle.

REFERENCES

1. Cesari M, Pahor M, Lauretani F, et al. Skeletal muscle and mortality results from the InCHIANTI Study. J Gerontol A Biol Sci Med Sci 2009;64:377–384.

2. Manini TM, Visser M, Won-Park S, et al. Knee extension strength cutpoints for maintaining mobility. Journal of the American Geriatrics Society 2007;55:451–457.

3. Newman AB, Kupelian V, Visser M, et al. Strength, but not muscle mass, is associated with mortality in the health, aging and body composition study cohort. J Gerontol A Biol Sci Med Sci 2006;61:72–77.

4. Visser M, Deeg DJ, Lips P, Harris TB, Bouter LM. Skeletal muscle mass and muscle strength in relation to lower-extremity performance in older men and women. J Am Geriatr Soc 2000;48:381–386.

5. Visser M, Simonsick EM, Colbert LH, et al. Type and intensity of activity and risk of mobility limitation: the mediating role of muscle parameters. J Am Geriatr Soc 2005;53: 762–770.

6. Tan BH, Fearon KC. Cachexia: prevalence and impact in medicine. Curr Opin Clin Nutr Metab Care 2008;11:400–407.

7. Manini TM, Clark BC. Dynapenia and Aging: An Update. The Journals of Gerontology Series A, Biological Sciences and Medical Sciences 2011.

8. Grimby G, Saltin B. The ageing muscle. Clinical Physiology 1983;3:209–218.

9. Maughan RJ, Watson JS, Weir J. Strength and cross-sectional area of human skeletal muscle. J Physiol 1983;338:37–49.

10. Hughes VA, Frontera WR, Wood M, et al. Longitudinal muscle strength changes in older adults: influence of muscle mass, physical activity, and health. J Gerontol A Biol Sci Med Sci 2001;56:B209–17.

11. Delmonico MJ, Harris TB, Visser M, et al. Longitudinal study of muscle strength, quality, and adipose tissue infiltration. Am J Clin Nutr 2009;90:1579–1585.

12. Goodpaster BH, Park SW, Harris TB, et al. The loss of skeletal muscle strength, mass, and quality in older adults: The Health, Aging and Body Composition Study. J Gerentol Med Sci 2006;61:1059–1064.

13. Marzetti E, Calvani R, Bernabei R, Leeuwenburgh C. Apoptosis in Skeletal Myocytes: A Potential Target for Interventions against Sarcopenia and Physical Frailty – A Mini-Review. Gerontology 2011.

14. Buchman AS, Boyle PA, Leurgans SE, Evans DA, Bennett DA. Pulmonary function, muscle strength, and incident mobility disability in elders. Proc Am Thorac Soc 2009;6:581–587.

15. Davis JW, Ross PD, Preston SD, Nevitt MC, Wasnich RD. Strength, physical activity, and body mass index: relationship to performance-based measures and activities of daily living among older Japanese women in Hawaii. J Am Geriatr Soc 1998;46:274–279.

16. Hairi NN, Cumming RG, Naganathan V, et al. Loss of Muscle Strength, Mass (Sarcopenia), and Quality (Specific Force) and Its Relationship with Functional Limitation and Physical Disability: The Concord Health and Ageing in Men Project. J Am Geriatr Soc 2010;58: 2055–2062.

17. Lauretani F, Russo CR, Bandinelli S, et al. Age-associated changes in skeletal muscles and their effect on mobility: an operational diagnosis of sarcopenia. J Appl Physiol 2003;95:1851–1860.

18. Rantanen T, Guralnik JM, Foley D, et al. Midlife hand grip strength as a predictor of old age disability. JAMA 1999;281:558–560.

19. Visser M, Goodpaster BH, Kritchevsky SB, et al. Muscle mass, muscle strength, and muscle fat infiltration as predictors of incident mobility limitations in well-functioning older persons. J Gerontol A Biol Sci Med Sci 2005;60:324–333.

20. Baumgartner RN, Koehler KM, Gallagher D, et al. Epidemiology of sarcopenia among the elderly in New Mexico. Am J Epidemiol 1998;147:755–763.

21. Cesari M, Kritchevsky SB, Leeuwenburgh C, Pahor M. Oxidative damage and platelet activation as new predictors of mobility disability and mortality in elders. Antioxidants & Redox Signaling 2006;8:609–619.

22. Delmonico MJ, Harris TB, Lee JS, et al. Alternative definitions of sarcopenia, lower extremity performance, and functional impairment with aging in older men and women. J Am Geriatr Soc 2007;55:769–774.

23. Janssen I. Influence of sarcopenia on the development of physical disability: the Cardiovascular Health Study. J Am Geriatr Soc 2006;54:56–62.

24. Janssen HC, Samson MM, Verhaar HJ. Vitamin D deficiency, muscle function, and falls in elderly people. Am J Clin Nutr 2002;75:611–615.

25. Newman AB, Haggerty CL, Goodpaster B, et al. Strength and muscle quality in a well-functioning cohort of older adults: the Health, Aging and Body Composition Study. J Am Geriatr Soc 2003;51:323–330.

26. Visser M, Harris TB, Langlois J, et al. Body fat and skeletal muscle mass in relation to physical disability in very old men and women of the Framingham Heart Study. J Gerontol A Biol Sci Med Sci 1998;53:M214–21.

27. Enoka RM. Muscle strength and its development. New perspectives. Sports Medicine 1988;6:146–168.

28. Enoka RM. Neural adaptations with chronic physical activity. J Biomech 1997;30:447–455.

29. McDonagh MJ, Hayward CM, Davies CT. Isometric training in human elbow flexor muscles. The effects on voluntary and electrically evoked forces. The Journal of Bone and Joint Surgery British volume 1983;65:355–358.

30. Seynnes OR, de Boer M, Narici MV. Early skeletal muscle hypertrophy and architectural changes in response to high-intensity resistance training. Journal of Applied Physiology 2007;102:368–373.

31. Enoka RM. Muscle strength and its development. Sports Med 1988;6:146–168.

32. Carroll TJ, Herbert RD, Munn J, Lee M, Gandevia SC. Contralateral effects of unilateral strength training: evidence and possible mechanisms. Journal of Applied Physiology 2006;101:1514–1522.

33. Lee M, Carroll TJ. Cross education: possible mechanisms for the contralateral effects of unilateral resistance training. Sports Medicine 2007;37:1–14.

34. Fimland MS, Helgerud J, Solstad GM, Iversen VM, Leivseth G, Hoff J. Neural adaptations underlying cross-education after unilateral strength training. Eur J Appl Physiol 2009;107:723–730.

35. Schieber MH. Dissociating Motor Cortex from the Motor. J Physiol 2011.

36. Avanzino L, Giannini A, Tacchino A, Pelosin E, Ruggeri P, Bove M. Motor imagery influences the execution of repetitive finger opposition movements. Neuroscience Letters 2009;466: 11–15.

37. Mendoza D, Wichman H. " Inner" darts: effects of mental practice on performance of dart throwing. Percept Mot Skills 1978;47:1195–1199.

38. Lejeune M, Decker C, Sanchez X. Mental rehearsal in table tennis performance. Percept Mot Skills 1994;79:627–641.

39. Yue G, Cole KJ. Strength increases from the motor program: comparison of training with maximal voluntary and imagined muscle contractions. Journal of Neurophysiology 1992;67:1114–1123.

40. Ranganathan VK, Siemionow V, Liu JZ, Sahgal V, Yue GH. From mental power to muscle power–gaining strength by using the mind. Neuropsychologia 2004;42:944–956.

41. Malouin F, Richards CL, Jackson PL, Dumas F, Doyon J. Brain activations during motor imagery of locomotor-related tasks: a PET study. Hum Brain Mapp 2003;19:47–62.

42. Clark BC, Fernhall B, Ploutz-Snyder LL. Adaptations in human neuromuscular function following prolonged unweighting: I. Skeletal muscle contractile properties and applied ischemia efficacy. Journal of Applied Physiology 2006;101:256–263.

43. Clark BC, Manini TM, Bolanowski SJ, Ploutz-Snyder LL. Adaptations in human neuromuscular function following prolonged unweighting: II. Neurological properties and motor imagery efficacy. Journal of Applied Physiology 2006;101:264–272.

44. Papadakis MA, Grady D, Black D, et al. Growth hormone replacement in healthy older men improves body composition but not functional ability. Ann Intern Med 1996;124:708–716.

45. Snyder PJ, Peachey H, Berlin JA, et al. Effects of testosterone replacement in hypogonadal men. J Clin Endocrinol Metab 2000;85:2670–2677.

46. Schroeder ET, He J, Yarasheski KE, et al. Value of measuring muscle performance to assess changes in lean mass with testosterone and growth hormone supplementation. Eur J Appl Physiol 2011.

47. Travison TG, Basaria S, Storer TW, et al. Clinical meaningfulness of the changes in muscle performance and physical function associated with testosterone administration in older men with mobility limitation. The Journals of Gerontology Series A, Biological Sciences and Medical Sciences 2011;66:1090–1099.

48. Bhasin S, Woodhouse L, Casaburi R, et al. Older men are as responsive as young men to the anabolic effects of graded doses of testosterone on the skeletal muscle. J Clin Endocrinol Metab 2005;90:678–688.

49. Gandevia SC. Spinal and supraspinal factors in human muscle fatigue. Physiol Rev 2001;81:1725–1789.

50. Ashe J. Force and the motor cortex. Behav Brain Res 1997;87:255–269.

51. Rekling JC, Funk GD, Bayliss DA, Dong XW, Feldman JL. Synaptic control of motoneuronal excitability. Physiol Rev 2000;80:767–852.

52. Taylor JL. Point: the interpolated twitch does/does not provide a valid measure of the voluntary activation of muscle. J Appl Physiol 2009;107:354–355.

53. Merton PA. Voluntary strength and fatigue. J Physiol 1954;123:553–564.

54. Clark BC, Issac LC, Lane JL, Damron LA, Hoffman RL. Neuromuscular plasticity during and following 3 wk of human forearm cast immobilization. J Appl Physiol 2008;105: 868–878.

55. Clark BC, Taylor JL, Hoffman RL, Dearth DJ, Thomas JS. Cast immobilization increases long-interval intracortical inhibition. Muscle & Nerve 2010;42:363–372.

56. Klass M, Baudry S, Duchateau J. Voluntary activation during maximal contraction with advancing age: a brief review. Eur J Appl Physiol 2007;100:543–551.

57. Brooke JD, Singh R, Wilson MK, Yoon P, McIlroy WE. Aging of human segmental oligosynaptic reflexes for control of leg movement. Neurobiology of Aging 1989;10:721–725.

58. Behm DG, Whittle J, Button D, Power K. Intermuscle differences in activation. Muscle Nerve 2002;25:236–243.

59. Russ DW, Towse TF, Wigmore DM, Lanza IR, Kent-Braun JA. Contrasting influences of age and sex on muscle fatigue. Medicine and Science in Sports and Exercise 2008;40:234–241.

60. Connelly DM, Rice CL, Roos MR, Vandervoort AA. Motor unit firing rates and contractile properties in tibialis anterior of young and old men. J Appl Physiol 1999;87:843–852.

61. Roos MR, Rice CL, Vandervoort AA. Age-related changes in motor unit function. Muscle Nerve 1997;20:679–690.

62. Harridge S, Kryger A, Stensgaard A. Knee extensor strength, activation, and size in very elderly peple following strength training. Muscle & Nerver 1999;22:831–839.

63. Jakobi JM, Rice CL. Voluntary muscle activation varies with age and muscle group. J Appl Physiol 2002;93:457–462.

64. Stevens JE, Stackhouse SK, Binder-Macleod SA, Snyder-Mackler L. Are voluntary muscle activation deficits in older adults meaningful? Muscle Nerve 2003;27:99–101.

65. Ward NS. Compensatory mechanisms in the aging motor system. Ageing Res Rev 2006;5:239–254.

66. Salat DH, Buckner RL, Snyder AZ, et al. Thinning of the cerebral cortex in aging. Cereb Cortex 2004;14:721–730.

67. Marner L, Nyengaard JR, Tang Y, Pakkenberg B. Marked loss of myelinated nerve fibers in the human brain with age. J Comp Neurol 2003;462:144–152.

68. Madden DJ, Whiting WL, Huettel SA, White LE, MacFall JR, Provenzale JM. Diffusion tensor imaging of adult age differences in cerebral white matter: relation to response time. Neuroimage 2004;21:1174–1181.

69. Carlsson A. Treatment of Parkinson's with L-DOPA. The early discovery phase, and a comment on current problems. J Neural Transm 2002;109:777–787.

70. Morgan DG, May PC, Finch CE. Dopamine and serotonin systems in human and rodent brain: effects of age and neurodegenerative disease. J Am Geriatr Soc 1987;35:334–345.

71. Bigham MH, Lidow MS. Adrenergic and serotonergic receptors in aged monkey neocortex. Neurobiol Aging 1995;16:91–104.

72. Bartus RT, Dean RL, 3rd, Beer B, Lippa AS. The cholinergic hypothesis of geriatric memory dysfunction. Science 1982;217:408–414.

73. Segovia G, Porras A, Del Arco A, Mora F. Glutamatergic neurotransmission in aging: a critical perspective. Mech Ageing Dev 2001;122:1–29.

74. Mora F, Segovia G, Del Arco A. Glutamate-dopamine-GABA interactions in the aging basal ganglia. Brain research reviews 2008;58:340–353.

75. Hayashi M, Yamashita A, Shimizu K. Somatostatin and brain-derived neurotrophic factor mRNA expression in the primate brain: decreased levels of mRNAs during aging. Brain Res 1997;749:283–289.

76. Volkow ND, Ding YS, Fowler JS, et al. Dopamine transporters decrease with age. J Nucl Med 1996;37:554–559.

77. Joseph JA, Berger RE, Engel BT, Roth GS. Age-related changes in the nigrostriatum: a behavioral and biochemical analysis. J Gerontol 1978;33:643–649.

78. Sale MV, Semmler JG. Age-related differences in corticospinal control during functional isometric contractions in left and right hands. J Appl Physiol 2005;99:1483–1493.

79. Heuninckx S, Wenderoth N, Debaere F, Peeters R, Swinnen SP. Neural basis of aging: the penetration of cognition into action control. J Neurosci 2005;25:6787–6796.

80. Naccarato M, Calautti C, Jones PS, Day DJ, Carpenter TA, Baron JC. Does healthy aging affect the hemispheric activation balance during paced index-to-thumb opposition task? An fMRI study. Neuroimage 2006;32:1250–1256.

81. Rowe JB, Siebner H, Filipovic SR, et al. Aging is associated with contrasting changes in local and distant cortical connectivity in the human motor system. Neuroimage 2006;32:747–760.

82. Fathi D, Ueki Y, Mima T, et al. Effects of aging on the human motor cortical plasticity studied by paired associative stimulation. Clin Neurophysiol 2009.

83. Sawaki L, Yaseen Z, Kopylev L, Cohen LG. Age-dependent changes in the ability to encode a novel elementary motor memory. Ann Neurol 2003;53:521–524.

84. Kobayashi M, Pascual-Leone A. Transcranial magnetic stimulation in neurology. Lancet Neurology 2003;2:145–156.

85. Kossev AR, Schrader C, Dauper J, Dengler R, Rollnik JD. Increased intracortical inhibition in middle-aged humans; a study using paired-pulse transcranial magnetic stimulation. Neuroscience letters 2002;333:83–86.

86. McGinley M, Hoffman RL, Russ DW, Thomas JS, Clark BC. Older adults exhibit more intracortical inhibition and less intracortical facilitation than young adults. Experimental Gerontology 2010;45:671–678.

87. Powers RK, Binder MD. Input-output functions of mammalian motoneurons. Rev Physiol Biochem Pharmacol 2001;143:137–263.

88. Henneman E, Somjen G, Carpenter DO. Excitability and inhibitability of motoneurons of different sizes. J Neurophysiol 1965;28:599–620.

89. Powers RK, Turker KS, Binder MD. What can be learned about motoneurone properties from studying firing patterns? Adv Exp Med Biol 2002;508:199–205.

90. Heckman CJ. Active conductances in motoneuron dendrites enhance movement capabilities. Exercise and sport sciences reviews 2003;31:96–101.

91. Rosenheimer JL. Factors affecting denervation-like changes at the neuromuscular junction during aging. Int J Dev Neurosci 1990;8:643–654.

92. Deschenes MR, Roby MA, Eason MK, Harris MB. Remodeling of the neuromuscular junction precedes sarcopenia related alterations in myofibers. Experimental Gerontology 2010;45:389–393.

93. Morita H, Shindo M, Yanagawa S, Yoshida T, Momoi H, Yanagisawa N. Progressive decrease in heteronymous monosynaptic Ia facilitation with human ageing. Experimental brain research Experimentelle Hirnforschung Experimentation cerebrale 1995;104:167–170.

94. Kamen G, Sison SV, Du CC, Patten C. Motor unit discharge behavior in older adults during maximal-effort contractions. J Appl Physiol 1995;79:1908–1913.

95. Christie A, Kamen G. Doublet discharges in motoneurons of young and older adults. J Neurophysiol 2006;95:2787–2795.

96. Lexell J, Taylor CC, Sjostrom M. What is the cause of the ageing atrophy? Total number, size and proportion of different fiber types studied in whole vastus lateralis muscle from 15- to 83-year-old men. Journal of the Neurological Sciences 1988;84:275–294.

97. Lee WS, Cheung WH, Qin L, Tang N, Leung KS. Age-associated decrease of type IIA/B human skeletal muscle fibers. Clinical Orthopaedics and Related Research 2006;450:231–237.

98. Jakobsson F, Borg K, Edstrom L. Fibre-type composition, structure and cytoskeletal protein location of fibres in anterior tibial muscle. Comparison between young adults and physically active aged humans. Acta Neuropathologica 1990;80:459–468.

99. Fry CS, Rasmussen BB. Skeletal Muscle Protein Balance and Metabolism in the Elderly. Current Aging Science 2011.

100. Cuthbertson D, Smith K, Babraj J, et al. Anabolic signaling deficits underlie amino acid resistance of wasting, aging muscle. The FASEB journal : official publication of the Federation of American Societies for Experimental Biology 2005;19:422–424.

101. Katsanos CS, Kobayashi H, Sheffield-Moore M, Aarsland A, Wolfe RR. Aging is associated with diminished accretion of muscle proteins after the ingestion of a small bolus of essential amino acids. The American Journal of Clinical Nutrition 2005;82:1065–1073.

102. Rasmussen BB, Wolfe RR, Volpi E. Oral and intravenously administered amino acids produce similar effects on muscle protein synthesis in the elderly. J Nutr Health Aging 2002;6: 358–362.

103. Katsanos CS, Kobayashi H, Sheffield-Moore M, Aarsland A, Wolfe RR. A high proportion of leucine is required for optimal stimulation of the rate of muscle protein synthesis by essential amino acids in the elderly. American Journal of Physiology Endocrinology and Metabolism 2006;291:E381–7.

104. Sheffield-Moore M, Paddon-Jones D, Sanford AP, et al. Mixed muscle and hepatic derived plasma protein metabolism is differentially regulated in older and younger men following resistance exercise. American Journal of Physiology Endocrinology and Metabolism 2005;288:E922–9.

105. Altun M, Besche HC, Overkleeft HS, et al. Muscle wasting in aged, sarcopenic rats is associated with enhanced activity of the ubiquitin proteasome pathway. J Biol Chem 2010;285:39597–39608.

106. Goodpaster BH, Carlson CL, Visser M, et al. Attenuation of skeletal muscle and strength in the elderly: The Health ABC Study. J Appl Physiol 2001;90:2157–2165.

107. Goodpaster BH, Kelley DE, Thaete FL, He J, Ross R. Skeletal muscle attenuation determined by computed tomography is associated with skeletal muscle lipid content. J Appl Physiol 2000;89:104–110.

108. Christie A, Kamen G. Short-term training adaptations in maximal motor unit firing rates and afterhyperpolarization duration. Muscle & Nerve 2010;41:651–660.

109. Han YS, Geiger PC, Cody MJ, Macken RL, Sieck GC. ATP consumption rate per cross bridge depends on myosin heavy chain isoform. Journal of Applied Physiology 2003;94:2188–2196.

110. He ZH, Bottinelli R, Pellegrino MA, Ferenczi MA, Reggiani C. ATP consumption and efficiency of human single muscle fibers with different myosin isoform composition. Biophysical Journal 2000;79:945–961.

111. Rivero JL, Talmadge RJ, Edgerton VR. Interrelationships of myofibrillar ATPase activity and metabolic properties of myosin heavy chain-based fibre types in rat skeletal muscle. Histochem Cell Biol 1999;111:277–287.

112. D'Antona G, Pellegrino MA, Adami R, et al. The effect of ageing and immobilization on structure and function of human skeletal muscle fibres. J Physiol 2003;552:499–511.

113. Thompson LV, Durand D, Fugere NA, Ferrington DA. Myosin and actin expression and oxidation in aging muscle. Journal of Applied Physiology 2006;101:1581–1587.

114. Clark BC. In Vivo Alterations in Skeletal Muscle Form and Function after Disuse Atrophy. Med Sci Sports Exerc 2009.

115. Klitgaard H, Zhou M, Schiaffino S, Betto R, Salviati G, Saltin B. Ageing alters the myosin heavy chain composition of single fibres from human skeletal muscle. Acta Physiol Scand 1990;140:55–62.

116. Carlsen RC, Walsh DA. Decrease in force potentiation and appearance of alpha-adrenergic mediated contracture in aging rat skeletal muscle. Pflugers Archiv : European Journal of Physiology 1987;408:224–230.

117. Geiger PC, Cody MJ, Macken RL, Sieck GC. Maximum specific force depends on myosin heavy chain content in rat diaphragm muscle fibers. Journal of Applied Physiology 2000;89:695–703.

118. Tomlinson BE, Irving D. The numbers of limb motor neurons in the human lumbosacral cord throughout life. J Neurol Sci 1977;34:213–219.

119. Larsson L, Li X, Frontera WR. Effects of aging on shortening velocity and myosin isoform composition in single human skeletal muscle cells. The American Journal of Physiology 1997;272:C638–49.

120. Hook P, Sriramoju V, Larsson L. Effects of aging on actin sliding speed on myosin from single skeletal muscle cells of mice, rats, and humans. Am J Physiol Cell Physiol 2001;280:C782–8.

121. Lowe DA, Thomas DD, Thompson LV. Force generation, but not myosin ATPase activity, declines with age in rat muscle fibers. Am J Physiol Cell Physiol 2002;283:C187–92.

122. Balagopal P, Ades P, Adey D, Nair K. Effect of resistance exercise on myosin heavy chair sysnthesis in the elderly people. FASEB J 1999;13:758.

123. Kawai M, Ishiwata S. Use of thin filament reconstituted muscle fibres to probe the mechanism of force generation. J Muscle Res Cell Motil 2006;27:455–468.

124. Capitanio D, Vasso M, Fania C, et al. Comparative proteomic profile of rat sciatic nerve and gastrocnemius muscle tissues in ageing by 2-D DIGE. Proteomics 2009;9:2004–2020.

125. Balogh J, Li Z, Paulin D, Arner A. Lower active force generation and improved fatigue resistance in skeletal muscle from desmin deficient mice. J Muscle Res Cell Motil 2003;24:453–459.

126. Ansved T, Wallner P, Larsson L. Spatial distribution of motor unit fibres in fast- and slow-twitch rat muscles with special reference to age. Acta Physiol Scand 1991;143:345–354.

127. Russ DW, Grandy JS. Increased desmin expression in hindlimb muscles of aging rats. J Cachex Sarcopenia Muscle 2011;2:175–180.

128. Boriek AM, Capetanaki Y, Hwang W, et al. Desmin integrates the three-dimensional mechanical properties of muscles. American Journal of Cell Physiology 2001;280:C46–52.

129. Di Biase V, Franzini-Armstrong C. Evolution of skeletal type e-c coupling: a novel means of controlling calcium delivery. The Journal of Cell Biology 2005;171:695–704.

130. Ma J, Pan Z. Junctional membrane structure and store operated calcium entry in muscle cells. Frontiers in Bioscience : a Journal and Virtual Library 2003;8:d242–55.

131. Berridge MJ. Calcium oscillations. J Biol Chem 1990;265:9583–9586.

132. Clapham DE. Calcium signaling. Cell 2007;131:1047–1058.

133. Rios E, Pizarro G, Stefani E. Charge movement and the nature of signal transduction in skeletal muscle excitation-contraction coupling. Annual Review of Physiology 1992;54:109–133.

134. Putney JW, Jr. The integration of receptor-regulated intracellular calcium release and calcium entry across the plasma membrane. Curr Top Cell Regul 1990;31:111–127.

135. Zhao X, Weisleder N, Thornton A, et al. Compromised store-operated Ca2+ entry in aged skeletal muscle. Aging Cell 2008;7:561–568.

136. Renganathan M, Delbono O. Caloric restriction prevents age-related decline in skeletal muscle dihydropyridine receptor and ryanodine receptor expression. FEBS Lett 1998;434:346–350.

137. Gonzalez E, Messi ML, Delbono O. The specific force of single intact extensor digitorum longus and soleus mouse muscle fibers declines with aging. The Journal of Membrane Biology 2000;178:175–183.

138. Boncompagni S, d'Amelio L, Fulle S, Fano G, Protasi F. Progressive disorganization of the excitation-contraction coupling apparatus in aging human skeletal muscle as revealed by electron microscopy: a possible role in the decline of muscle performance. The journals of gerontology Series A, Biological Sciences and Medical Sciences 2006;61:995–1008.

139. Renganathan M, Messi ML, Delbono O. Dihydropyridine receptor-ryanodine receptor uncoupling in aged skeletal muscle. J Membr Biol 1997;157:247–253.

140. Margreth A, Damiani E, Bortoloso E. Sarcoplasmic reticulum in aged skeletal muscle. Acta Physiol Scand 1999;167:331–338.

141. Wang ZM, Messi ML, Delbono O. L-Type Ca(2+) channel charge movement and intracellular Ca(2+) in skeletal muscle fibers from aging mice. Biophys J 2000;78:1947–1954.

142. Delbono O. Molecular mechanisms and therapeutics of the deficit in specific force in ageing skeletal muscle. Biogerontology 2002;3:265–270.

143. Wang ZM, Messi ML, Delbono O. L-Type Ca(2+) channel charge movement and intracellular Ca(2+) in skeletal muscle fibers from aging mice. Biophysical Journal 2000;78:1947–1954.

144. Cheng W, Altafaj X, Ronjat M, Coronado R. Interaction between the dihydropyridine receptor Ca2+ channel beta-subunit and ryanodine receptor type 1 strengthens excitation-contraction coupling. Proc Natl Acad Sci U S A 2005;102:19225–19230.

145. Schredelseker J, Di Biase V, Obermair GJ, et al. The beta 1a subunit is essential for the assembly of dihydropyridine-receptor arrays in skeletal muscle. Proc Natl Acad Sci U S A 2005;102:17219–17224.

146. Taylor JR, Zheng Z, Wang ZM, Payne AM, Messi ML, Delbono O. Increased CaVbeta1A expression with aging contributes to skeletal muscle weakness. Aging Cell 2009;8:584–594.

147. Payne AM, Jimenez-Moreno R, Wang ZM, Messi ML, Delbono O. Role of Ca2+, membrane excitability, and Ca2+ stores in failing muscle contraction with aging. Exp Gerontol 2009;44:261–273.

148. Thomas JS, Ross AJ, Russ DW, Clark BC. Time to task failure of trunk extensor muscles differs with load type. Journal of Motor Behavior 2011;43:27–29.

149. Russ DW, Grandy JS, Toma K, Ward CW. Ageing, but not yet senescent, rats exhibit reduced muscle quality and sarcoplasmic reticulum function. Acta Physiologica 2011;201:391–403.

150. Andersson DC, Betzenhauser MJ, Reiken S, et al. Ryanodine receptor oxidation causes intracellular calcium leak and muscle weakness in aging. Cell Metabolism 2011;14:196–207.

151. Ferrington DA, Krainev AG, Bigelow DJ. Altered turnover of calcium regulatory proteins of the sarcoplasmic reticulum in aged skeletal muscle. J Biol Chem 1998;273:5885–5891.

152. Brandt NR, Franklin G, Brunschwig JP, Caswell AH. The role of mitsugumin 29 in transverse tubules of rabbit skeletal muscle. Archives of Biochemistry and Biophysics 2001;385:406–409.

153. Wieslander A, Linden T, Musi B, Carlsson O, Deppisch R. Biological significance of reducing glucose degradation products in peritoneal dialysis fluids. Perit Dial Int 2000;20 Suppl 5:S23–7.

154. Kurebayashi N, Takeshima H, Nishi M, Murayama T, Suzuki E, Ogawa Y. Changes in Ca2+ handling in adult MG29-deficient skeletal muscle. Biochem Biophys Res Commun 2003;310:1266–1272.

155. Weisleder N, Brotto M, Komazaki S, et al. Muscle aging is associated with compromised Ca2+ spark signaling and segregated intracellular Ca2+ release. The Journal of Cell Biology 2006;174:639–645.

156. Thornton AM, Zhao X, Weisleder N, et al. Store-operated Ca(2+) entry (SOCE) contributes to normal skeletal muscle contractility in young but not in aged skeletal muscle. Aging 2011;3:621–634.

157. Musaro A, Dobrowolny G, Rosenthal N. The neuroprotective effects of a locally acting IGF-1 isoform. Experimental Gerontology 2007;42:76–80.

158. Payne AM, Messi ML, Zheng Z, Delbono O. Motor neuron targeting of IGF-1 attenuates age-related external Ca2+-dependent skeletal muscle contraction in senescent mice. Experimental Gerontology 2007;42:309–319.

159. Boesze-Battaglia K, Schimmel R. Cell membrane lipid composition and distribution: implications for cell function and lessons learned from photoreceptors and platelets. The Journal of Experimental Biology 1997;200:2927–2936.

160. Ferrington DA, Jones TE, Qin Z, Miller-Schlyer M, Squier TC, Bigelow DJ. Decreased conformational stability of the sarcoplasmic reticulum Ca-ATPase in aged skeletal muscle. Biochimica et Biophysica Acta 1997;1330:233–247.

161. Kido A, Tanaka N, Stein RB. Spinal excitation and inhibition decrease as humans age. Can J Physiol Pharmacol 2004;82:238–248.

162. Kamen G. Aging, resistance training, and motor unit discharge behavior. Can J Appl Physiol 2005;30:341–351.

163. Scaglioni G, Ferri A, Minetti AE, et al. Plantar flexor activation capacity and H reflex in older adults: adaptations to strength training. J Appl Physiol 2002;92:2292–2302.

164. Narici MV, Maganaris CN. Adaptability of elderly human muscles and tendons to increased loading. J Anat 2006;208:433–443.

165. Delbono O. Regulation of excitation contraction coupling by insulin-like growth factor-1 in aging skeletal muscle. J Nutr Health Aging 2000;4:162–164.

166. Clark BC, Manini TM. Sarcopenia =/= dynapenia. J Gerontol A Biol Sci Med Sci 2008;63:829–834.

167. Harridge SD, Kryger A, Stensgaard A. Knee extensor strength, activation, and size in very elderly people following strength training. Muscle Nerve 1999;22:831–839.

168. Wilder MR, Cannon J. Effect of age on muscle activation and twitch properties during static and dynamic actions. Muscle Nerve 2009;39:683–691.

169. Cannon J, Kay D, Tarpenning KM, Marino FE. Comparative effects of resistance training on peak isometric torque, muscle hypertrophy, voluntary activation and surface EMG between young and elderly women. Clin Physiol Funct Imaging 2007;27:91–100.

170. Knight CA, Kamen G. Adaptations in muscular activation of the knee extensor muscles with strength training in young and older adults. J Electromyogr Kinesiol 2001;11:405–412.

171. De Serres SJ, Enoka RM. Older adults can maximally activate the biceps brachii muscle by voluntary command. Journal of Applied Physiology 1998;84:284–291.

172. Bilodeau M, Henderson TK, Nolta BE, Pursley PJ, Sandfort GL. Effect of aging on fatigue characteristics of elbow flexor muscles during sustained submaximal contraction. J Appl Physiol 2001;91:2654–2664.

173. Klein CS, Rice CL, Marsh GD. Normalized force, activation, and coactivation in the arm muscles of young and old men. J Appl Physiol 2001;91:1341–1349.

174. Yue GH, Ranganathan VK, Siemionow V, Liu JZ, Sahgal V. Older adults exhibit a reduced ability to fully activate their biceps brachii muscle. J Gerontol A Biol Sci Med Sci 1999;54:M249–53.

175. Hunter SK, Todd G, Butler JE, Gandevia SC, Taylor JL. Recovery from supraspinal fatigue is slowed in old adults after fatiguing maximal isometric contractions. J Appl Physiol 2008;105:1199–1209.

176. Yoon T, De-Lap BS, Griffith EE, Hunter SK. Age-related muscle fatigue after a low-force fatiguing contraction is explained by central fatigue. Muscle Nerve 2008;37:457–466.

177. Kent-Braun JA, Alexander VN. Specifice strength and voluntary muscle activation in young and elderly women and men. J Appl Physiol 1999;87:22–29.

178. Connelly DM, Rice CL, Roos MR, Vandervoort AA. Motor unit firing rates and contractile properties in tibialis anterior of young and old men. Journal of Applied Physiology 1999;87:843–852.

179. Lanza IR, Russ DW, Kent-Braun JA. Age-related enhancement of fatigue resistance is evident in men during both isometric and dynamic tasks. J Appl Physiol 2004;97:967–975.

180. Klass M, Baudry S, Duchateau J. Aging does not affect voluntary activation of the ankle dorsiflexors during isometric, concentric, and eccentric contractions. J Appl Physiol 2005;99:31–38.

181. Simoneau E, Martin A, Van Hoecke J. Muscular performances at the ankle joint in young and elderly men. J Gerontol A Biol Sci Med Sci 2005;60:439–447.

182. Chung LH, Callahan DM, Kent-Braun JA. Age-related resistance to skeletal muscle fatigue is preserved during ischemia. J Appl Physiol 2007;103:1628–1635.

CHAPTER 7

Is Sarcopenia a Geriatric Syndrome?

Jean-Pierre Michel
Honorary Professor of Medicine, Geneva University, Switzerland

Alfonso J. Cruz-Jentoft
Servicio de Geriatría, Hospital Universitario Ramón y Cajal, Madrid, Spain

INTRODUCTION

In 1988, during a meeting devoted to 'Ageing-Diet-Health and Diseases', Irwin H. Rosenberg affirmed that 'over the decades of life, there was probably no decline in structure and function more dramatic than the decline in lean body mass or muscle mass' [1]. A decade later, he proposed to use the term 'sarcopenia' (from the Greek words 'sarx' and 'penia', in English 'loss of flesh') to describe the loss of skeletal muscle mass among older people [2].

Since the publication of the first naming of this clinical condition, numerous authors have been discussing, completing or radically changing its definition and span. Nowadays, discussions are mostly focused on a better understanding of the physiopathology, the early recognition of risk factors, an integrative approach on clinical presentations, complications and prevention treatment or reversibility of the loss of skeletal muscle mass and function. Many of these topics are considered in other chapters of this book.

Geriatric syndromes have been defined as health conditions common in older persons that result from the accumulated effect of multiple predisposing factors and that may be precipitated by an acute insult [3]. Geriatric syndromes are relevant because they may be the presenting manifestation of multiple underlying diseases and conditions; they cause morbidity by themselves; and are treatable when a multidimensional approach is used. Screening for geriatric syndromes is more effective than using medical diagnosis in identifying frail older subjects at risk for mortality and nursing home utilization [4].

Geriatric syndromes have recently been reconsidered and redefined [5,6]. They have been shown to be a useful construct for tackling atypical presentations and other specific manifestations of disease in old age. In this chapter we will try to demonstrate that sarcopenia

Sarcopenia, First Edition. Edited by Alfonso J. Cruz-Jentoft and John E. Morley.
© 2012 John Wiley & Sons, Ltd. Published 2012 by John Wiley & Sons, Ltd.

can be considered as a geriatric syndrome, which opens the door to an integrative approach to its management and prevention.

The concept of frailty is also being revised in recent times [7–14]. Frailty has also been considered to be a geriatric syndrome [15], and is closely linked to sarcopenia and muscle function [16,17] as described in Chapter 11. We will thus explore if sarcopenia, as a geriatric syndrome, can be an equivalent of physical frailty.

EVOLUTION OF THE SARCOPENIA DEFINITIONS WITH TIME

Rosenberg's 1997 definition of sarcopenia as 'an involuntary loss of skeletal muscle mass that occurs with advancing age' [2] appeared just after WJ Evans's important statement affirming that the loss of muscle mass was a normal age related muscle wasting well counterbalanced by gains in fatty tissue [18]. Soon, it was stated that the loss of mass was related to the loss of muscle quality [19] and muscle strength [20]. Physiopathological explanations of these phenomenons followed: loss of individual myofibrils mainly through fast-twitch type II fibers [21], diminished synthesis of muscle proteins and altered mitochondrial function [22]. But it was only recently that both non age-related factors such as bed rest [23], sedentary life and a less than optimal diet [24], were proposed as possible or combined causes of sarcopenia.

On the other hand, the functional impacts of sarcopenia (mobility disorders, falls and disability) were stressed in evolving definitions [25], reinforcing the close relationships between sarcopenia and frailty [26–29]. This link between these two medical conditions is even more stressed by the recent European consensus definition of sarcopenia, where sarcopenia was described as 'a *syndrome* characterized by progressive and generalized loss of skeletal muscle mass, strength and function with a risk of adverse outcomes, such as physical disability, poor quality of life, and death' [30]. It is important to notice that, in comparison with the American definition [31,32], the European definition neither includes age (which is replaced by muscle functioning) nor mobility impairment, because the European working group also proposed different stages of severity of sarcopenia, where the presarcopenia stage (pure loss of muscle mass) is not directly linked to mobility disorders [30].

CAN SARCOPENIA BE INCLUDED IN THE NEWLY DEFINED GERIATRIC SYNDROMES?

Can sarcopenia be considered as a disease?

A disease is a clinical entity that can be unequivocally defined by its aetiology and pathogenesis and is presented as a single symptom or clinical sign or a well-known combination of clinical signs [6]. With the present knowledge, defining sarcopenia as a single disease is unacceptable: it does not have a unique and clear pathophysiological and clinical picture [33]. In fact, many diseases or combinations of diseases may be conveyed in the clinical picture of sarcopenia, and age related sarcopenia can be present in the absence of disease. Moreover, variability in muscle mass and strength increases with age, and many individuals may not reach the point where these changes have clinical consequences [34]. Many diseases or injuries, as well as changes in lifestyles and living habits, can amplify or reduce the incidence of sarcopenia [35]. Therefore, although sarcopenia is frequently an age-related phenomenon, it cannot be considered a mere consequence of ageing. The complexity of sarcopenia is not captured by defining it as a disease.

Can sarcopenia be considered as a classical syndrome?

First translated in English by Galien in 1541, the word syndrome ('running together') means a concurrence of constant patterns of abnormal symptoms and signs that occur together and constitute a picture of the disease with a single underlying cause [6]. The Cochrane Library and most medical textbooks list numerous classical syndromes such as acute chest pain, acute coronary, Behcet, burning mouth, carpal tunnel, Cushing and many others. In each of these cases the etiology and/or the pathogenesis are not always well known, but in every case the clinical symptoms or set of signs are well defined [6]. Moreover, the specific morbid process causes multiple phenomenologies which are more or less expressed but always present. For example, cortisol excess leads to moon faces, Buffalo neck, truncal obesity, proximal muscle weakness, skin thinning / bruisability and osteoporosis. In any case, the reduction of the cortisol excess will cure or allege all the symptoms and signs of the classical syndrome [36].

Classical syndromes imply a single and linear pathogenesis, even when unknown. A structured patho-genetic pathway can be defined or expected. This is not the case [35,33], as multiple interacting pathways are involved in the pathogenesis of sarcopenia. Different paths may lead into a common clinical picture. Therefore, sarcopenia cannot be considered as a classical syndrome. Moreover, no single intervention (physical, nutritional or medicinal) can completely restore the muscle quality (mass, strength and function), as would be expected when a classical syndrome is treated.

Can sarcopenia be considered as a true geriatric syndrome?

The term 'geriatric syndrome' has been commonly used in the geriatric literature for decades to define complex clinical conditions that are common in older persons and do not fit into discrete disease categories such delirium, dementia, depression, urinary incontinence, dizziness, failure to thrive, falls or gait disorders. The concept of 'geriatric syndrome' is well understood by any professional working in geriatric medicine, and most geriatric textbooks include a series of chapters on their diagnosis and management. However, it is surprising how sparse the literature is in conceptualizing what geriatric syndromes are.

The scientific definition of geriatric syndromes has recently been explored and updated, with the support of 20 years of knowledge brought by many recent randomized control trials [5]. Geriatric syndromes correspond to observable characteristics at the physical, morphologic and biochemical levels of an individual as determined by the genotype and the environment [37]. Moreover, the term 'geriatric syndrome' is now used to capture clinical conditions in older persons that do not fit into 'disease categories', but are highly prevalent in old age, multifactorial, associated with multiple co-morbidities and poor outcomes such as increased disabilities and decreased quality of life [5]. The conceptual understanding of a geriatric problem as a geriatric syndrome has been shown to be feasible and useful [38].

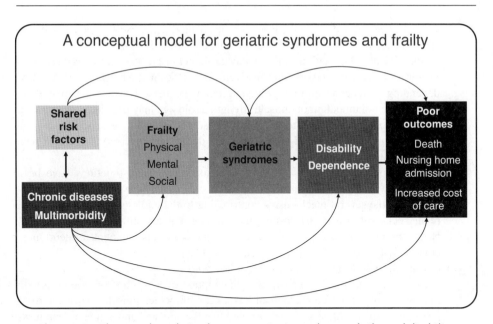

Figure 7.1 The complex relation between geriatric syndromes, frailty and disability.

A unifying concept of geriatric syndromes to understand the link between diseases, disability and poor outcomes is evolving (Figure 7.1). As previously discussed [39] we believe that sarcopenia fits with this current definition of a geriatric syndrome, for the following reasons:

1. Sarcopenia is highly prevalent: muscle wasting is present in 30% of the 65+ population and more than 50% of the population over the age of 80 years [40–43]. In a recent study performed on 157 residents of a Turkish nursing home, with a mean age of 73.1 ± 6.7 years, the prevalence of sarcopenia only estimated by bio-impedance analysis reached 85.4% [44]. An Italian study using the European definition that uses muscle mass and strength found that sarcopenia was present in 32.8% of the residents, with a prevalence of 68% in male residents [45].
2. Sarcopenia is a unified manifestation of multiple causations [36,6].The identified risk or causative factors of sarcopenia are:
   (a) *Constitutional factors including genetic susceptibility*. It is well recognized that age and gender modify the prevalence of sarcopenia [46] and that many genetic aspects influence muscle metabolism and turnover along the lifespan [35,47]. A common feature between cell physiology of ageing and exercise is that in both situations, mitochondria are critical in normal cell functioning [48,49]. Mitochondrial synthesis is stimulated by PGC-1α [50] through the PGC-1α-NRF1-TFAM pathway allowing the duplication of mitochondrial DNA molecules. This pathway is impaired in ageing, but mitochondrial biogenesis can be stimulated by exercises (more in young than in old adults) [48,49,51,52]. The developmental aspects of sarcopenia are fully detailed in Chapter 8.

(b) As mentioned above, the *ageing process* itself modifies muscle turnover, with increased catabolic stimuli, and decreased anabolic stimuli [53–55].

Subclinical inflammation can also play a role in muscle wasting; Tumor Necrosis Factor-α (TNFα) both favors and negatively affects the muscle regenerative capacity, depending on its concentration, which is time dependent. Thus the negative effect of systemic inflammation on muscle strength at old age may only become apparent when it exceeds a certain threshold and persists for a prolonged period [56,57]. In clinical settings, rheumatoid arthritis disease duration is inversely associated with hand grip strength [58].

Many hormonal changes affecting the muscle mass and functions have been described with aging [59,60].

Among the several mechanisms contributing to the etiology of sarcopenia, age-related denervation at the neuro-muscular junction appears before myo-fiber atrophy. However, this process appears to be delayed in cases of high amounts of neuromuscular activity [20,33,61–63] and is detailed in Chapters 3 and 5.

(c) *Certain life habits or changes in living conditions*

Sarcopenia results from inadequate dietary intake of energy and/or protein, as with malabsorption, gastrointestinal disorders, or use of medications that cause anorexia [30]. The ABC health study demonstrated that the adjusted appendicular lean mass (aLM) loss is in close relation with the energy-adjusted total protein intake [64].

When low protein intake is associated with disuse or poor physical exercise throughout life [65], use of alcohol [66] and tobacco [67] the risk and severity of sarcopenia is much higher. Moreover, it is now well proven that bed rest has a very deleterious effect in old adults [68]. Twelve healthy older adults (mean age = 67 y.o. and 50% women), agreed to remain in bed continuously for 10 days (except for toileting) and to follow a strict eucaloric diet (RDA, including 0.8 g of protein/kg/d). The comparison between their basal and post bed rest status showed a decrease of muscle protein synthesis reaching 30% ([95CI, −7% −54%]), as well as a reduction of the whole body mass (−1.50 Kg [95CI, −0.62 −2.48 kg]), the low extremity lean mass (−0.95 Kg [95CI, −0.42 −1.48 kg]) and strength (−19 Newton [95CI, −11 −30]), while the fat body mass stayed stable. −0.07 kg mass ([95CI, −0.67 −0.53 kg] [23,68].

So it is now established that prolonged bed rest immobility [23] and deconditioning increase sarcopenia, as weightlessness [69,70].

(d) Numerous *chronic clinical conditions* have a strong potential to induce, coincide or accelerate the sarcopenia process [71].

Peripheral artery disease, diabetes and obesity as well as hypoxic diseases, liver failure, chronic kidney disease, HIV/AIDS and cancers are part of the long list of diseases and behavior conditions contributing to myocyte and myofibrillar protein loss [34,72]. This list would not be complete without mentioning Alzheimers disease, cognitive impairment and mood disturbances which raised the difficult question of the relationship between reduced body mass and brain atrophy [73].

3. The consequences of sarcopenia are mainly impaired mobility, inability in daily living, disability and increased mortality. These consequences depend on the severity of sarcopenia. Muscle wasting also impairs other physiological functions, including glucose regulation, hormone production, and cellular communication [71]. Moreover, muscle tissues provide the body's only major reserve of readily available amino acids [74]. Thus

inadequate muscle mass prior to the onset of a disease condition may be dangerous in patients who need a large protein reservoir to recover [71]. As a result, sarcopenic patients prior to disease diagnosis or surgery may face impaired recovery and increased mortality [75].

These various consequences linked closely sarcopenia and the physical frailty components previously mentioned.

Therefore, it can be stated that sarcopenia corresponds to a multifactorial health condition that occurs when the accumulated effects of impairments in multiple systems render an older person vulnerable to situational challenges [37] and indeed sarcopenia seems to be amenable to being considered as a geriatric syndrome, according to the current scientific definition [5]. It occurs in old age, provokes mobility disorders and leads to poor outcomes: functional disturbances and poor quality of life. Indeed, it can be argued that mood or cognitive disturbances are not always included in sarcopenia definitions, but the prevalence of these conditions and their links with sarcopenia do support the hypothesis that all geriatric syndromes have shared risk factors [76,77].

IF SARCOPENIA IS A GERIATRIC SYNDROME, WHAT IS THE RELATION TO PHYSICAL FRAILTY?

The consequences of sarcopenia correspond perfectly to those of the currently used definition of a geriatric syndrome [5]. They are linked to poor outcomes, notably increased vulnerability which is a dynamic process of negative adaptation in the face of adversity or external stressors [78]. As proposed by LP Fried, sarcopenia plays a crucial etiological role in the frailty process itself [14], being also a key player of its latent phase and explaining numerous phenomenologies of the frailty status [7]. Moreover frailty leads to dramatic consequences as repeated falls, multiple and various traumas, functional decline, disability, multiple emergency visits, and hospital stay, cross infections, loss of independence, nursing home admission, poor quality of life and ultimately death [79–82] (see Chapter 11).

Although frailty is a more complex problem that includes physical, functional, mental and social aspects, physical frailty is closely linked to sarcopenia [83]. Recent research on the frailty syndrome is focusing on physical frailty, [84] but definitions based on phenotype or on accumulations of deficits (see Chapter 11) are still unpractical for clinical use. Sarcopenia, being the link between physical frailty and disability (Figure 7.1) and being closer to the musculoskeletal system (the organ system with the function of mobility), may be a more useful construct, especially when considered as a geriatric syndrome, for clinical diagnosis and intervention.

CONCLUSION

Sarcopenia meets all the different criteria for naming 'geriatric syndrome' a medical condition which does not fit with the term of disease [5], including:

- high prevalence;
- shared risk factors: older age, impaired mobility, functioning and altered cognition;
- dramatic consequences such as frailty, disability and higher mortality.

Sarcopenia, when considered as a geriatric syndrome using the most recent definitions of 'geriatric syndromes', is the essential component of physical frailty, and may be considered as a solid construct of the key item 'physical frailty'.

REFERENCES

1. Rosenberg, I., Summary comments: Epidemiological and methodological problems in determining nutritional status of older persons. Am J Clin Nutr, 1989. 50: p. 1231–1233.

2. Rosenberg, I., Sarcopenia: Origins and clinical relevance. J Nutr, 1997. 127: p. 990–1S.

3. Tinetti, M., Approach to the clinical care of the older patient, in Principles of Geriatric Medicine & Gerontology., B.J. Hazzard WR, Halter JB, Ouslander JG, Tinetti ME (eds), Editor. 2003, McGraw-Hill: New York. p. 95–98.

4. Winograd, C.H., et al., Screening for frailty: criteria and predictors of outcomes. J Am Geriatr Soc, 1991. 39(8): p. 778–784.

5. Inouye, S.K., et al., Geriatric syndromes: clinical, research, and policy implications of a core geriatric concept. J Am Geriatr Soc, 2007. 55(5): p. 780–791.

6. Olde Rikkert, M.G., et al., Geriatric syndromes: medical misnomer or progress in geriatrics? Neth J Med, 2003. 61(3): p. 83–87.

7. Fried, L., Watson, J., Frailty and failure to thrive:, in *Principles of Geriatric Medicine and Gerontology (Ed 4), H.J.* In: Ettinger WH, Ouslander JG Eds, Editor. 1998, Mc Graw Hill Health professions divisions: New York. p. 1387–1402.

8. Rockwood, K., et al., A brief clinical instrument to classify frailty in elderly people. Lancet, 1999. 353(9148): p. 205–206.

9. Fried, L.P., et al., Preclinical mobility disability predicts incident mobility disability in older women. J Gerontol A Biol Sci Med Sci, 2000. 55(1): p. M43–52.

10. Rockwood, K., D.B. Hogan, and C. MacKnight, Conceptualisation and measurement of frailty in elderly people. Drugs Aging, 2000. 17(4): p. 295–302.

11. Fried, L.P., et al., Frailty in older adults: evidence for a phenotype. J Gerontol A Biol Sci Med Sci, 2001. 56(3): p. M146–56.

12. Fried, L.P., et al., Untangling the concepts of disability, frailty, and comorbidity: implications for improved targeting and care. J Gerontol A Biol Sci Med Sci, 2004. 59(3): p. 255–263.

13. Rockwood, K., A. Mogilner, and A. Mitnitski, Changes with age in the distribution of a frailty index. Mech Ageing Dev, 2004. 125(7): p. 517–519.

14. Fried, L.P., et al., From bedside to bench: research agenda for frailty. Sci Aging Knowledge Environ, 2005. 2005(31): p. pe24.

15. Ahmed, N., R. Mandel, and M.J. Fain, Frailty: an emerging geriatric syndrome. Am J Med, 2007. 120(9): p. 748–753.

16. Theou, O., et al., An exploration of the association between frailty and muscle fatigue. Appl Physiol Nutr Metab, 2008. 33(4): p. 651–665.

17. Frisoli, A., Jr., et al., Severe osteopenia and osteoporosis, sarcopenia, and frailty status in community-dwelling older women: results from the Women's Health and Aging Study (WHAS) II. Bone, 2011. 48(4): p. 952–957.

18. Evans, W.J., What is sarcopenia? J Gerontol A Biol Sci Med Sci, 1995. 50 Spec No: p. 5–8.

19. Schwartz, R.S., Sarcopenia and physical performance in old age: introduction. Muscle Nerve Suppl, 1997. 5: p. S10–2.

20. Morley, J.E., et al., Sarcopenia. J Lab Clin Med, 2001. 137(4): p. 231–243.

21. Vandervoort, A.A., Aging of the human neuromuscular system. Muscle Nerve, 2002. 25(1): p. 17–25.

22. Greenlund, L.J. and K.S. Nair, Sarcopenia–consequences, mechanisms, and potential therapies. Mech Ageing Dev, 2003. 124(3): p. 287–299.

23. Kortebein, P., et al., Functional impact of 10 days of bed rest in healthy older adults. J Gerontol A Biol Sci Med Sci, 2008. 63(10): p. 1076–1081.

24. Paddon-Jones, D., et al., Role of dietary protein in the sarcopenia of aging. Am J Clin Nutr, 2008. 87(5): p. 1562S–1566S.

25. Goodpaster, B.H., et al., The loss of skeletal muscle strength, mass, and quality in older adults: the health, aging and body composition study. J Gerontol A Biol Sci Med Sci, 2006. 61(10): p. 1059–1064.

26. Morley, J.E., Anorexia, sarcopenia, and aging. Nutrition, 2001. 17(7–8): p. 660–663.

27. Bales, C.W. and C.S. Ritchie, Sarcopenia, weight loss, and nutritional frailty in the elderly. Annu Rev Nutr, 2002. 22: p. 309–323.

28. Janssen, I., S.B. Heymsfield, and R. Ross, Low relative skeletal muscle mass (sarcopenia) in older persons is associated with functional impairment and physical disability. J Am Geriatr Soc, 2002. 50(5): p. 889–896.

29. Vanitallie, T.B., Frailty in the elderly: contributions of sarcopenia and visceral protein depletion. Metabolism, 2003. 52(10 Suppl 2): p. 22–26.

30. Cruz-Jentoft, A.J., et al., Sarcopenia: European consensus on definition and diagnosis: Report of the European Working Group on Sarcopenia in Older People. Age Ageing. 39(4): p. 412–423.

31. Fielding, R.A., et al., Sarcopenia: an undiagnosed condition in older adults. Current consensus definition: prevalence, etiology, and consequences. International working group on sarcopenia. J Am Med Dir Assoc. 12(4): p. 249–256.

32. Morley, J.E., et al., Sarcopenia with limited mobility: an international consensus. J Am Med Dir Assoc. 12(6): p. 403–409.

33. Clark, B.C. and T.M. Manini, Sarcopenia $=/=$ dynapenia. J Gerontol A Biol Sci Med Sci, 2008. 63(8): p. 829–834.

34. Sayer, A.A., et al., The developmental origins of sarcopenia: using peripheral quantitative computed tomography to assess muscle size in older people. J Gerontol A Biol Sci Med Sci, 2008. 63(8): p. 835–840.

35. Rolland, Y., et al., Sarcopenia: its assessment, etiology, pathogenesis, consequences and future perspectives. J Nutr Health Aging, 2008. 12(7): p. 433–450.

36. Flacker, J.M., What is a geriatric syndrome anyway? J Am Geriatr Soc, 2003. 51(4): p. 574–576.

37. Tinetti, M.E., et al., Shared risk factors for falls, incontinence, and functional dependence. Unifying the approach to geriatric syndromes. Jama, 1995. 273(17): p. 1348–1353.

38. Tinetti, M.E., C.S. Williams, and T.M. Gill, Dizziness among older adults: a possible geriatric syndrome. Ann Intern Med, 2000. 132(5): p. 337–344.

39. Cruz-Jentoft, A.J., et al., Understanding sarcopenia as a geriatric syndrome. Curr Opin Clin Nutr Metab Care. 13(1): p. 1–7.

40. Baumgartner, R.N., et al., Epidemiology of sarcopenia among the elderly in New Mexico. Am J Epidemiol, 1998. 147(8): p. 755–763.

41. Cawthon, P.M., et al., Frailty in older men: prevalence, progression, and relationship with mortality. J Am Geriatr Soc, 2007. 55(8): p. 1216–1223.

42. Iannuzzi-Sucich, M., K.M. Prestwood, and A.M. Kenny, Prevalence of sarcopenia and predictors of skeletal muscle mass in healthy, older men and women. J Gerontol A Biol Sci Med Sci, 2002. 57(12): p. M772–7.

43. Newman, A.B., et al., Sarcopenia: alternative definitions and associations with lower extremity function. J Am Geriatr Soc, 2003. 51(11): p. 1602–1609.

44. Bahat, G., et al., Prevalence of sarcopenia and its association with functional and nutritional status among male residents in a nursing home in Turkey. Aging Male. 13(3): p. 211–214.

45. Landi, F., et al., Sarcopenia and Mortality among Older Nursing Home Residents. J Am Med Dir Assoc, 2011.

46. Cesari, M. and M. Pahor, Target population for clinical trials on sarcopenia. J Nutr Health Aging, 2008. 12(7): p. 470–478.

47. Gautel, M., The sarcomere and the nucleus: functional links to hypertrophy, atrophy and sarcopenia. Adv Exp Med Biol, 2008. 642: p. 176–191.

48. Wenz, T., Mitochondria and PGC-1alpha in Aging and Age-Associated Diseases. J Aging Res. 2011: p. 810619.

49. Iversen, N., et al., Mitochondrial biogenesis and angiogenesis in skeletal muscle of the elderly. Exp Gerontol. 46(8): p. 670–678.

50. Arnold, A.S., A. Egger, and C. Handschin, PGC-1alpha and myokines in the aging muscle – a mini-review. Gerontology. 57(1): p. 37–43.

51. Waters, D.L., et al., Mitochondrial function in physically active elders with sarcopenia. Mech Ageing Dev, 2009. 130(5): p. 315–319.

52. Huang, J.H. and D.A. Hood, Age-associated mitochondrial dysfunction in skeletal muscle: Contributing factors and suggestions for long-term interventions. IUBMB Life, 2009. 61(3): p. 201–214.

53. Ventadour, S. and D. Attaix, Mechanisms of skeletal muscle atrophy. Curr Opin Rheumatol, 2006. 18(6): p. 631–635.

54. Yarasheski, K.E., Exercise, aging, and muscle protein metabolism. J Gerontol A Biol Sci Med Sci, 2003. 58(10): p. M918–22.

55. Combaret, L., et al., Skeletal muscle proteolysis in aging. Curr Opin Clin Nutr Metab Care, 2009. 12(1): p. 37–41.

56. Jensen, G.L. and R. Roubenoff, Introduction: nutrition and inflammation: Research Makes The Connection–Intersociety Research Workshop, Chicago, February 8-9, 2008. JPEN J Parenter Enteral Nutr, 2008. 32(6): p. 625.

57. Degens, H., The role of systemic inflammation in age-related muscle weakness and wasting. Scand J Med Sci Sports. 20(1): p. 28–38.

58. Beenakker, K.G., et al., Patterns of muscle strength loss with age in the general population and patients with a chronic inflammatory state. Ageing Res Rev. 9(4): p. 431–436.

59. Cappola, A.R., et al., Association of IGF-I levels with muscle strength and mobility in older women. J Clin Endocrinol Metab, 2001. 86(9): p. 4139–4146.

60. Brennan, M.D., et al., The impact of overt and subclinical hyperthyroidism on skeletal muscle. Thyroid, 2006. 16(4): p. 375–380.

61. Dreyer, H.C. and E. Volpi, Role of protein and amino acids in the pathophysiology and treatment of sarcopenia. J Am Coll Nutr, 2005. 24(2): p. 140S–145S.

62. Deschenes, M.R., et al., Remodeling of the neuromuscular junction precedes sarcopenia related alterations in myofibers. Exp Gerontol. 45(5): p. 389–393.

63. Clark, D.J., et al., Muscle performance and physical function are associated with voluntary rate of neuromuscular activation in older adults. J Gerontol A Biol Sci Med Sci. 66(1): p. 115–121.

64. Houston, D.K., et al., Dietary protein intake is associated with lean mass change in older, community-dwelling adults: the Health, Aging, and Body Composition (Health ABC) Study. Am J Clin Nutr, 2008. 87(1): p. 150–155.

65. Timiras, P.S., Disuse and aging: same problem, different outcomes. J Gravit Physiol, 1994. 1(1): p. P5–7.

66. Maddalozzo, G.F., et al., Alcohol alters whole body composition, inhibits bone formation, and increases bone marrow adiposity in rats. Osteoporos Int, 2009. 20(9): p. 1529–1538.

67. Petersen, A.M., et al., Smoking impairs muscle protein synthesis and increases the expression of myostatin and MAFbx in muscle. Am J Physiol Endocrinol Metab, 2007. 293(3): p. E843–8.

68. Zhang, P., X. Chen, and M. Fan, Signaling mechanisms involved in disuse muscle atrophy. Med Hypotheses, 2007. 69(2): p. 310–321.

69. di Prampero, P.E., Factors limiting maximal performance in humans. Eur J Appl Physiol, 2003. 90(3–4): p. 420–429.

70. Lemoine, J.K., et al., Muscle proteins during 60-day bedrest in women: impact of exercise or nutrition. Muscle Nerve, 2009. 39(4): p. 463–471.

71. Buford, T.W., et al., Models of accelerated sarcopenia: critical pieces for solving the puzzle of age-related muscle atrophy. Ageing Res Rev. 9(4): p. 369–383.

72. Pfisterer, M.H., et al., The impact of detrusor overactivity on bladder function in younger and older women. J Urol, 2006. 175(5): p. 1777–1783; discussion 1783.

73. Burns, J.M., et al., Reduced lean mass in early Alzheimer disease and its association with brain atrophy. Arch Neurol. 67(4): p. 428–433.

74. Genaro Pde, S. and L.A. Martini, Effect of protein intake on bone and muscle mass in the elderly. Nutr Rev, 2010. 68(10): p. 616–623.

75. Prado, C.M., et al., Sarcopenia as a determinant of chemotherapy toxicity and time to tumor progression in metastatic breast cancer patients receiving capecitabine treatment. Clin Cancer Res, 2009. 15(8): p. 2920–2926.

76. Burns, J.M., et al., Reduced lean mass in early Alzheimer disease and its association with brain atrophy. Arch Neurol, 2010. 67(4): p. 428–433.

77. Kim, N.H., et al., Depression is associated with sarcopenia, not central obesity, in elderly korean men. J Am Geriatr Soc, 2011. 59(11): p. 2062–2068.

78. Kuh, D., A life course approach to healthy aging, frailty, and capability. J Gerontol A Biol Sci Med Sci, 2007. 62(7): p. 717–721.

79. Evans, W.J., et al., Frailty and muscle metabolism dysregulation in the elderly. Biogerontology. 11(5): p. 527–536.

80. Landi, F., et al., Sarcopenia and Mortality among Older Nursing Home Residents. J Am Med Dir Assoc.

81. Rolland, Y., et al., Treatment strategies for sarcopenia and frailty. Med Clin North Am. 95(3): p. 427–438, ix.

82. Weber, J., S. Gillain, and J. Petermans, [Sarcopenia: a physical marker of frailty]. Rev Med Liege. 65(9): p. 514–520.

83. Abellan van Kan, G., et al., The assessment of frailty in older adults. Clin Geriatr Med, 2010. 26(2): p. 275–286.

84. Xue, Q.L., The frailty syndrome: definition and natural history. Clin Geriatr Med, 2011. 27(1): p. 1–15.

CHAPTER 8

Adverse Outcomes and Functional Consequences of Sarcopenia

David R. Thomas

Division of Geriatric Medicine, Saint Louis University, Saint Louis, MO, USA

For the last two decades, considerable interest has been directed to the loss of muscle mass that occurs with aging, defined as sarcopenia. Previous work demonstrated that the excretion of urinary creatinine, a measure of tissue creatine content and total muscle mass, decreases by nearly 50% between the ages of 20 and 50 years, and occurs in both sedentary and active aging adults [1]. In addition, maximal oxygen consumption (VO_{2max}) declines with age at a rate of 3.8% per decade beginning at the age of 30 years [2]. After correction for muscle mass, there is no important decline in VO_{2max} with aging, indicating that the change in muscle mass is the significant contributing factor [3].

The complexity of estimating muscle mass in individuals has limited studies to small observations. The current ability to easily measure body composition by dual energy X-ray absorptiometry (DEXA) or by bioelectrical impedence analysis (BIA) has allowed evaluation of muscle mass in large epidemiological populations.

The results of this technology have shown that the frequency of sarcopenia in older adults is surprisingly high. Baumgartner and colleagues [4] found that 14% of men younger than 70 years, 20% of men aged 70 to 74 years, 27% of men aged 75 to 80 years, and 53% of men older than 80 years had sarcopenia as measured by dual energy X-ray absorptiometry (DEXA). In women, sarcopenia was found in 25%, 33%, 36%, and 43% in the same age groups.

Measurements of muscle mass by Jansen using bioelectrical impedance (BIA) in the National Health and Nutrition Examination Survey, divided skeletal muscle mass adjusted for height into Normal, Class I sarcopenia (skeletal muscle index within one to two standard deviations of young adult values), and Class II sarcopenia (skeletal muscle index below two standard deviations of young adult values. The prevalence of Class I sarcopenia was greater than 59% in women and greater than 45% in men over the age of 60 years. For

Sarcopenia, First Edition. Edited by Alfonso J. Cruz-Jentoft and John E. Morley.
© 2012 John Wiley & Sons, Ltd. Published 2012 by John Wiley & Sons, Ltd.

Table 8.1 Example Definitions of Adverse Outcomes Associated with Sarcopenia

Outcome	Definition
	Disability Outcome
Major disability	ADL disability (needing assistance with rising from a bed or chair, bathing or showering, or dressing), needing equipment to ambulate, and the presence of a mobility disability (inability to walk one quarter of a mile or climb 10 steps.).
Physical disability	Response to two questions: 1) 'Because of any impairment or health problem, do you need the help of other persons with personal care needs, such as eating, bathing, dressing, or getting around the home?' and 2) 'Because of any impairment or health problem, do you need the help of other persons in handling routine needs, such as everyday household chores, doing necessary business, shopping, or getting around for other purposes?'
Loss of Independence	Activities of Daily Living limitations
	Physical Performance Outcomes
Functional (or mobility) impairment	Limitations in mobility performance (e.g, walking 0.25 mile (0.402 km), climbing 10 stairs, lifting/ carrying 10 pounds (4.54 kg), or standing from a chair).
Physical functioning	Timed 6 meter walk Timed 7 meter walk Timed chair rise without using the arms to push off, five consecutive times Timed get-up-and-go test
	Muscle Strength Outcomes
Muscle strength	Knee extension strength (maximal isokinetic force) Quadriceps strength Hand grip strength dynamometers
Muscle power	Force per unit of time
Muscle quality	Muscle strength per unit of muscle mass

Class II sarcopenia, the prevalence was greater than 10% in older women and 7% in older men [5].

The high frequency of low muscle mass found in aging populations indicated that this may be a predictor of functional decline. Subsequent work confirmed the association of adverse outcomes with low lean body mass. Examples of outcomes and their definitions are shown in Table 8.1.

RELATIONSHIP OF LOW MUSCLE MASS AND ADVERSE OUTCOMES

In observational studies, a skeletal muscle mass more than two standard deviations below young sex-matched controls, is strongly associated with physical disability. In men with

Table 8.2 Reported Adverse
Consequences of Sarcopenia

Disability
Functional impairment
Decreased physical performance
Loss of independence
Frailty Index
Falls
Hospitalization
Mortality
Loss of muscle strength

Observed adverse outcomes in clinical
studies. See text for references.

sarcopenia, an approximately four-fold increase in the risk of disability in at least three of the Instrumental Activities of Daily Living, a two to three-fold increase in the risk of having a balance disorder, and a two-fold greater likelihood of having to use a cane or walker has been observed. In women, an approximately four-fold increase in the risk of disability in at least three of the instrumental activities of daily living has been reported [6]. In other observations, the likelihood of functional impairment and physical disability was approximately twice as great in the older men and three times as great in the older women with severe sarcopenia than in the older men and women with a normal skeletal muscle index [5].

The amount of skeletal muscle mass loss is also strongly associated with physical disability. In men, a four-fold higher likelihood of physical disability was observed in the lowest category of skeletal muscle mass and a three-fold likelihood of physical disability in the middle category of skeletal muscle mass. In women, a three-fold higher likelihood for physical disability was observed in the lowest category of skeletal muscle mass, but no higher likelihood of physical disability was seen in women in the middle and highest categories of skeletal muscle mass [7].

Total muscle cross sectional area decreases by approximately 40% between the ages of 20 and 60 years [8,9]. In the InCHIANTI population, the calf muscle cross-sectional area in men and women had an almost linear relationship with handgrip strength, knee extension, and lower extremity muscle power in participants with sarcopenia [10].

Sarcopenia in older adults has been related to falls [4,5,11], functional impairment [12,13], loss of independence [14], increased mortality [15], and has been postulated to be a major factor in the strength decline with aging [16–18] (Table 8.2). Sarcopenia has also been suggested as a contributor to the frailty syndrome. When low skeletal fat mass was substituted for weight loss in the Fried frailty index, men who were defined as frail exhibited a two-fold increase in mortality [19].

This conceptual model of sarcopenia posits that a low skeletal muscle mass leads to a decrease in muscle strength. A decrease in strength affects physical performance and is thought to precede physical disability [20]. Thus, sarcopenia is predictive of physical disability and other adverse outcomes [21].

While the association of sarcopenia and poor functional outcomes is strong, further investigation has suggested that the relationship is more complex. For example, after adjustment for age, race, body mass index, health, and comorbidity, the strength of the association of severe sarcopenia with measures of physical performance is weakened. Among 12 functional measures in men, severe sarcopenia was related only to tandem standing performance and self-reported limitation in stooping or kneeling. In women, severe sarcopenia was associated with difficulty climbing 10 stairs, lifting/carrying 10 pounds, stooping/crouching/kneeling, standing from a chair, and performing household chores. Only severe sarcopenia was associated with future disability, whereas moderate sarcopenia conveys no apparent risk compared to persons with normal muscle mass [22].

In the Framingham Heart Study, total body and lower-extremity muscle mass by dual-energy X-ray absorptiometry was not associated with disability [23]. In other trials, skeletal muscle mass was not associated with physical performance or self-reported functional limitations [24]. Most recent prospective studies have found weak or no associations between sarcopenia, defined by skeletal muscle mass, and functional status.

RELATIONSHIP OF DECREASED MUSCLE STRENGTH AND ADVERSE OUTCOMES

Muscle strength decreases by 20 to 40% with aging [25–27]. Isokinetic muscle strength declines by 14% per decade in knee extensors and 16% per decade for knee flexors in both men and women. The rate of decline in strength is greater in older subjects [8].

Among men and women in the lowest quartile of muscle strength, subjects were two-fold more likely to develop mobility limitations compared with those in the highest quartile of muscle strength [28]. In other studies, leg extension strength is directly associated with poor physical performance [29].

Muscle strength is measured in various ways, including isokinetic force, power, and muscle quality. Strength is measured by the magnitude of force generation, whereas power is work done per unit time. Muscle power is probably a more important muscular predictor of physical function than strength alone [30]. In healthy older people, power is lost faster than strength [31–33]. Muscle quality refers to strength per unit of cross-sectional area or strength per unit of muscle mass and is considered a more meaningful indicator of muscle function than strength alone [17]. However, accurate measurement of power or muscle quality requires complex, expensive equipment and technical skills, which are not readily available in clinical practice.

Men experience a 16% loss of isokinetic leg muscle torque (strength), and women experience a 13% loss of strength with aging [34]. The decrease in muscle strength was 2-5 times greater than the loss of muscle cross-sectional area, both in those who lost weight and in those who did not lose weight. Weight gain did not prevent the loss of muscle strength despite a small increase in muscle cross-sectional area. This suggests that a loss of muscle strength in older adults is greater than loss in muscle cross-sectional area, which suggests a decrease in muscle quality.

Using knee extension isokinetic torque, handgrip, lower extremity muscle power, and calf muscle area to define sarcopenia, the prevalence of sarcopenia increases with age in both men and women. The age-associated increase in prevalence was maximum for muscle power and minimum for calf-muscle area [10]. However, measures of lower extremity muscle power were no better than measures of either handgrip strength or knee extension torque in predicting poor mobility, defined either as walking speed less than 0.8 meters/second or inability to walk at least 1 kilometer without developing symptoms. This suggests that handgrip strength, easily measured by a simple dynometer, can be clinically useful in predicting future mobility loss.

INTERACTION OF LOW SKELETAL MUSCLE MASS AND DECREASED MUSCLE STRENGTH

When both low skeletal muscle mass and muscle strength are included as variables to predict future adverse outcomes, the associations change. To test for this interaction, three clusters of variables were used to observe their effect on disability after six years of follow up: An Adiposity component (fat mass, weight, and muscle density); a Lean Body Size and Strength component (lean mass, weight, and strength); and a Physical Performance component (walking speed and chair stand performance). The Adiposity and Performance factors, but not Lean Body Size, predicted future disability [35]. This suggests that while both strength and lean body mass decline with age, the effect may not be collinear.

The loss of leg strength in older women (approximately 3% per year) and in older men (approximately 4% per year) is greater than the annualized rates of leg lean mass (approximately 1% per year). In addition, persons who maintained or even gained lean muscle mass were not able to prevent their loss of strength. This more rapid decline in strength than in muscle mass suggests a decline in muscle quality [36].

In studies measuring strength and muscle mass, the change in muscle mass with aging was poorly associated with change in muscle strength and accounted for less than 5% of the variation in the change in strength. Although the amount of change in muscle mass was related to the change in strength over time, strength declined in spite of maintenance of muscle mass or even a gain in muscle mass [37]. This suggests that muscle strength does not depend solely on muscle mass, and the relationship between strength and mass is not linear [7].

In subjects older than 70 years, poor lower extremity performance was predicted by leg muscle strength but not leg muscle mass [38]. Low muscle strength, but not low lean body mass, is a strong predictor of mortality in older adults [39]. Hand grip strength is a predictor of all-cause mortality which is not explained by muscle size or other body composition measures [40].

Sarcopenia, defined by calf skeletal muscle area and fat mass alone, was not a significant risk factor for mortality in community-dwelling older adults, On the other hand, physical performance, defined by walking speed, was a powerful predictor of mortality [41]. Skeletal muscle mass does not predict one year mortality in older nursing home residents [42].

Impaired quadriceps strength is associated with mortality, but adjustment for muscle cross-sectional area or regional lean mass had only a slight additive effect on mortality. Muscle size, determined by either cross-sectional area or DEXA regional lean mass, is not strongly related to mortality. Low muscle mass did not explain the strong association of strength with mortality, suggesting that muscle strength is more important than muscle mass in estimating mortality risk [43]. Interestingly, grip strength had a similar predictive value compared to quadriceps strength. Muscle strength measures of different body compartments are correlated, and grip strength measured in standard conditions with a handheld dynamometer can be a reliable surrogate for more complicated measures of muscle strength in the lower arms or legs.

Isometric hand grip strength is strongly related with lower extremity muscle power, knee extension torque and calf cross-sectional muscle area. Low handgrip strength is a clinical marker of poor mobility and a better predictor of clinical outcomes than low muscle mass [44]. There is also a linear relationship between baseline handgrip strength and future disability in Activities of Daily Living [45].

Older persons in the lowest quartile of muscle mass are more likely to have future hospitalizations than those in the highest quartile. Similarly, persons with the weakest grip strength are more likely to be hospitalized. Measures of physical performance, including knee strength, walking pace, and repeated chair stands, were also associated with future hospitalizations. However, lean muscle mass and muscle area were not associated with future risk of hospitalization, suggesting that muscle strength and function may be more important than lean body mass alone [46]. In these analyses, lean mass was not independently associated with greater risk of hospitalization. This data also suggests that operational definitions of sarcopenia that rely solely on muscle mass may not be as clinically useful as definitions that include measures of strength or performance.

In a study of older women, sarcopenia was not associated with physical difficulties in the absence of obesity. Only women who were obese or who had obesity and sarcopenia had impairment in physical functions. There was a two-fold increase in difficulty climbing stairs and other measures of physical function compared to non-obese controls [47].

In the Health, Aging, and Body Composition study, muscle mass did not predict mobility limitation, defined as two consecutive self-reports of any difficulty walking one-quarter mile or climbing 10 steps, when muscle strength entered the model [28].

In older adults prospectively followed for six years, the change in leg strength showed little relationship to the change in leg muscle mass. Individuals who maintained leg strength exhibited change in muscle mass that was similar to individuals who had strength decline greater than 3% per year [48].

Other observational studies investigating both low muscle mass and poor muscle strength consistently showed a strong association between muscle strength and function in older persons, with no or much weaker associations between muscle mass and function [10].

CLINICAL STRATEGY BASED ON ADVERSE CONSEQUENCES

The initial definition of sarcopenia focused on the loss of lean muscle mass (Figure 8.1). Intuitively, the loss of lean body mass should result in loss of muscle strength and function. However, recent work suggests that loss of muscle strength may precede or follow the loss of lean muscle mass, and is more strongly linked to adverse consequences than lean muscle mass alone.

The loss of muscle mass observed in aging populations may not predict future adverse outcomes such as the absence of loss in muscle strength. This recognition from clinical observations has forced the inclusion of muscle strength into the definition of sarcopenia. Thus, both a loss of muscle mass and muscle strength are necessary to diagnose sarcopenia [36,49]. As the definition of sarcopenia continues to evolve, abnormalities in physical performance have been suggested as an additional diagnostic criteria [50].

The observation that lean muscle mass is not always independently associated with adverse health outcomes has suggested a further refinement in the current definition. Some investigators have proposed that the loss of muscle strength (with or without loss of muscle

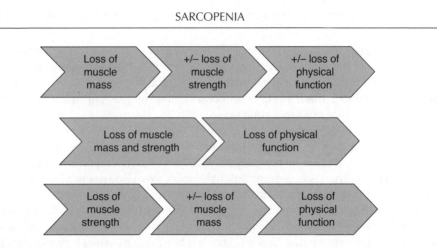

Figure 8.1 Top: Loss of muscle mass may or may not be associated with loss of strength. In the absence of loss of muscle strength, there may be no loss of physical function. Middle: Combined consensus definition of sarcopenia. Bottom: Loss of muscle strength may or may not be associated with loss of muscle mass, but is predictive of loss of physical function.

mass) be defined as dynapenia and separated from the more limited term sarcopenia, which implies only the loss of lean muscle mass [51]. This has resulted from a recognition that muscle strength may be a more robust predictor of adverse outcomes than muscle mass alone.

In clinical practice, the assessment of lean muscle mass requires an additional evaluation using DEXA, BIA, or radiological evaluation of muscle cross-sectional area [52]. Measures of physical performance, particularly walking speed, grip strength, or chair stands, are more suited to clinical settings and require no special equipment. Since these clinical measures may predict adverse clinical consequences as well as or better than measures of lean muscle mass, screening can be achieved much more easily in practice settings.

Sarcopenia without impairment in muscle strength may be a normal expression of aging. The loss of muscle strength with aging may depend on other factors, including altered hormonal status, decreased physical activity, decreased total caloric and protein intake, inflammatory mediators, and factors leading to altered protein synthesis. The loss of muscle strength suggests a decline in muscle quality, including loss of skeletal muscle fibers due to decreased numbers of motor neurons.

The presence of decreased muscle strength and/or physical function is a more robust predictor of adverse outcomes. The clinical implication of dynapenia suggests that older persons who have low muscle strength (decreased handgrip strength or difficulty walking quarter mile or climbing 10 steps without resting) should be considered for further evaluation of low muscle mass. The combined effect of a loss of muscle strength and muscle mass would allow calculation of muscle quality, which may improve prediction of future adverse clinical outcomes.

This conceptual definition may be useful in directing therapy. Interventions to improve lean muscle mass may not improve muscle strength. For example, three years of testosterone replacement in hypogonadal men resulted in a 3 kg average increase in lean body mass without a significant change in either maximal knee extension or flexion strength [53]. Six months growth hormone supplementation increased lean body mass 4% without significant changes in knee extension or hand grip strength [54]. Other studies have shown improvement in lean body mass and number of leg presses [55], but not physical function [56]. A combination of growth hormone and testosterone increased total lean body mass by 2.2 kg and improved maximum voluntary muscle strength by 14% [57].

A key element in improving outcomes may lie in interventions to increase muscle strength and power. Resistance exercise produces an increase in muscular strength and improvement in balance, but is independent of any change in body composition [58]. Even in the frail elderly, resistance training exercise increases muscle mass and strength [59], but whether this improves functional outcomes is not known. The effect of resistance exercise training declines rapidly after cessation of exercise.

SUMMARY

The observation that skeletal muscle mass declines with aging in high numbers of older persons and is associated with adverse outcomes is well established. The observation that muscle strength, power, and quality declines with aging is also widely observed. Increasingly, studies suggest that a decline in muscle strength is a more robust predictor of future adverse outcomes than loss of muscle mass alone.

In clinical settings, less complex measures of physical function, such as decreased handgrip strength or difficulty arising from a chair or difficulty walking quarter mile or climbing 10 steps without resting, suggest an accurate way to predict future adverse outcomes. Interventions to improve both muscle mass and muscle strength may be targets for preventing future disability, but will require additional prospective interventional clinical trials.

REFERENCES

1. Hughes VA, Frontera WR, Roubenoff R, et al. (2002) Longitudinal changes in body composition in older men and women: role of body weight changes and physical activity. Am J Clin Nutr 76:473–481.
2. Astrand I, Astrand PO, Hallback I, et al. (1973) Reduction in maximal oxygen uptake with age. J Appl Phys 35(5):649–654.
3. Fleg JL, Lakatta EG. (1985) Loss of muscle mass is a major determinant of the age related decline in maximal aerobic capacity. Circulation 72S:464.
4. Baumgartner RN, Waters DL, Gallagher D, et al. (1999) Predictors of skeletal muscle mass in elderly men and women. Mech Ageing Dev 107:123–136.
5. Janssen I, Heymsfield SB, and Ross R. (2002) Low Relative Skeletal Muscle Mass (Sarcopenia) in Older Persons Is Associated with Functional Impairment and Physical Disability. J Am Geriatr Soc 50:889–896.
6. Baumgartner RN, Koehler KM, Gallagher D, et al. (1998) Epidemiology of sarcopenia among the elderly in New Mexico. Am J Epidemiol 147:755–763.
7. Janssen I, Baumgartner RN, Ross R, Rosenberg IH, Roubenoff R. (2004) Skeletal muscle cut-points associated with elevated physical disability risk in older men and women. Am J Epidemiol 159(4):413–421.
8. Doherty TJ, Vandervoort AA, and Brown WF. (1993) Effects of ageing on the motor unit: a brief review. Can J Appl Physiol 18:331–358.

9. Vandervoort AA. (2002) Aging of the human neuromuscular system. Muscle Nerve 25:17–25.

10. Lauretani F, Russo CR, Bandinelli S, et al. (2003) Age-associated changes in skeletal muscles and their effect on mobility: an operational diagnosis of sarcopenia. J Appl Phys 95(5):1851–1860.

11. Lord SR, Ward JA, Williams P, Anstey KJ. (1994) Physiological factors associated with falls in older community-dwelling women. J Am Geriatr Soc. 42:1110–1117.

12. Visser M, Kritchevsky SB, Goodpaster BH, et al. (2002) Leg muscle mass and composition in relation to lower extremity performance in men and women aged 70 to 79: the Health, Aging and Body Composition study. J Am Geriatr Soc. 50:897–904.

13. Evans WJ, Campbell WW. (1993) Sarcopenia and age-related changes in body composition and functional capacity. J Nutr. 123:465–468.

14. Rantanen T, Avlund K, Suominen H, Schroll M, Frandin K, Pertti E. (2002) Muscle strength as a predictor of onset of ADL dependence in people aged 75 years. Aging Clin Exp Res. 14:10–15.

15. Bigaard J, Frederiksen K, Tjonneland A, et al. (2004) Body fat and fat-free mass and all cause mortality. Obesity Research 12:1042–1049.

16. Doherty TJ. (2003) Invited review: Aging and sarcopenia. J Appl Physiol. 95:1717–1727.

17. Roubenoff R, Hughes VA. (2000) Sarcopenia: current concepts. J Gerontol Med Sci. 55A:M716–M724.

18. Newman AB, Haggerty CL, Goodpaster B, et al. (2003) Strength and muscle quality in a well-functioning cohort of older adults: the Health, Aging and Body Composition study. J Am Geriatr Soc. 51:323–330.

19. Cawthon PM, Marshall LM, Michael Y et al. (2007) Frailty in older men: prevalence, progression, and relationship with mortality. J Am Geriatr Soc 55:1216–1223.

20. Nagi SZ. (1976) An epidemiology of disability among adults in the United States. Milbank Mem Fund Q Health Soc 54:439–467.

21. Thomas DR. (2007) Loss of skeletal muscle mass in aging: examining the relationship of starvation, sarcopenia and cachexia. Clinical Nutrition 26(4):389–399.

22. Janssen I. (2006) Influence of sarcopenia on the development of physical disability: the Cardiovascular Health Study. J Am Geriatr Soc 54:56–62.

23. Visser M, Harris TB, Langlois J, et al. (1998) Body fat and skeletal muscle mass in relation to physical disability in very old men and women of the Framingham Heart Study. J Gerontol A Biol Sci Med Sci 53:M214–21.

24. Jankowski CM, Gozansky WS, Van Pelt RE, et al. (2008) Relative contributions of adiposity and muscularity to physical function in community-dwelling older adults. Obesity (Silver Spring) 16:1039–1044.

25. Larsson L, Grimby G, and Karlsson J. (1979) Muscle strength and speed of movement in relation to age and muscle morphology. J Appl Physiol 46:451–456.

26. Murray MP, Duthie EH Jr, Gambert SR, Sepic SB, and Mollinger LA. (1985) Age-related differences in knee muscle strength in normal women. J Gerontol A Biol Sci Med Sci 40:275–280.

27. Young A, Stokes M, and Crowe M. (1985) The size and strength of the quadriceps muscles of old and young men. Clin Physiol 5:145–154.

28. Visser M, Goodpaster BH, Kritchevsky SB, et al. (2005) Muscle mass, muscle strength, and muscle fat infiltration as predictors of incident mobility limitations in well-functioning older persons. J Gerontol A Biol Sci Med Sci 60:324–333.

29. Bouchard DR, Janssen I. (2010) Dynapenic-obesity and physical function in older adults. J Gerontol A Biol Sci Med Sci 65(1):71–77.

30. Bassey EJ, Fiatarone MA, O'Neill EF, Kelly M, Evans WJ, and Lipsitz LA. (1992) Leg extensor power and functional performance in very old men and women. Clin Sci 82:321–327.

31. Bean JF, Kiely DK, Herman S et al. (2002) The relationship between leg power and physical performance in mobility-limited older people. J Am Geriatr Soc 50:461–467.

32. Suzuki T, Bean JF, Fielding RA. (2001) Muscle power of the ankle flexors predicts functional performance in community-dwelling older women. J Am Geriatr Soc 49:1161–1167.

33. Foldvari M, Clark M, Laviolette LC et al. (2000) Association of muscle power with functional status in community-dwelling elderly women. J Gerontol A Biol Sci Med Sci 55:M192–9.

34. Delmonico MJ. Harris TB. Visser M. Park SW. Conroy MB. Velasquez-Mieyer P. Boudreau R. Manini TM. Nevitt M. Newman AB. Goodpaster BH. Health, Aging, and Body. (2009) Longitudinal study of muscle strength, quality, and adipose tissue infiltration. American Journal of Clinical Nutrition. 90(6):1579–1585.

35. Cawthon PM. Fox KM. Gandra SR. Delmonico MJ. Chiou CF. Anthony MS. Caserotti P. Kritchevsky SB. Newman AB. Goodpaster BH. Satterfield S. Cummings SR. Harris TB. Health, Aging and Body Composition Study. (2011) Clustering of strength, physical function, muscle, and adiposity characteristics and risk of disability in older adults. Journal of the American Geriatrics Society. 59(5):781–787.

36. Goodpaster BH, Park SW, Harris TB et al. (2006) The loss of skeletal muscle strength, mass, and quality in older adults: The health, aging and body composition study. J Gerontol A Biol Sci Med Sci 61:1059–1064.

37. Hughes VA. Frontera WR. Wood M. Evans WJ. Dallal GE. Roubenoff R. Fiatarone Singh MA. (2001) Longitudinal muscle strength changes in older adults: influence of muscle mass, physical activity, and health. Journals of Gerontology Series A-Biological Sciences & Medical Sciences. 56(5):B209–17.

38. Visser M, Newman AB, Nevin MC, et al. (2000) Skeletal muscle mass and muscle strength in relation to lower-extremity performace in older men and women. J Am Geriatr Soc 48:381–386.

39. Newman AB, Kupelian V, Visser M, et al. (2006) Sarcopenia: alternative definition and association with lower extremity function. J Am Geriatr Soc 54:56–62.

40. Gale CR, Martyn CN, Cooper C, et al. (2007) Grip strength, body composition and mortality. Int J Epidemiol 36:228–235.

41. Cesari M. Pahor M. Lauretani F. Zamboni V. Bandinelli S. Bernabei R. Guralnik JM. Ferrucci L. (2009) Skeletal muscle and mortality results from the InCHIANTI Study. Journals of Gerontology Series A-Biological Sciences & Medical Sciences. 64(3):377–384.

42. Kimyagarov S. Klid R. Levenkrohn S. Fleissig Y. Kopel B. Arad M. Adunsky A. (2010) Body mass index (BMI), body composition and mortality of nursing home elderly residents. Archives of Gerontology & Geriatrics. 51(2):227–230.

43. Newman AB, Kupelian V, Visser M, Simonsick EM, Goodpaster BH, Kritchevsky SB, Tylavsky FA, Rubin SM, Harris TB. (2006) Strength, but not muscle mass, is associated with mortality in the health, aging and body composition study cohort. Journals of Gerontology Series A-Biological Sciences & Medical Sciences. 61(1):72–77.

44. Laurentani F, Russo C, Bandinelli S et al. (2003) Age-associated changes in skeletal muscles and their effect on mobility: an operational diagnosis of sarcopenia. J Appl Physiol 95:1851–1860.

45. Al Snih S, Markides K, Ottenbacher K et al. (2004) Hand grip strength and incident ADL disability in elderly Mexican Americans over a seven-year period. Aging Clin Exp Res. 16:481–486.

46. Cawthon PM. Fox KM. Gandra SR. Delmonico MJ. Chiou CF. Anthony MS. Sewall A. Goodpaster B. Satterfield S. Cummings SR. Harris TB. Health, Aging and Body Composition Study. (2009) Do muscle mass, muscle density, strength, and physical function similarly influence risk of hospitalization in older adults? Journal of the American Geriatrics Society. 57(8):1411–1419.

47. Rolland Y, Lauwers-Cances V, Cristini C, Abellan van Kan G, Janssen I, Morley JE, Vellas B. (2009) Difficulties with physical function associated with obesity, sarcopenia, and sarcopenic-obesity in community-dwelling elderly women: the EPIDOS (EPIDemiologie de l'OSteoporose) Study. Am J Clin Nutr 89:1895–1900.

48. Manini TM, Chen H, Angleman S, et al. (2006) The role of disease in initial differences and longitudinal trajectories of muscle strength and quality among older adults. Gerontologist 46:153.

49. Delmonico MJ, Harris TB, Lee JS et al. (2007) Alternative definitions of sarcopenia, lower extremity performance, and functional impairment with aging in older men and women. J Am Geriatr Soc 55:769–774.

50. Cruz-Jentoft AJ, Baeyens JP,. Bauer JM, Boirie Y, Cederholm T, Landi F, Martin FC, Michel JP, Rolland Y,. Schneider SM, Topinková E, Vandewoude M, Mauro Zamboni M. (2010) Sarcopenia: European consensus on definition and diagnosis. Age and Ageing 39:412–423.

51. Clark BC and Manini TM. (2010) Functional consequences of sarcopenia and dynapenia in the elderly. Current Opinion in Clinical Nutrition and Metabolic Care 13:271–276.

52. Thomas DR. (2010) Sarcopenia. Clinics in Geriatric Medicine. 26(2):331–46.

53. Snyder PJ, Peachey H, Berlin JA, et al. (2000) Effects of testosterone replacement in hypogonadal men. J Clin Endocrinol Metab. 85:2670–2677.

54. Papadakis MA, Grady D, Black D, et al. (1996) Growth hormone replacement in healthy older men improves body composition but not functional ability. Ann Intern Med 124:708–716.

55. Bhasin S, Woodhouse L, Casaburi R, et al. (2005) Older men are as responsive as young men to the anabolic effects of graded doses of testosterone on the skeletal muscle. J Clin Endocrinol Metab. 90:678–688.

56. Storer TW. Woodhouse L. Magliano L. Singh AB. Dzekov C. Dzekov J. Bhasin S. (2008) Changes in muscle mass, muscle strength, and power but not physical function are related to testosterone dose in healthy older men. Journal of the American Geriatrics Society. 56(11):1991–1999.

57. Sattler FR. Castaneda-Sceppa C. Binder EF. Schroeder ET. Wang Y. Bhasin S. Kawakubo M. Stewart Y. Yarasheski KE. Ulloor J. Colletti P. Roubenoff R. Azen SP. (2009) Testosterone and growth hormone improve body composition and muscle performance in older men. Journal of Clinical Endocrinology & Metabolism. 94(6):1991–2001.

58. Swanenburg J, de Bruin ED, Stauffacher M, et al. (2007) Effects of exercise and nutrition on postural balance and risk of falling in elderly people with decreased bone mineral density: randomized controlled trial pilot study. Clin Rehabil 21:523–534.

59. Hagerman FC, Walsh SJ, Staron RS, et al. (2000) Effects of high-intensity resistance training on untrained older men. I. Strength, cardiovascular, and metabolic responses. J Gerontol A Biol Sci Med Sci 55:B336.

CHAPTER 9

A Lifecourse Approach to Sarcopenia

Avan Aihie Sayer

*Academic Geriatric Medicine, MRC Lifecourse Epidemiology Unit,
University of Southampton, Southampton, UK*

INTRODUCTION

There is growing support for a lifecourse approach to understanding sarcopenia both in terms of identifying major health consequences and in terms of recognizing important influences operating from conception to death [1]. Sarcopenia is the loss of skeletal muscle mass and function with age. It is a common condition and although there is ongoing debate about how it should best be characterized, its association with serious future disability, morbidity and mortality, as well as significant healthcare costs, is well documented.

Adult determinants of sarcopenia have been extensively described. However there remains considerable unexplained variation in skeletal muscle between older individuals which might be explained in part by the observation that muscle mass and function in later life reflect not only the rate of loss but also the peak attained earlier in life. In terms of aetiology, a lifecourse approach includes identifying the determinants of peak muscle mass and function as well as the determinants of loss, and birth cohorts are a key resource for such studies. A lifecourse approach to sarcopenia has important clinical relevance with regard to the prediction, prevention and development of novel therapeutic agents for sarcopenia.

This chapter will provide background to the lifecourse approach and describe the value of birth cohorts. It will present the epidemiological evidence linking sarcopenia to a range of adverse health consequences. Then, with regard to aetiology, it will provide an overview of lifecourse influences prior to focusing on the evidence for size at birth, early nutrition and current understanding about underlying cellular and molecular mechanisms. The final section will summarize how a lifecourse approach to sarcopenia is of importance to clinical practice.

A LIFECOURSE APPROACH

The impetus for a lifecourse approach has come from a series of epidemiological studies demonstrating the relationship between small size at birth and an increased risk of

---

Sarcopenia, First Edition. Edited by Alfonso J. Cruz-Jentoft and John E. Morley.
© 2012 John Wiley & Sons, Ltd. Published 2012 by John Wiley & Sons, Ltd.

age-related disease in later life. Initial observations came from geographical studies. Forsdahl reported that the prevalence of arteriosclerotic heart disease correlated with past infant mortality in the 20 counties of Norway, and was the first to suggest that a poor standard of living in childhood and adolescence was a risk factor in heart disease [2].

A subsequent landmark study showed that differences in rates of death from coronary heart disease in different parts of England and Wales paralleled previous differences in death rates among newborn babies [3]. This led to the Barker developmental origins of health and disease hypothesis that adverse environmental influences *in utero* and during infancy, permanently change the body's structure, physiology and metabolism increasing susceptibility to disease in later life. This link between early environmental influences, growth and development, and long term consequences for human health, ageing and disease is called programming; a process whereby a stimulus or insult acting at a critical period of development has lasting or lifelong significance [4].

The developmental origins of health and disease is thought to be a subset of the broader biological process of developmental plasticity by which organisms adapt to the environment experienced. Developmental plasticity involves a single genotype producing alternative forms of structure or function in response to early environmental conditions and it appears to have evolved because it is adaptive. It promotes Darwinian fitness by enhancement of survival and reproductive success through enabling a range of phenotypes better suited to both the prevailing environmental conditions and the anticipated future conditions [5].

The biologic basis for invoking developmental plasticity as an influence on the risk of disease derives from animal studies in which dietary, endocrine, or physical challenges at various times from conception until weaning induce persistent changes in cardiovascular and metabolic function of the offspring. The most commonly used animal models involve a prenatal nutrient imbalance which can be induced by a reduction in overall maternal food intake or by protein restriction in an isocaloric diet. Other models include non-nutritional interventions such as glucocorticoid exposure or placental restriction to impact on early growth and development [6].

There is growing evidence that epigenetic mechanisms are responsible for tissue-specific gene expression during differentiation and that these mechanisms underlie the processes of developmental plasticity. Examples of epigenetic mechanisms include coordinated changes in the methylation of cytidine-guanosine (CpG) nucleotides in the promoter regions of specific genes, changes in chromatin structure through histone acetylation and methylation, and post-transcriptional control by microRNA. Cues for plasticity operate particularly during early development and they may affect a single organ or system, but generally they induce integrated changes in the mature phenotype [7].

In mammals, an adverse intrauterine environment, including suboptimal nutrition, results in an integrated range of responses, suggesting the involvement of a few key regulatory genes that reset the developmental trajectory in expectation of poor postnatal conditions. Mismatch between the anticipated and the actual mature environment exposes the organism to risks of adverse consequences. For humans, it is suggested that prediction is inaccurate for many individuals because of changes in the postnatal environment toward energy-dense nutrition and low energy expenditure, contributing to the epidemic of age-related disease [8].

More recently the focus has been extended beyond prenatal and infant life to encompass influences on growth and development through childhood and adolescence, as well as those operating subsequently in adult life. This lifecourse approach uses a multi-disciplinary framework to understand the importance of time and timing in inter-relationships between exposures and outcomes at the individual and population levels [9].

USE OF BIRTH COHORTS

Birth cohorts are key to studies involving a lifecourse approach. They include retrospective and prospective longitudinal study designs and can encompass the collection of information on individuals from birth to death as well as information across generations. For example some recent birth cohorts include description of individuals during gestation as well as description of their mothers prior to and during pregnancy. The use of prospective and retrospective birth cohorts allows influences on skeletal muscle growth, development and ageing to be studied across the lifecourse.

Retrospective birth cohorts involve the use of historical records of information from early in life. The Barker hypothesis was established with the use of data from the county of Hertfordshire UK where a large set of historical records were discovered. In the early twentieth century, there was widespread concern about the physical deterioration of the British people. In 1911, Ethel Margaret Burnside (Hertfordshire's first 'chief health visitor and lady inspector of midwives') assembled a team of midwives and nurses charged with improving the health of children in Hertfordshire. A midwife attended women during childbirth and recorded the birth weight of their offspring on a card. A health visitor subsequently went to each baby's home throughout its infancy and recorded its illnesses, development and method of infant feeding. The baby was then weighed again at one year of age. This information was transcribed into ledgers at the Hertfordshire county office. The ledgers cover all births in Hertfordshire from 1911 until the National Health Service was formed in 1948.

The Hertfordshire Ageing Study was established in 1995 to examine the developmental origins of ageing utilizing the historical records of early growth and collecting longitudinal data on ageing phenotypes across a range of body systems in men and women born 1920–1930 [10]. Subsequently the larger Hertfordshire Cohort Study was set up to evaluate the combined effects of genetic and early environmental influences as well as adult diet and lifestyle on health, ageing and disease in people born 1931–1939 [11]. Both studies have included characterization of skeletal muscle in older people allowing a lifecourse approach to the study of sarcopenia.

The United Kingdom also has a number of national prospective birth cohorts with younger individuals. The National Survey of Health and Development is a socially stratified sample of all births that occurred during one week in March 1946 across England, Scotland and Wales. This cohort of 5362 men and women has been followed up prospectively across life from birth onwards, the most recent data collection being completed with the participants aged 60 – 64 years [12]. A further national birth cohort has included individuals born in 1958 [13].

A more recent development in prospective birth cohorts is the description of individuals during gestation as well as description of the mothers prior to conception. An excellent example of this is the Southampton Women's Survey which has recruited over 12,500 women aged 20–34 years living in the city of Southampton UK and interviewed them to assess health, body composition, lifestyle and diet [14]. They have been followed in subsequent pregnancies and their offspring followed through childhood, with the aim of prospectively identifying the influence of the pre-conceptional and antenatal environment on the growth and development of the foetus, infant and child. The Avon Longitudinal Study of Parents and Children is another major prospective population study including over 11,000 infants followed through pregnancy and born at term 1991–1992, although data on maternal characteristics prior to conception is not available in this study [15].

LIFECOURSE CONSEQUENCES OF SARCOPENIA

The definition of sarcopenia, initially restricted to the loss of skeletal muscle mass with age, has widened to include age-related loss of muscle strength and/or reduced physical performance [16]. A number of studies from the US have shown that measures of skeletal muscle such as grip strength are powerful predictors of future mortality and disability independent of co-morbidity and we have extended these findings to the UK.

Utilizing data from the UK Department of Health and Social Security National Nutrition Survey, we were able to investigate the relationship between grip strength, body composition and cause-specific and total mortality in 800 men and women aged 65 years and over [17]. Random samples of older men and women living in eight areas of Britain were surveyed 1973–1974 to assess the nutritional state of older people and this included assessment of grip strength and body composition. Survival analysis was used to determine mortality over 24 years of follow up (Figure 9.1). Poorer grip strength was significantly associated with increased mortality from all causes, from cardiovascular disease and from cancer in men after adjustment for potential confounding factors, including body composition.

More recently a systematic review and meta-analysis have been carried out by Cooper and colleagues looking at the relationship between objectively measured physical capability measures and mortality using published and unpublished data [18]. Although heterogeneity was detected, consistent evidence was found of associations between all four measures of physical capability (grip strength, walking speed, chair rises and standing balance) and mortality. Those people who performed less well in these tests were found to be at higher risk of 'all cause mortality' is a specific epidemiological concept and not the same as 'all causes of mortality'.

The summary hazard ratio for mortality comparing the weakest with the strongest quarter of grip strength (14 studies, 53476 participants) was 1.67 (95% confidence interval 1.45 to 1.93) after adjustment for age, sex, and body size. The summary hazard ratio for mortality comparing the slowest with the fastest quarter of walking speed (five studies, 14 692 participants) was 2.87 (2.22 to 3.72) after similar adjustments. Whereas studies of the associations of walking speed, chair rising, and standing balance with mortality had only been done in older populations (average age over 70 years), the association of grip strength with mortality was also found in younger populations (five studies had an average age under 60 years).

There is also interest in the association between measures of sarcopenia and morbidity, in particular type 2 diabetes, in light of the evidence that type 2 diabetes is associated with impaired physical performance. We were able to test the hypothesis that glucose tolerance, muscle strength and physical function would be linked in people with and without type 2 diabetes utilizing data from 1391 community-dwelling men and women aged 59–73 years of age participating in the Hertfordshire Cohort Study [19]. A graded association was demonstrated between increased glucose level, weaker muscle strength and impaired physical function, not only in older people with diabetes or impaired glucose tolerance,

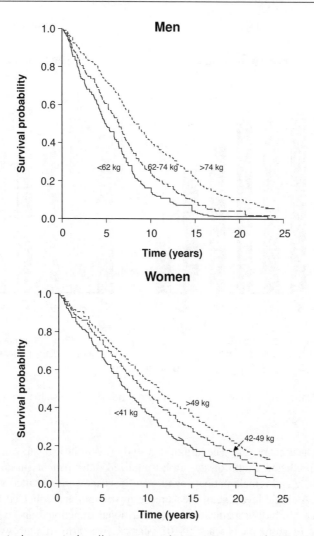

Figure 9.1 Survival curves in for all-cause mortality in 452 men and 348 women according to grip strength. Reprinted with permission from Gale CR, Martyn CN, Cooper C, Sayer AA. Grip strength, body composition, and mortality. Int J Epidemiol 2007;36(1):228–235.

but also in those without either diagnosis (Figure 9.2). This may reflect a link between the metabolic and mechanical functions of muscle.

Further work on participants in the Hertfordshire Cohort Study has established a link between grip strength as a marker of sarcopenia and health-related quality of life (HRQoL), as assessed by the eight domain scores of the Short Form 36 questionnaire, including general health and physical functioning [20]. Subjects in the lowest sex-specific fifth of the distribution were classified as having 'poor' status for each domain. Lower grip strength was associated with reduced HRQoL in both men and women. This did not appear to be explained by age, size, physical activity or co-morbidity.

The findings linking grip strength with mortality, morbidity and quality of life provided the rationale for a small clinical study to investigate the relationship between grip strength

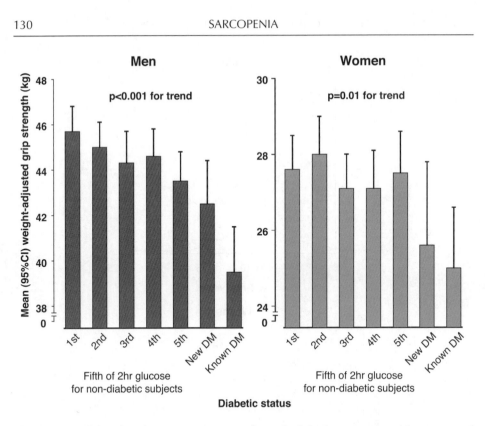

Figure 9.2   Relationship between grip strength and diabetic status in older men and women [19].

and receipt of healthcare [21]. The aim of this study was to investigate whether admission grip strength predicted length of stay in hospitalized older patients in an acute medical setting. 120 male and female patients aged over 75 years were recruited within 48 hours of admission. A single investigator measured grip strength and collected information on age, gender, co-morbidity, medication, and nutritional, functional and case-mix scores. The age range of participants was 75–101 years. Lower grip strength was significantly associated with worse nutritional status, impaired functional status and a reduced likelihood of discharge home, providing preliminary evidence that there would be a benefit from measuring grip strength in routine clinical practice (Figure 9.3).

LIFECOURSE DETERMINANTS OF SARCOPENIA

Adult determinants of sarcopenia including age, gender, size and level of physical activity have been extensively described and the beneficial effect, in particular of exercise interventions, to slow the age-related loss of muscle has been well documented. However it is recognized that sarcopenia is not solely due to reduced levels of physical activity in older people as some loss of muscle mass and strength is experienced even by elite athletes maintaining very high levels of exercise into later life [22]. Twin studies suggest a heritable component and a recent genome-wide association study identified *TRHR* as an important

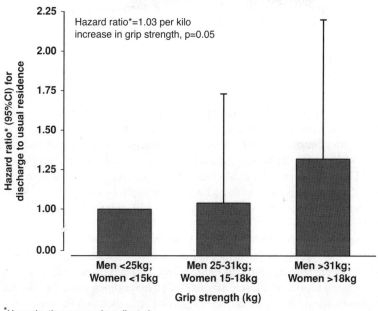

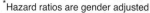

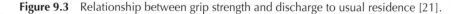

*Hazard ratios are gender adjusted

Figure 9.3 Relationship between grip strength and discharge to usual residence [21].

gene for lean body mass [23]. Nevertheless there remains considerable unexplained variation in muscle mass and strength between older people of the same age which may reflect the importance not only of the current rate of loss but also the peak attained earlier in life (Figure 9.4) [24].

Early growth and development of muscle are important determinants of peak muscle mass and strength which are achieved in early adulthood and generally remain stable until the fifth decade. Over the age of 50 years, muscle mass is lost at a rate of 1–2% per year and strength at 1.5–3.0% per year. To date most observational and interventional epidemiological studies have focused on factors modifying decline in later life but a lifecourse approach

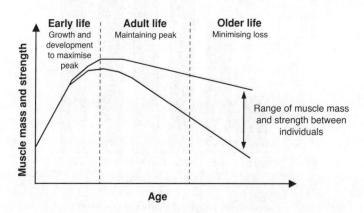

Figure 9.4 A lifecourse approach to sarcopenia [24].

to sarcopenia additionally focuses attention on the determinants of peak muscle mass and function attained in early adulthood.

SIZE AT BIRTH

The link between birth weight and muscle strength in older people was first observed in the Hertfordshire Ageing Study, a retrospective cohort study of men and women born in Hertfordshire UK between 1920 and 1930 and still living there 60–70 years later [25]. They had historical health visitor records of weight at birth and one year and were traced through the National Health Service Central Registry in Southport UK. Following a home interview, 717 people attended a local clinic for measurement of current size and markers of ageing in different body systems including grip strength. Lower birth weight and weight at one year were significantly associated with lower grip strength in later life, independent of adult size (Figure 9.5).

This finding has now been replicated in the Hertfordshire Cohort Study where participants were born 1931–1939[26] and also in the National Survey of Health and Development where the participants were born in 1946 [27]. More recent work has demonstrated a similar effect size of birth weight on adult muscle strength in young women aged 20–34 years taking part in the Southampton Women's Survey suggesting an association between early size and peak muscle strength rather than decline [28]. Currently, work is underway to identify the relationship between early growth and grip strength in the women's offspring.

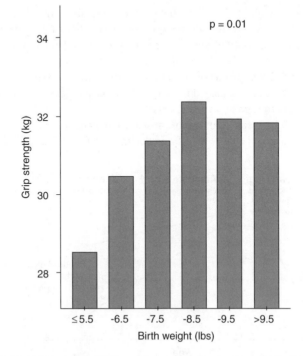

Figure 9.5   Relationship between birth weight and adult grip strength: findings from the Hertfordshire Ageing Study [25].

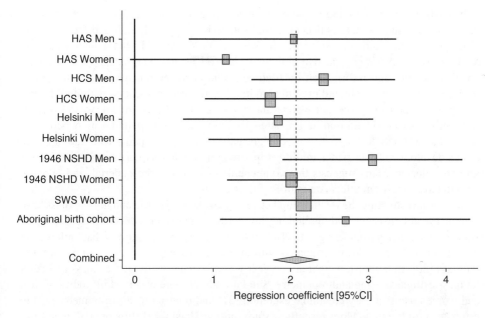

Figure 9.6 Systematic review [24].

A systematic review of the published evidence for an association between lower birth weight and reduced grip strength in later life has allowed the derivation of a pooled estimate for the association between birth weight and grip strength in absolute terms [24]. Ten independent articles were found describing the relationship between birth weight and grip strength in later life. Four of these studied small groups of low birth weight versus normal birth weight individuals and only followed participants to childhood or early adulthood; all demonstrated lower grip strength amongst lower birth weight individuals. The remaining six studies considered the full range of birth weight with follow-up ages ranging from 16 to 73 years of age.

A forest plot showed remarkable homogeneity of association between birth weight and grip strength (Figure 9.6) with a pooled estimate of a 2.06kg increase in grip strength per kilogram increase in birth weight (95%CI 1.77, 2.35). Effect sizes were homogenous for men and women and no individual study unduly influenced the pooled estimate. The studies considered different potential confounders, so no pooled adjusted estimate of effect size could be obtained. Adult size typically attenuated, but did not remove, the birth weight versus grip strength relationship.

The data from existing epidemiological studies also allow consideration of the effect of birth weight on grip strength relative to the effect of other major determinants of strength such as age. For example grip strength increased by 2.42 kg per kilogram of birth weight in men aged 59–71 years taking part in the Hertfordshire Cohort Study (HCS). This association accounted for 2.2% of the variance in adult grip strength which is comparable to the 3.6% of variance in grip strength explained by age. It is likely that birth weight also contributes to the 16.2% of variance in grip strength accounted for by adult height as there is evidence for tracking of size throughout life.

It has been possible to add to these findings with a more detailed lifecourse approach using the longitudinal data collected in the National Survey of Health and Development [29]. Grip strength and body size were measured in 1406 men and 1444 women who were 53 years old and had prospective childhood data on weight, height, motor milestones, cognitive ability and information on lifetime social class, current physical activity and health status. Birth weight and pre-pubertal height gain were associated with midlife grip strength, independently of later weight and height gain. Pubertal growth was also independently associated with midlife grip strength. For men, weight gain during puberty was beneficial, whereas for women it was height gain. Those participants with earlier infant motor development had better midlife grip strength which was partly explained by the growth trajectory. This suggests that components of prenatal, pre-pubertal, and pubertal growth have long-term effects on midlife grip strength.

Studies investigating the relationship between growth in early life and muscle mass have demonstrated consistent findings linking low birth weight with reduced muscle mass. A study of older men participating in the Hertfordshire Cohort Study showed that birth weight was significantly positively associated with fat-free mass but not with measures of adult fat mass [30]. In contrast, weight at one year was associated with fat-free mass and adult fat mass estimated using anthropometry. Similar findings were observed in studies of men and women using urinary creatinine excretion [31] and dual x-ray absorptiometry [32] to estimate muscle mass. More recently a study on the Helsinki Birth Cohort Finland has replicated the relationships between small size at birth, lower muscle mass and reduced grip strength in older people [33]. Studies of birth weight and muscle mass in earlier stages of life demonstrate similar findings for children, teenagers and young adults.

It is now also possible to measure muscle size directly using peripheral quantitative computed tomography (pQCT) and we were able to assess this in 313 men and 318 women from the Hertfordshire Cohort Study [34]. Birth weight was strongly positively related to forearm muscle area in the men and women and there were similar but weaker associations between birth weight and calf muscle area. These relationships were all attenuated by adjustment for adult size. The findings are consistent with the tracking of muscle size across the lifecourse.

EARLY NUTRITION

The effect of early nutrition on long term human health is challenging to ascertain but can be studied in a number of ways. For example the Dutch Famine Birth Cohort has used a natural experiment approach where survivors from the Dutch Famine Winter (1944–1945) have been followed up to determine the long term effects of exposure to famine in utero. The findings suggest that poor early nutrition has long term adverse effects on health with the type and timing of the nutrient deprivation being important. For example, exposure to famine at any stage of gestation has been associated with glucose intolerance and exposure in early gestation has been associated with obesity although there has been some inconsistency in the findings.

An alternative approach is to use historical records of infant feeding as there is a growing literature that links greater duration and exclusivity of breastfeeding to beneficial effects on adult health outcomes. Muscle growth in the neonatal period may be sensitive to variations in early nutrition but little is known about long-term effects of infant feeding on muscle strength. The relationship between type of milk feeding in infancy and muscle strength in adult life was examined in 2,983 community-dwelling older men and women participating in the Hertfordshire Cohort Study. Information about milk feeding for each participant was abstracted from the historical records. 60% (1783) of the participants were breastfed only, 31% (926) were breast & bottle-fed, 9% (274) were bottle-fed only. There were no differences in type of milk feeding between men and women, or according to social class at birth. In men but not women, grip strength was related to the type of milk feeding, such that greater exposure to breast milk in infancy was associated with greater grip strength in adult life (P=0.023). These data suggest that differences in nutritional exposure in the early postnatal period may have lifelong implications for muscle strength in men.

Retrospective cohort studies such as the Hertfordshire Cohort Study allow the efficient study of influences operating over a long period but do not have sufficiently detailed early data to identify specific early nutritional influences. However these questions can be addressed in prospective cohorts such as the Southampton Women's Survey. Data from 448 mother-offspring pairs in the Southampton Women's Survey have been used to examine parental influences on neonatal body composition, ascertained by dual x-ray absorptiometry [35]. Taller women and those with higher parity had offspring with increased birth weight, fat and lean mass, whereas women who smoked during pregnancy had smaller babies, with reduced fat and lean mass. Maternal walking speed was negatively associated with birth weight and fat mass positively predicted neonatal total and proportionate fat but was negatively correlated with proportionate lean mass. Future analyses will focus on the influence of maternal diet on neonatal body composition and childhood grip strength.

CELLULAR AND MOLECULAR MECHANISMS

Skeletal muscle growth and development

Muscle fibre number is a critical determinant of muscle mass and strength at all stages of life. For human skeletal muscle, it appears that fibre number is set at 24 weeks of gestation and fibres are incapable of replication thereafter. Hence subsequent growth, maintenance and repair is believed to occur through muscle fibre hypertrophy rather than hyperplasia, achieved by recruitment of myoblasts derived from embryonic stem cells at approximately 6 weeks of gestation. Fibre hypertrophy appears to be particularly important for muscle growth in the neonatal period when skeletal muscle is the fastest growing protein mass due to accelerated rates of protein synthesis accompanied by the rapid accumulation of muscle nuclei. These observations suggest that key periods during early life may influence the formation of myofibres and recruitment of myoblasts with long-term consequences for muscle mass and strength [36].

Developmental plasticity of skeletal muscle: animal models

Animal models provide excellent evidence to support the concept of developmental plasticity of skeletal muscle. Developmental plasticity is exploited in the farming industry where manipulation of the diet of livestock is routinely used to maximize muscle growth and therefore meat yield. In polytocous species, such as the pig, there is natural intra-litter variation in birth weight affording the opportunity to investigate the association between birth weight and skeletal muscle development. Low birth weight piglets tend to have a reduced number of larger muscle fibres and demonstrate an inability to exhibit postnatal catch-up growth. At slaughter, carcasses have low lean mass and increased fat content [37–39].

Prenatal myogenesis and growth are complex, highly integrated processes under the control of a range of genetic and environmental factors and there is a close interplay between nutritional supply/utilization and regulation by hormones and growth factors which can be targeted for growth manipulation. A recent study showed that peri-implantation and late gestation maternal undernutrition differentially affected skeletal muscle development in fetal sheep [40]. There was evidence of reduced slow-twitch myofibre and capillary density in the fetal triceps but not the soleus after undernutrition at both time points. This reduction in fibre density, which may have been a consequence of decreased capillary density, was associated with higher insulin receptor, GLUT-4 and type 1 insulin growth factor receptor mRNA levels, suggesting a redistribution of resources at the expense of specific peripheral tissues as a consequence of undernutrition.

Other studies involving experimental manipulation of early nutrition have also shown that prenatal maternal diet restriction is associated with reduced neonatal muscle weight in a range of animal models. In particular, maternal undernutrition appears to have a predominant effect on the growth and development of secondary fibres whereas the major influence on primary fibre number appears to be genetic and there is evidence that these effects on muscle persist [41].

The maternal somatotropic axis plays a significant role in coordinating nutrient partitioning and utilization between maternal, placental and fetal tissues. Maternal nutrition may alter nutrient concentrations and in turn the expression of growth regulating factors such as insulin-like growth factors (IGFs) and insulin-like growth factor binding proteins (IGFBPs) in the blood and tissues, whilst growth hormone (GH) acts in parallel via changing IGFs/IGFBPs and nutrient availability. Indeed the infusion of growth hormone into pregnant sows can increase both birth weight and fibre number [42–44]. The GH-IGF axis remains very important after birth and a study in rodents found that muscle from small neonatal rats secreted significantly more IGFBPs and less IGF than average sized littermates. This differential expression, if maintained postnatally, could potentially account for the persistence of small muscle size throughout life and have consequences for lifelong muscle function.

Proteomic analyses of the gastrocnemius from small and normal weight newborn piglets have demonstrated major adaptations in proteins associated with reduced muscle size at birth [45]. These proteins relate primarily to macronutrient metabolism, particularly protein synthesis and degradation, antioxidant function and immune response as well as to cellular structure. Akt is a protein kinase essential for metabolism and survival which acts downstream of both the IGF-1 and insulin receptors. Signalling through Akt following the binding of IGF-1 to its receptor, is positively associated with muscle protein synthesis. Myofibre contraction has also recently been demonstrated to stimulate Akt signalling as well as GLUT4 translocation, both central regulators of glucose homeostasis.

mTOR is another important protein kinase. It regulates translation and its expression increases with muscle hypertrophy and vice versa suggesting an important role in determining muscle mass. Nutrition, insulin and IGF-I all activate the Akt/mTOR pathway and reduced mTOR concentrations may underlie the association between undernutrition, alteration in the GH-IGF axis and impaired skeletal muscle development. Sirtuins may also be important. There is evidence that SIRT1 is central to the ability of adult skeletal muscle fibres to sense and react to nutrient availability and it has been postulated that sirtuin expression might also be affected by nutrient restriction in utero or early childhood.

Developmental plasticity of skeletal muscle: human studies

There has been less work linking early environmental influences with changes in human muscle at a molecular or cellular level. One small study involving 27 adult women looked at the relationship between size at birth and skeletal muscle morphology but did not find significant associations [46]. In contrast, a more recent study focused on a group of 40 young men and showed that those with low birth weight had altered skeletal muscle fibre composition as well as specific changes in muscle insulin-signalling protein expression [47].

This work is now being taken forward in studies of older adults to investigate mechanisms underlying the developmental origins of sarcopenia. One of the main challenges is collecting tissue to carry out this basic science research but recently the Hertfordshire Sarcopenia Study [48] has demonstrated that it is both feasible and acceptable to carry out muscle biopsy in older men taking part in an established epidemiological study [49]. This study was able to investigate whether low birth weight was associated with altered skeletal muscle morphology in older men. It involved 99 men with historical records of birth weight aged 68–76 years who consented for detailed characterization of muscle, including a biopsy of the vastus lateralis [50]. Tissue was processed for immunohistochemical studies and analyzed to determine myofibre density, area, and score.

Muscle fibre score was significantly reduced in those with lower birth weight. In addition there was a trend for reduced myofibre density and increased myofibre area in those with lower birth weight although these differences were not statistically significant. These findings provide preliminary evidence that developmental influences on human muscle morphology may be similar to those demonstrated in animal models and explain the widely reported associations between lower birth weight and sarcopenia. Larger studies including older women as well as older men are now needed and understanding of mechanisms can be taken forward with detailed molecular as well as cellular characterization.

RELEVANCE OF A LIFECOURSE APPROACH TO CLINICAL PRACTICE

Taking a lifecourse approach to sarcopenia is relevant to clinical practice for several reasons. It provides an opportunity to identify individuals at risk of sarcopenia earlier in the lifecourse. It also suggests that the window for instituting beneficial interventions such as increasing physical activity or optimizing nutritional intake should be widened to include all stages of life. Furthermore, knowledge of underlying mechanisms, particularly at the cellular and molecular level has the potential to inform the development of novel therapeutic agents to treat sarcopenia.

CONCLUSION

There is growing support for a lifecourse approach to understanding sarcopenia both in terms of identifying major health consequences and in terms of recognizing important influences operating from conception to death. There is consistent evidence that sarcopenia is associated with increased disability, morbidity and mortality, as well as significant healthcare costs. In terms of aetiology, a lifecourse approach includes identifying the determinants of peak muscle mass and function as well as the determinants of loss and birth cohorts are a key resource for such studies. A lifecourse approach to sarcopenia has important clinical relevance with regard to the prediction, prevention and development of novel therapeutic agents for sarcopenia.

REFERENCES

1. Sayer AA. Sarcopenia. BMJ 2010;341:c4097.
2. Forsdahl A. Are poor living conditions in childhood and adolescence an important risk factor for arteriosclerotic heart disease? Brit J Prev Soc Med 1977;31:91–95.
3. Barker DJP, Osmond C. Infant mortality, childhood nutrition and ischaemic heart disease in England and Wales. Lancet 1986;1:1077–1081.
4. Lucas A. Programming by early nutrition in man. In: Bock GR, Whelan J, editors. The childhood environment and adult disease. Ciba Foundation Symposium 156. Chichester: John Wiley; 1991. 38–50.
5. Bateson P, Barker D, Clutton-Brock T, Deb D, D'Udine B, Foley RA et al. Developmental plasticity and human health. Nature 2004;430(6998):419–421.
6. Tarry-Adkins JL, Ozanne SE. Mechanisms of early life programming: current knowledge and future directions. Am J Clin Nutr 2011.
7. Burdge GC, Hanson MA, Slater-Jefferies JL, Lillycrop KA. Epigenetic regulation of transcription: a mechanism for inducing variations in phenotype (fetal programming) by differences in nutrition during early life? Br J Nutr 2007;97(6):1036–1046.
8. Gluckman PD, Hanson MA, Bateson P, Beedle AS, Law CM, Bhutta ZA et al. Towards a new developmental synthesis: adaptive developmental plasticity and human disease. Lancet 2009;373(9675):1654–1657.
9. Ben-Shlomo Y, Kuh D. A life course approach to chronic disease epidemiology: conceptual models, empirical challenges and interdisciplinary perspectives. Int J Epidemiol 2002;31(2):285–293.
10. Syddall HE, Simmonds SJ, Martin HJ, Watson C, Dennison EM, Cooper C et al. Cohort profile: The Hertfordshire Ageing Study (HAS). Int J Epidemiol 2010;39(1):36–43.
11. Syddall HE, Sayer AA, Dennison EM, Martin HJ, Barker DJ, Cooper C. Cohort Profile: The Hertfordshire Cohort Study. Int J Epidemiol 2005.
12. Wadsworth M, Kuh D, Richards M, Hardy R. Cohort Profile: The 1946 National Birth Cohort (MRC National Survey of Health and Development). Int J Epidemiol 2006;35(1):49–54.
13. Power C, Elliott J. Cohort profile: 1958 British birth cohort (National Child Development Study). Int J Epidemiol 2006;35(1):34–41.
14. Inskip HM, Godfrey KM, Robinson SM, Law CM, Barker DJ, Cooper C. Cohort profile: The Southampton Women's Survey. Int J Epidemiol 2006;35:42–48.
15. Golding J, Pembrey M, Jones R. ALSPAC–the Avon Longitudinal Study of Parents and Children. I. Study methodology. Paediatr Perinat Epidemiol 2001;15(1):74–87.

16. Cruz-Jentoft AJ, Baeyens JP, Bauer JM, Boirie Y, Cederholm T, Landi F et al. Sarcopenia: European consensus on definition and diagnosis: Report of the European Working Group on Sarcopenia in Older People. Age Ageing 2010;39(4):412–423.

17. Gale CR, Martyn CN, Cooper C, Sayer AA. Grip strength, body composition, and mortality. Int J Epidemiol 2007;36(1):228–235.

18. Cooper R, Kuh D, Hardy R. Objectively measured physical capability levels and mortality: systematic review and meta-analysis. BMJ 2010; 341:c4467.

19. Sayer AA, Dennison EM, Syddall HE, Gilbody HJ, Phillips DI, Cooper C. Type 2 diabetes, muscle strength, and impaired physical function: the tip of the iceberg? Diabetes Care 2005;28(10):2541–2542.

20. Sayer AA, Syddall HE, Martin HJ, Dennison EM, Roberts HC, Cooper C. Is grip strength associated with health-related quality of life? Findings from the Hertfordshire Cohort Study. Age Ageing 2006;35(4):409–415.

21. Kerr A, Syddall HE, Cooper C, Turner GF, Briggs RS, Sayer AA. Does admission grip strength predict length of stay in hospitalised older patients? Age Ageing 2006;35(1):82–84.

22. Faulkner JA, Davis CS, Mendias CL, Brooks SV. The aging of elite male athletes: age-related changes in performance and skeletal muscle structure and function. Clin J Sport Med 2008;18(6):501–507.

23. Liu XG, Tan LJ, Lei SF, Liu YJ, Shen H, Wang L et al. Genome-wide association and replication studies identified TRHR as an important gene for lean body mass. Am J Hum Genet 2009;84(3):418–423.

24. Sayer AA, Syddall H, Martin H, Patel H, Baylis D, Cooper C. The developmental origins of sarcopenia. J Nutr Health Aging 2008;12(7):427–432.

25. Sayer AA, Cooper C, Evans JR, Rauf A, Wormald RP, Osmond C et al. Are rates of ageing determined in utero? Age Ageing 1998;27(5):579–583.

26. Sayer AA, Syddall HE, Gilbody HJ, Dennison EM, Cooper C. Does sarcopenia originate in early life? Findings from the Hertfordshire Cohort Study. J Gerontol 2004;59A:930–934.

27. Kuh D, Bassey J, Hardy R, Aihie Sayer A, Wadsworth M, Cooper C. Birth weight, childhood size, and muscle strength in adult life: evidence from a birth cohort study. Am J Epidemiol 2002;156(7):627–633.

28. Inskip HM, Godfrey KM, Martin HJ, Simmonds SJ, Cooper C, Aihie Sayer A. Size at birth and its relation to muscle strength in young adult women. J Int Med 2007; In press.

29. Kuh D, Hardy R, Butterworth S, Okell L, Wadsworth M, Cooper C et al. Developmental origins of midlife grip strength: findings from a birth cohort study. J Gerontol A Biol Sci Med Sci 2006;61(7):702–706.

30. Sayer AA, Syddall HE, Dennison EM, Gilbody HJ, Duggleby SL, Cooper C et al. Birth weight, weight at 1 y of age, and body composition in older men: findings from the Hertfordshire Cohort Study. Am J Clin Nutr 2004;80(1):199–203.

31. Phillips DIW. Relation of fetal growth to adult muscle mass and glucose tolerance. Diab Med 1995;12:686–690.

32. Gale CR, Martyn CN, Kellingray S, Eastell R, Cooper C. Intrauterine programming of adult body composition. J Clin Endocrinol Metab 2001;86(1):267–272.

33. Yliharsila H, Kajantie E, Osmond C, Forsen T, Barker DJ, Eriksson JG. Birth size, adult body composition and muscle strength in later life. Int J Obes (Lond) 2007;31(9): 1392–1399.

34. Sayer AA, Dennison EM, Syddall HE, Jameson K, Martin HJ, Cooper C. The developmental origins of sarcopenia: using peripheral quantitative computed tomography to assess muscle size in older people. J Gerontol A Biol Sci Med Sci 2008;63(8):835–840.

35. Harvey NC, Poole JR, Javaid MK, Dennison EM, Robinson S, Inskip HM et al. Parental deter-
    minants of neonatal body composition. J Clin Endocrinol Metab 2007;92(2):523–526.

36. Sayer AA, Stewart C, Patel H, Cooper C. The developmental origins of sarcopenia: from epi-
    demiological evidence to underlying mechanisms. J Devel Orig Health Dis 2010;1(3):150–157.

37. Rehfeldt C, Kuhn G. Consequences of birth weight for postnatal growth performance and carcass
    quality in pigs as related to myogenesis. J Anim Sci 2006;84 Suppl:E113–E123.

38. Gondret F, Lefaucheur L, Juin H, Louveau I, Lebret B. Low birth weight is associated with
    enlarged muscle fiber area and impaired meat tenderness of the longissimus muscle in pigs. J
    Anim Sci 2006;84(1):93–103.

39. Rehfeldt C, Tuchscherer A, Hartung M, Kuhn G. A second look at the influence of birth weight
    on carcass and meat quality in pigs. Meat Sci 2008;78(3):170–175.

40. Costello PM, Rowlerson A, Astaman NA, Anthony FW, Aihie SA, Cooper C et al. Peri-
    implantation and late gestation maternal undernutrition differentially affect fetal sheep skeletal
    muscle development. J Physiol 2008;586(9):2371–2379.

41. Maltin CA, Delday MI, Sinclair KD, Steven J, Sneddon AA. Impact of manipulations of myoge-
    nesis in utero on the performance of adult skeletal muscle. Reproduction 2001;122(3):359–374.

42. Rehfeldt C, Fiedler I, Weikard R, Kanitz E, Ender K. It is possible to increase skeletal muscle
    fibre number in utero. Biosci Rep 1993;13(4):213–220.

43. Rehfeldt C, Kuhn G, Vanselow J, Furbass R, Fiedler I, Nurnberg G et al. Maternal treatment with
    somatotropin during early gestation affects basic events of myogenesis in pigs. Cell Tissue Res
    2001;306(3):429–440.

44. Rehfeldt C, Nissen PM, Kuhn G, Vestergaard M, Ender K, Oksbjerg N. Effects of maternal nutri-
    tion and porcine growth hormone (pGH) treatment during gestation on endocrine and metabolic
    factors in sows, fetuses and pigs, skeletal muscle development, and postnatal growth. Domest
    Anim Endocrinol 2004;27(3):267–285.

45. Wang J, Chen L, Li D, Yin Y, Wang X, Li P et al. Intrauterine growth restriction affects
    the proteomes of the small intestine, liver, and skeletal muscle in newborn pigs. J Nutr
    2008;138(1):60–66.

46. Thompson CH, Sanderson AL, Sandeman D, Stein C, Borthwick A, Radda GK et al. Fetal
    growth and insulin resistance in adult life: role of skeletal muscle morphology. Clin Sci (Colch)
    1997;92(3):291–296.

47. Jensen CB, Storgaard H, Madsbad S, Richter EA, Vaag AA. Altered skeletal muscle fiber
    composition and size precede whole-body insulin resistance in young men with low birth weight.
    J Clin Endocrinol Metab 2007;92(4):1530–1534.

48. Patel HP, Syddall HE, Martin HJ, Stewart CE, Cooper C, Sayer AA. Hertfordshire Sarcopenia
    Study: design and methods. BMC Geriatrics 2010;10:43.

49. Patel H, Syddall HE, Martin HJ, Cooper C, Stewart C, Sayer AA. The feasibility and acceptability
    of muscle biopsy in epidemiological studies: findings from the Hertfordshire Sarcopenia Study
    (HSS). J Nutr Health Aging 2011;15(1):10–15.

50. Patel H, Jameson K, Syddall H, Martin H, Stewart C, Cooper C et al. Developmental Influences,
    Muscle Morphology, and Sarcopenia in Community-Dwelling Older Men. J Gerontol A Biol Sci
    Med Sci 2012 Jan;67(1):82–87.

CHAPTER 10

Cachexia and Sarcopenia

Maurizio Muscaritoli, Simone Lucia and Filippo Rossi Fanelli

Department of Clinical Medicine, Sapienza, University of Rome, Italy

INTRODUCTION

Modern medicine is mainly featured by both an increasing specialization leading to significant improvement in diagnosis, treatment and cure of diseases and its dealing with the progressive aging of the general population, leading to a higher prevalence of elderly patients, with polymorbidity and polypharmacy. Average life span has dramatically increased and age-related diseases have become of major public interest, particularly in western countries where medical progress, combined with high standards of living and hygiene have significantly reduced the main causes of death of the previous eras (e.g. infections).

The scientific community and society are wondering how to deal and to manage this increasing prevalence of elderly people in order to improve or at least maintain individual and social wellness. We are now witness to new and interesting talks about the nature, features and consequences of aging; several theories are attempting to better explain its mechanisms, but several pathogenic aspects still remain unclear and philosophical aspects yet unsolved.

Over time, physicians and philosophers have assigned to aging different meanings: they considered it as a disease, like in the Ancient Greek and Roman history, or as a time of wisdom, or as a mid-way stage between health and illness. Human aging has also been viewed as the declining function of most body systems due to intrinsic and extrinsic mechanisms as well as the progressive accumulation of damaged tissue and the progressive loss of normal tissue. According to its four main features, aging is defined by Bernard Strehler *universal* (as it occurs in all members), *intrinsic* (as it seems not to be influenced by environmental variables), *progressive* (as it is gradual and cumulative) and *deleterious* (as it could not be reversed) [1].

The main question is whether we should consider human aging as a physiological or a pathological state, and the answer is still unclear, as both views might be correct [2]. The path to discriminate between the two conditions should start from the definition of health: elderly people who have a good physical, psychological and social life could be defined 'healthy' even if they have a certain degree of cognitive dysfunction, hypertension, sarcopenia, osteoporosis, insulin resistance or other age-related organ dysfunction. The

Sarcopenia, First Edition. Edited by Alfonso J. Cruz-Jentoft and John E. Morley.
© 2012 John Wiley & Sons, Ltd. Published 2012 by John Wiley & Sons, Ltd.

term 'successful aging' was created to describe such a kind of aging and current public health efforts point in this direction.

AGING AND MUSCLE

One of the several changes which occurs with aging is the progressive loss of muscle mass and function, i.e. sarcopenia. After the age of fifty, approximately 1–2% per year of muscle mass is lost, with this age-related reduction in muscle mass and strength being accompanied by intramuscular fat accumulation, muscle atrophy (especially the type IIa fibers), decreased satellite cell proliferation and differentiation capacity, and reduction in motor unit number. This muscle remodeling results in changes in muscle architecture that is believed to play a key role in the loss of muscle force and power characteristic of advanced age [3,4].

Depending on the definition considered, the prevalence of sarcopenia has been estimated at 5–13% in 60–70-year-old subjects, while in people >80 years its reported prevalence ranges from 11 to 50%. However, although precise data on the age-specific prevalence of sarcopenia is still lacking, it is estimated that sarcopenia affects roughly >50 million people worldwide and that >200 million people will be affected in the next 40 years [5].

Sarcopenia of the elderly represents an onerous healthcare cost: in the United States $18.5 billion were attributable to sarcopenia in 2000 (about 1.5% of total healthcare costs). The cost of sarcopenia will represent in the future a significant economic burden for healthcare systems [5].

Recently, the view has consolidated that, in order to implement the concept of sarcopenia in both clinical practice and research, an operational definition and diagnostic criteria were strongly needed. During the last few years, several efforts have been made to reach a consensus on its definition [6]: in 2010, the European Working Group on Sarcopenia in Older People (EWGSOP) developed a practical clinical definition and consensus diagnostic criteria that could be useful for research and clinical purposes. According to this definition sarcopenia is defined as 'a syndrome characterized by progressive and generalized loss of skeletal muscle mass and strength with a risk of adverse outcomes such as physical disability, poor quality of life and death'. The experts recommend that both low muscle mass and low muscle function (strength and performance) must be documented to allow for the diagnosis of sarcopenia [7]. The definition and the diagnostic criteria of sarcopenia are discussed in depth in Chapter 6 of this book.

Sarcopenia promotes poor outcomes such as mobility disorders, disability, poor quality of life, death and is therefore considered as a geriatric syndrome [8]. Geriatric syndromes are groups of specific signs and symptoms that occur more often in the elderly and can impact patient morbidity and mortality. Considering sarcopenia a geriatric syndrome has major educational and clinical implications, since it may help to address it with a multidimensional and multidisciplinary approach providing additional benefit to older patients.

Muscle loss is, however, not specific to age-related sarcopenia. Starvation and malnutrition [9], bed rest, prolonged physical inactivity, denervation [10,11], are also associated with relevant segmental or systemic skeletal muscle atrophy. Age-related sarcopenia must therefore be distinguished from other forms of muscle depletion, in particular from cachexia of chronic diseases.

CACHEXIA IN CHRONIC DISEASES

The term cachexia is derived from the Greek words *kakòs* (bad) and *héxis* (condition). Cachexia was recently defined as 'a complex metabolic syndrome associated with underlying illness and characterized by loss of muscle mass with or without loss of fat mass. The prominent feature of cachexia is weight loss in adults' [12].

Cachexia is related to underlying illness such as cancer, chronic obstructive pulmonary disease (COPD), chronic kidney disease (CKD), chronic liver failure (CLF) chronic infections or chronic heart hailure (CHF) [13]. Although often underestimated and frequently neglected, its prevalence is high, ranging from 5–15% in CHF to 60–80% in advanced cancer.

Cachexia should be differentiated from starvation, age-related loss of muscle mass, primary depression, malabsorption and hyperthyroidism [14,15,16], and should rather be considered a metabolic syndrome, originating from the complex interplay between chronic disease, host metabolism and the imbalance between pro-inflammatory (such as IL-1, IL-6, TNF-α, IFN γ) and anti inflammatory (e.g. IL-4, IL-12, IL-15) cytokines. This interaction also implies an abnormal production of neuropeptides and hormones, at least in part responsible for anorexia, the main metabolic alterations seen in cachexia, such as insulin resistance, increased lipolysis and lipid oxidation, increased protein turnover [17,18]. Although cachexia is not fully reversible by conventional nutrition support, reduced nutrient availability (because of reduced intake, impaired absorption and/or increased losses, or a combination of these) [14] may be a relevant component and play a relevant role in the pathogenesis of cachexia. Indeed, it is noteworthy that while not all malnourished patients are cachectic, all cachectic patients are invariably malnourished.

Irrespective of the underlying causative illness, the progressive loss of muscle mass and function is by far the most clinically relevant phenotypic feature of cachexia. Progressive skeletal muscle mass loss negatively affects muscle strength, respiratory function, functional status, disability risk and QoL [19,20] and independently predicts morbidity and mortality [21,22,23].

An imbalance between anabolic and catabolic rates at the muscle level is responsible for accelerated muscle loss, with increased muscle protein degradation playing the prominent role. Upregulation of the main muscle proteolytic systems (i.e. ATP-dependent ubiquitin-proteasome system, the calcium activated calpain system and lysosomal systems) has been largely documented in cancer-related cachexia [24].

Decreased anabolic response due to hyperexpression of negative regulators of muscle mass (e.g. Myostatin), hypoexpression of positive regulators (e.g. MyoD) and impaired IGF-1 signaling, have also been documented in cachexia of chronic diseases [25,26,27].

Systemic inflammation is believed to be causally involved in the derangement of the whole musclular machinery typical of cachexia, but hormones [28,29], tumor derived factors such as proteolysis-inducing factor (PIF) [30], bed rest, and disease-related inadequate nutrient intake [31] may well contribute to the devastating picture of cachexia.

To overcome the limits related to a descriptive definition of this multifactorial syndrome, a set of diagnostic criteria for cachexia in both the clinical and the research setting has been developed [12]. These criteria are reported in Table 10.1.

Another recent significant advancement in the cachexia field is represented by its staging. The European Society of Clinical Nutrition and Metabolism (ESPEN), Special Interest Groups (SIGs) on 'cachexia-anorexia in chronic wasting diseases' and 'nutrition in geriatrics' have recently proposed a staging of cachexia of chronic diseases [14].

Table 10.1 Diagnostic criteria for cachexia (modified from Evans et al. [12])

* Weight loss > 5% in 12 months or less (edema-free) or
* BMI <20 kg/m^2

Plus at least 3 of the following criteria:
* Decreased muscle strength
* Fatigue
* Anorexia
* Low fat-free mass index
* Abnormal biochemistry:
  * Increased inflammatory markers (CRP>5.0 mg/l, IL-6 >4.0 pg/ml)
  * Anemia (Hb <12 g/dL)
  * Low serum albumin (<3.2 g/dL)

The staging of cachexia was felt necessary, based on a number of reasons: i) late-stage cachexia is substantially untreatable with currently available tools; ii) staging may facilitate identification of early markers of cachexia; iii) staging may increase the awareness of conditions potentially leading to cachexia; iiii) staging may favor the initiation of preventative rather than therapeutic strategies for cachexia and support the pursuit of good timing and treatment modalities.

The panel also agreed that staging of cachexia into many grades might generate confusion among health professionals and caregivers, potentially leading to delayed diagnosis. Therefore it has been proposed that cachexia of chronic diseases should be graded into cachexia and pre-cachexia.

While the panel definition of cachexia does not substantially differ from the one reported above [12], the diagnostic criteria for pre-cachexia were originally developed by the ESPEN-SIGs.

Pre-cachexia includes patients with a chronic disease (i.e. cancer, COPD, CHF, CKD, CLF, AIDS, etc) [13,14,32], minimal or small weight loss, a chronic or recurrent systemic inflammatory response and anorexia. Inflammation is indicated by higher-than-normal values of inflammatory markers like C-reactive protein. Decreased spontaneous food intake may be revealed by visual analogue scales (VAS), specific questionnaires [33] and/or reduced intake below 70% estimated needs. The section AC/S-12 of the FAACT questionnaire [34] was suggested by the SIG to be employed to assess anorexia-related symptoms.

Pre-cachexia is therefore defined based on the presence of the following criteria [14]: a) underlying chronic diseases; b) by unintentional weight loss ≤5% of usual body weight during the last 6 months; c) chronic or recurrent systemic inflammatory response (e.g. elevated serum levels of C-reactive protein); d) and anorexia or anorexia-related symptoms.

It is likely that the definition and the diagnostic criteria of pre-cachexia will allow for large multicenter epidemiological and intervention studies aimed at preventing or delaying changes in body composition and nutritional complications linked to chronic diseases.

In this perspective, a new, operational consensus definition and classification of cancer cachexia has been recently developed based on a Delphy process. Cancer cachexia is defined as 'multifactorial syndrome characterized by an ongoing loss of skeletal muscle mass (with or without loss of fat mass) that cannot be fully reversed by conventional nutritional support and leads to progressive functional impairment'. Cancer cachexia is seen as a continuum with three stagings of clinical relevance, i.e. pre-cachexia, cachexia and refractory cachexia.

Cancer pre-cachexia is therefore defined by the presence of involuntary weight loss ≤5%, anorexia and metabolic changes. Cancer cachexia defined by weight loss ≥5% over past

6 months in absence of simple starvation or the combination of ongoing weight loss >2% with BMI <20 or sarcopenia.

Refractory cachexia can be substantially unresponsive to therapy as a result of very advanced cancer (pre-terminal) or the presence of rapidly progressive cancer unresponsive to antineoplastic treatments. Refractory cachexia is characterized by a low performance status (WHO score 3 or 4) and a life expectancy of less than 3 months [35]. In patients with refractory cachexia, the risks of nutritional support likely outweigh their possible benefits.

After a period of validation, this new classification should provide a mechanism for the introduction of new interventions aimed at improving prevention and treatment of cancer-related cachexia.

AGING, COMORBIDITIES AND LOSS OF MUSCLE: IS IT SARCOPENIA OR CACHEXIA?

The assessment of comorbidities (simply counting the number of concurrent diseases in addition to the index patient's disease or with more valid and reliable methods like Charlson Index, the CIRS, the ICED and the Kaplan Index) [36–39] represents an essential part of a proper diagnostic and therapeutic process, particularly in the elderly, where multimorbidity and polipharmacy are frequent and could limit performance, impair activities of daily living and impinge QoL, even in the absence of wasting and sarcopenia (e.g. in the presence of osteoarthritis, obesity, pain) [40,41]. Comorbidities must be differentiated from disability, that represents the difficulty or the dependency in carrying out activities essential to independent living, and from frailty, that can be defined as an aggregate of subclinical losses of reserve due to physiological systems' alterations and leading to an increased vulnerability to stressors [42].

Although there is no consensus regarding definition of '*comorbidity*', a useful description may be the one given by Fried et al: 'comorbidity is the presence of two or more medically diagnosed diseases in the same individual, with the diagnosis of each contributing disease based on established, widely recognized criteria'[42].

The presence of comorbidities increases significantly with age, mainly because the rate of chronic conditions increases with age. Indeed, the prevalence of chronic conditions continues to increase and it is estimated that by 2020 nearly 50% of the US population will have at least one chronic condition. It is estimated that as much as 45% of the general population and 88% of all the population aged 65 years and older has one chronic condition or more. However, most elderly present with multiple chronic conditions: in 2000, 57 million Americans were estimated to have multiple chronic conditions and the number is projected to increase to 81 million by 2020 [43,44]. European data indicate that most elderly patients aged 65–79 years present with 4.9 comorbidities, while subjects aged >80 have 5.4 comorbidities [45].

Persons with multiple chronic conditions have more rapid decline in health status and a greater likelihood of disability. Therefore, it is clear that comorbidities contribute to increase frailty in the elderly [46]. Hypertension, coronary artery disease (CAD), diabetes, CKD and COPD are the most prevalent chronic conditions affecting elderly people.

Not only is the process of aging associated with increased risk of chronic conditions, but also with physiological changes at the organ level which may, in turn lead to major derangements in body metabolism. Let us consider, as an example, the changes in renal function occurring with normal aging. In most of the cross-sectional studies, the glomerular filtration rate (GFR) descent began around age 30 to 40, irrespective of gender. The average rate of decline varies, but it averages about 0.8 mL/min/1.73 m^2/ year after age 30. Some have suggested that the decline accelerates after about age 65 to 70 [47,48,49]. GFR decline is independent of hypertension or cardiovascular impairment, occurring even in indigenous native societies where hypertension is completely absent [50].

Epidemiologic data suggest that the majority of elderly US adults have at least a mild reduction in GFR (<90 ml/min/1.73 m^2), and that nearly one-quarter of those older than 70 years have a GFR lower than 60 ml/min/1.73 m^2 [51,52]. In terms of GFR ranges for specific ages, an average 85-year-old male would be expected to have a GFR around 55–60 mL/min/1.73 m^2, depending on his GFR at age 30.

The National Kidney Foundation classifies all patients who have a GFR lower than 60 ml/ min/ 1.73 m^2 as having chronic kidney disease. As a consequence, most 'healthy' elderly patients will present with CKD, a condition associated with inflammation, metabolic alterations and loss of muscle mass and function [53,54].

The question then arises whether, in such patients, inflammation and muscle functional decline should be considered the consequence of aging *per se* or, rather the effect of a superimposed chronic comorbidity, which in turn impairs physical activity, or a combination of both. In daily clinical practice, it is not infrequent for a clinician to deal with patients aged >75 years with hypertension, mild to moderate CHF, type 2 diabetes, dyslipidemia, COPD, osteoarthritis (in addition to the age-related CKD), treated with polypharmacy. In this patient, whilst the likelihood of sarcopenia is high, the individual role of aging, superimposed chronic conditions and inflammation in its pathogenesis cannot be ascertained. In fact, as summarized in Tables 10.2 and 10.3, both inflammation and decreased muscle mass and function are hallmarks of chronic diseases. Inflammation is an adaptive response to intrinsic and extrinsic stimuli that attempts to preserve homeostatic state, to remove the injurious stimuli and to initiate the healing process, even though it may have a negative impact on metabolic homeostasis in acute and chronic diseases.

Table 10.2 Inflammation is a common feature of most prevalent chronic diseases

Chronic Disease	Inflammation	References
COPD	YES	Yao H et al (2009)[55]; Cornwell WD et al (2010)[56]
CKD	YES	Rifkin DE et al (2009)[53]; Witasp A et al (2010)[57]
CANCER	YES	Mantovani et al (2008)[58]; Grivennikov SI et al (2010)[59]
CHF	YES	Fu M (2009)[60]; Parish RC et al (2008)[61]
T2DM	YES	Donath MY et al (2011)[62]; Hotamisligil GS (2006)[63]
MetS	YES*	Espinola-Klein C et al (2011)[64]; Monteiro R (2010)[65]

Abbreviations: COPD = Chronic Obstructive Pulmonary Disease; CKD = Chronic Kidney Disease; CHF = Chronic Heart Failure; T2DM = Type 2 Diabetes; MetS = Metabolic Syndrome
*few evidences

Table 10.3 Loss of muscle mass and function is a common feature in most prevalent chronic diseases

Chronic Disease	Muscle Mass Loss	Muscle Function Loss	References
COPD	YES	YES	Seymour JM et al (2010)[66]; Schols AM et al (2002)[67]
CKD	YES	YES	Workeneh BTet al (2010)[54]; Leal VO et al (2011)[68]
CANCER	YES	YES	Fearon et al (2011)[35]
CHF	YES	YES	von Haehling S & Anker SD (2010)[13]; Narici MV et al (2010)[3]
T2DM	YES	YES	Park SW et al (2007, 2009)[69, 70]; Krause MP et al (2011)[71]
MetS	YES*	YES*	Lim KI et al (2010)[72]; Yang EJ et al (2011)[73]

Abbreviations: COPD = Chronic Obstructive Pulmonary Disease; CKD = Chronic Kidney Disease; CHF = Chronic Heart Failure; T2DM = Type 2 Diabetes; MetS = Metabolic Syndrome
*few evidences

Systemic low grade of inflammation, also called inflammaging, has been largely recognized as a feature of the aging process [74]. Whether inflammaging is the consequence of aging *per se* or the effect of chronic comorbidities remains, to date, to be fully elucidated [75]. Increased pro-inflammatory cytokines may also be the consequence of increased fat mass during aging. The excess of pro-inflammatory cytokines acts synergistically to promote loss of muscle mass and function. In this clinical picture, also referred to as sarcopenic obesity [76], the accumulation of the intramuscular fat and connective tissue (*myosteatosis*) is inversely related to the level of physical activity and negatively affects insulin sensitivity on muscles. The vicious cycle of linking inflammation and fat accumulation in aging is depicted in Figure 10.1.

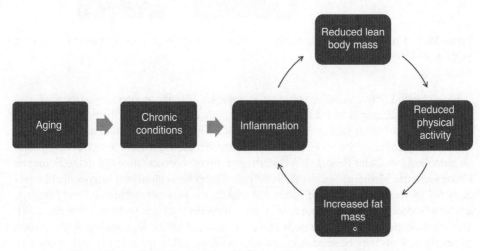

Figure 10.1 The vicious cycle of inflammation and fat accumulation.

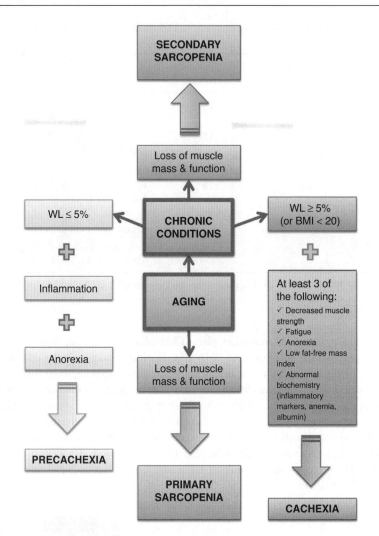

Figure 10.2 Comprehensive diagnostic algorithm for sarcopenia, pre-cachexia and cachexia in aging and chronic diseases.

Based on the above considerations, it is apparent that the geriatric syndrome of sarcopenia is multifactorial and that it can result from a combination of the process of aging with a number of other factors including chronic comorbidities, inflammation, nutritional deficiencies, sedentary life-style, inactivity. For these reasons the European Working Group on Sarcopenia in Older People (EWGSOP), a group of representatives from the European Union Geriatric Medicine Society (EUGMS), has proposed classifying sarcopenia into primary (or age-related), when age solely can explain the loss of muscle mass and function, and into 'secondary' when sarcopenia is the consequence of one or more other cause [7]. This classification fits well with daily clinical practice, where a decision-making approach to elderly patients may be needed to distinguish primary (i.e. age-related) from secondary (i.e. disease-related) causes.

A unifying algorithm guiding in the diagnosis of sarcopenia of aging and chronic diseases is depicted in Figure 10.2. As shown in the figure, independently of age, chronic conditions may lead to pre-cachexia (left green blocks) or cachexia (right red blocks), depending on degree of weight loss and the combination of concomitant biochemical and metabolic alterations. The process of aging (center blocks) may lead to sarcopenia *per se* or due to the combination with superimposed chronic comorbidities associated with loss of muscle mass and function. Consequently, elderly patients may well also be pre-cachectic or cachectic, provided that the diagnostic criteria are fulfilled.

CONCLUSION

Although cachexia has been long considered a late and ineluctable event complicating the natural history of many chronic diseases such as cancer, chronic heart failure, COPD, chronic renal failure, etc., the most recent clinical and experimental evidences indicate that those mechanisms ultimately leading to the severe wasting of cachexia are operating early during the natural history of disease, suggesting that appropriate interventions might be effective in preventing or delaying the onset of this syndrome.

The consensus definition of the clinical syndrome of cachexia, its staging and the development of diagnostic criteria for both cachexia and pre-cachexia in chronic diseases represent a major achievement in clinical medicine which, until recently, was barely conceivable. This will allow for early recognition, prevention and timely-appropriate treatments aimed at least at delaying the onset of this devastating condition.

The progressive knowledge of the biochemical and molecular mechanisms underlying cachexia is showing that cachexia and sarcopenia share analogies in both the pathogenic mechanisms and the phenotypic features. Indeed, loss of muscle mass and strength is a hallmark of both these clinical entities and cachexia may be one of the conditions underlying sarcopenia. Although frequently overlapping and often indistinguishable from one another, especially in the elderly, these conditions are not the same. It is only the accurate patient's multidimensional and clinical evaluation that may guide the clinician through their differential diagnosis and the most appropriate therapeutic options. Given the several commonalities between cachexia and sarcopenia, it is likely that new therapeutic approaches, combining nutritional support, conventional drugs and targeting of molecular pathways may be effective in both conditions.

REFERENCES

1. Strehler BL. (1997) Time, Cells, and Aging. Academic Press, New York, USA.

2. Goto M. (2008) Inflammaging (inflammation + aging): A driving force for human aging based on an evolutionarily antagonistic pleiotropy theory? Biosci Trends. 2(6), 218–230.

3. Narici MV, Maffulli N. (2010) Sarcopenia: characteristics, mechanisms and functional significance. Br Med Bull 95, 139–159.

4. Thomas DR. (2007) Loss of skeletal muscle mass in aging: examining the relationship of starvation, sarcopenia and cachexia. Clin Nutr. 26(4), 389–399.

5. Janssen I, Shepard DS, Katzmarzyk PT, et al. (2004) The healthcare costs of sarcopenia in the United States. J Am Geriatr Soc. 52(1), 80–85.

6. Cederholm TE, Bauer JM, Boirie Y, et al. (2011) Toward a definition of sarcopenia. Clin Geriatr Med. 27(3), 341–353. doi: 10.1016/j.cger.2011.04.001.

7. Cruz-Jentoft AJ, Baeyens JP, Bauer JM, et al. (2010) European Working Group on Sarcopenia in Older People. Sarcopenia: European consensus on definition and diagnosis: Report of the European Working Group on Sarcopenia in Older People. Age Ageing 39(4), 412–423.

8. Cruz-Jentoft AJ, Landi F, Topinková E, et al. (2010) Understanding sarcopenia as a geriatric syndrome. Curr Opin Clin Nutr Metab Care. 13(1), 1–7.

9. Barendregt K, Soeters PB, Allison SP. (2004) Influence of malnutrition on physiological function. In: Sobotka L, editor. Basics in clinical nutrition. 3rd ed. Galen, p.18–20.

10. Biolo G, Ciocchi B, Stulle M, et al. (2005) Metabolic consequences of physical inactivity. J Ren Nutr 15(1), 49–53.

11. Biolo G, Heer M, Narici M, et al. (2003) Microgravity as a model of ageing. Curr Opin Clin Nutr Metab Care 6(1) 31–40.

12. Evans WJ, Morley JE, Argilés J, et al. (2008) Cachexia: a new definition. Clin Nutr 27(6), 793–799.

13. von Haehling S, Anker SD. (2010) Cachexia as a major underestimated and unmet medical need: facts and numbers. J Cachex Sarcopenia Muscle 1(1), 1–5.

14. Muscaritoli M, Anker SD, Argilés J, et al. (2010) Consensus definition of sarcopenia, cachexia and pre-cachexia: joint document elaborated by Special Interest Groups (SIG) 'cachexia-anorexia in chronic wasting diseases' and 'nutrition in geriatrics'. Clin Nutr 29(2), 154–159.

15. Marín Caro MM, Laviano A, Pichard C. (2007) Nutritional intervention and quality of life in adult oncology patients. Clin Nutr 26(3), 289–301.

16. Fearon KC. (1992) The mechanisms and treatment of weight loss in cancer. Proc Nutr Soc 51(2), 251–265.

17. Tisdale MJ. (2009) Mechanisms of cancer cachexia. Physiol Rev 89(2), 381–410.

18. Krasnow SM, Marks DL. (2010) Neuropeptides in the pathophysiology and treatment of cachexia. Curr Opin Support Palliat Care 4(4), 266–271.

19. Schols A, Broekhuizen R, Weling-Scheepers CA, et al. (2005) Body composition and mortality in chronic obstructive pulmonary disease. Am J Clin Nutr 82, 53–59.

20. Mantovani G. (2006) Cachexia related to multiple cause. In: Mantovani G, editor. *Cachexia and wasting: a modern approach*. Springer, p. 161–162.

21. Vigano A, Donaldson N, Higginson IJ, et al. (2004) Quality of life and survival prediction interminal cancer patients: a multicenter study. Cancer 101(5), 1090–1098.

22. Vigano A, Dorgan M, Buckingham J, et al. (2000) Survival prediction in terminal cancer patients:a systematic review of the medical literature. Palliat Med 14(5), 363–374.

23. Tisdale MJ. (2010) Cancer cachexia. Curr Opin Gastroenterol 26(2), 146–151.

24. Costelli P, Baccino FM. (2003) Mechanisms of skeletal muscle depletion in wasting syndromes: role of ATP-ubiquitin-dependent proteolysis. Curr Opin Clin Nutr Metab Care 6(4), 407–412.

25. Aversa Z, Bonetto A, Penna F, et al. (2011) Changes in Myostatin Signaling in Non-Weight-Losing Cancer Patients. Ann Surg Oncol. Apr 26. [Epub ahead of print]

26. Penna F, Bonetto A, Muscaritoli M, et al. (2010) Muscle atrophy in experimental cancer cachexia: is the IGF-1 signaling pathway involved? Int J Cancer 127(7), 1706–1717.

27. Aversa Z, Bonetto A, Costelli P, et al. (2011) β-hydroxy-β-methylbutyrate (HMB) attenuates muscle and body weight loss in experimental cancer cachexia. Int J Oncol 38(3), 713–720. doi: 10.3892/ijo.2010.885.

28. Goldspink G. (2006) Impairment of IGF-I gene splicing and MGF expression associated with muscle wasting. Int J Biochem Cell Biol 38(3), 481–489.

29. Saini A, Al-Shanti N, Stewart CE. (2006) Waste management – cytokines, growth factors and cachexia. Cytokine Growth Factor Rev 17(6), 475–486.

30. Tisdale MJ. (2003) The "cancer cachectic factors". Support Care Cancer 11(2), 73–78.

31. Barendregt K, Soeters PB, Allison SP, et al. (2004) Simple and stress starvation. In: Sobotka L, editor. Clinical nutrition, 3rd ed. Galen, p. 107–113.

32. Tan BH, Fearon KC. (2008) Cachexia: prevalence and impact in medicine. Curr Opin Clin Nutr Metab Care 11(4), 400–407.

33. Laviano A, Meguid MM, Rossi Fanelli F. (2003) Cancer anorexia: clinical implications, pathogenesis, and therapeutic strategies. Lancet Oncol 4, 686–694.

34. Ribaudo JM, Cella D, Hahn EA, et al. (2000) Re-validation and shortening of the Functional Assessment of Anorexia/Cachexia Therapy (FAACT) questionnaire. Qual Life Res 9, 1137–1146.

35. Fearon K et al. (2011) Definition and classification of cancer cachexia: an international consensus. Lancet Oncol 12(5), 489–495.

36. Rochon PA, Katz JN, Morrow LA, et al. (1996) Comorbid illness is associated with survival and length of hospital stay in patients with chronic disability. A prospective comparison of three comorbidity indices. Med Care 34(11), 1093–1101.

37. Gross PA, Stein MR, van Antwerpen C, et al. (1991) Comparison of severity of illness indicators in an intensive care unit. Arch Intern Med 151(11), 2201–2205.

38. Stineman MG, Escarce JJ, Tassoni CJ, et al. (1998) Diagnostic coding and medical rehabilitation length of stay: their relationship. Arch Phys Med Rehabil 79(3), 241–248.

39. de Groot V, Beckerman H, Lankhorst GJ, et al. (2003) How to measure comorbidity. a critical review of available methods. J Clin Epidemiol 56(3), 221–229.

40. Lee JS, Auyeung TW, Kwok T, et al. (2007) Associated factors and health impact of sarcopenia in older chinese men and women: a cross-sectional study. Gerontology 53(6), 404–410.

41. Rolland Y, Czerwinski S, Abellan Van Kan G, et al. (2008) Sarcopenia: its assessment, etiology, pathogenesis, consequences and future perspectives. J Nutr Health Aging 12(7), 433–450.

42. Fried LP, Ferrucci L, Darer J, et al. (2004) Untangling the concepts of disability, frailty, and comorbidity: implications for improved targeting and care. J Gerontol A Biol Sci Med Sci 59(3), 255–263.

43. Hoffman C, Rice D, Sung HY. (1996) Persons with chronic conditions. Their prevalence and costs. JAMA 276(18), 1473–1479.

44. Wu SY, Green A. (2000) Projection of Chronic Illness Prevalence and Cost Inflation. Washington DC, RAND Health.

45. Bocognano A, Durnesni JS, Frerot L, et al. (1999) Santè, soins et protection sociale en 1998. CREDES Edition.

46. Fried LP, Bandeen-Roche K, Kasper JD, et al. (1999) Association of comorbidity with disability in older women: the Women's Health and Aging Study. J Clin Epidemiol 52, 27–37.

47. Davies DF, Shock NW. (1950) Age changes in glomerular filtration rate, effective renal plasma flow, and tubular excretory capacity in adult males. J Clin Invest 29, 496–507.

48. Wesson LG Jr. (1969) Renal hemodynamics in physiological states. In Physiology of the Human Kidney. New York: Grune and Stratton, 96–108.

49. Macías-Núñez JF, López-Novoa JM. (2008) Physiology of the healthy aging kidney. In: Macías-Núñez JF, Cameron JS, Oreopoulos DM, eds. The Aging Kidney in Health and Disease. New York: Springer, 93–112.

50. Hollenberg NK, Rivera A, Meinking T, et al. (1999) Age, renal perfusion, and function in island-dwelling indigenous Kuna Amerinds of Panama. Nephron 82, 131–138.

51. Hoang K, Tan JC, Derby G, et al. (2003) Determinants of glomerular hypofiltration in aging humans. Kidney Int 64, 1417–1424.

52. National Kidney Foundation Kidney Disease Outcomes Quality Initiative. (2002) Clinical Practice Guidelines for Chronic Kidney Disease: Evaluation, Classification, and Stratification. Am J Kidney Dis (suppl 1) 39, s1-s266.

53. Rifkin DE, Sarnak MJ. (2009) Does inflammation fuel the fire in CKD? Am J Kidney Dis 53(4), 572–575.

54. Workeneh BT, Mitch WE. (2010) Review of muscle wasting associated with chronic kidney disease. Am J Clin Nutr 91(4), 1128S–1132S.

55. Yao H, Rahman I. (2009) Current concepts on the role of inflammation in COPD and lung cancer. Curr Opin Pharmacol 9(4), 375–383.

56. Cornwell WD, Kim V, Song C, et al. (2010) Pathogenesis of inflammation and repair in advanced COPD. Semin Respir Crit Care Med 31(3), 257–266.

57. Witasp A, Carrero JJ, Heimbürger O, et al. (2011) Increased expression of pro-inflammatory genes in abdominal subcutaneous fat in advanced chronic kidney disease patients. J Intern Med 269(4), 410–9. doi: 10.1111/j.1365-2796.2010.02293.x.

58. Mantovani A, Allavena P, Sica A, et al. (2008) Cancer-related inflammation. Nature 454(7203), 436–444.

59. Grivennikov SI, Greten FR, Karin M. (2010) Immunity, inflammation, and cancer. Cell 140(6), 883–899.

60. Fu M. (2009) Inflammation in chronic heart failure: what is familiar, what is unfamiliar? Eur J Heart Fail 11(2), 111–112.

61. Parish RC, Evans JD. (2008) Inflammation in chronic heart failure. Ann Pharmacother 42(7), 1002–1016.

62. Donath MY, Shoelson SE. (2011) Type 2 diabetes as an inflammatory disease. Nat Rev Immunol 11(2), 98–107.

63. Hotamisligil GS. (2006) Inflammation and metabolic disorders. Nature 444(7121), 860–867.

64. Espinola-Klein C, Gori T, Blankenberg S, et al. (2011) Inflammatory markers and cardiovascular risk in the metabolic syndrome. Front Biosci 16, 1663–1674.

65. Monteiro R, Azevedo I. (2010) Chronic inflammation in obesity and the metabolic syndrome. Mediators Inflamm, doi: 10.1155/2010/289645. Epub 2010 Jul 14.

66. Seymour JM, Spruit MA, Hopkinson NS, et al. (2010) The prevalence of quadriceps weakness in COPD and the relationship with disease severity. Eur Respir J 36(1), 81–8.

67. Schols AM. Pulmonary cachexia. Int J Cardiol. 2002 Sep;85(1): 101–110.

68. Leal VO, Mafra D, Fouque D, Anjos LA. (2011) Use of handgrip strength in the assessment of the muscle function of chronic kidney disease patients on dialysis: a systematic review. Nephrol Dial Transplant 26(4), 1354–1360.

69. Park SW, Goodpaster BH, Lee JS, et al. (2009) Health, Aging, and Body Composition Study. Excessive loss of skeletal muscle mass in older adults with type 2 diabetes. Diabetes Care 32(11), 1993–1997.

70. Park SW, Goodpaster BH, Strotmeyer ES, et al. (2007) Health, Aging, and Body Composition Study. Accelerated loss of skeletal muscle strength in older adults with type 2 diabetes: the health, aging, and body composition study. Diabetes Care 30(6), 1507–1512.

71. Krause MP, Riddell MC, Hawke TJ. (2011) Effects of type 1 diabetes mellitus on skeletal muscle: clinical observations and physiological mechanisms. Pediatr Diabetes 12(4 Pt 1), 345–64. doi: 10.1111/j.1399-5448.2010.00699.x.

72. Lim KI, Yang SJ, Kim TN, et al. (2010) The association between the ratio of visceral fat to thigh muscle area and metabolic syndrome: the Korean Sarcopenic Obesity Study (KSOS). Clin Endocrinol (Oxf), 73(5), 588–94. doi: 10.1111/j.1365-2265.2010.03841.x.

73. Yang EJ, Lim S, Lim JY, et al. (2011) Association between muscle strength and metabolic syndrome in older Korean men and women: the Korean Longitudinal Study on Health and Aging. Metabolism Aug 24. [Epub ahead of print]

74. Franceschi C, Bonafè M, Valensin S, et al. (2000) Inflamm-aging. An evolutionary perspective on immunosenescence. Ann N Y Acad Sci 908, 244–254.

75. Roubenoff R. (2003) Catabolism of aging: is it an inflammatory process? Curr Opin Clin Nutr Metab Care 6(3), 295–299.

76. Zamboni M, Mazzali G, Fantin F, et al. (2008) Sarcopenic obesity: a new category of obesity in the elderly. Nutr Metab Cardiovasc Dis 18(5), 388–395.

CHAPTER 11

Sarcopenia and Frailty

Cornel C. Sieber

*Institute for Biomedicine of Ageing, Friedrich-Alexander-University
Erlangen-Nürnberg, Germany*

INTRODUCTION

Since the term sarcopenia was coined and became commonplace in the late 1980s and early 1990s [1,2], there has been continuous interest in research on the age-associated decrease of muscle mass and muscle strength. Nevertheless, studies elucidating the clinical aspects of sarcopenia – including the overlap with the frailty syndrome – have been performed with a relevant time-lag.

Although popular among geriatricians and even non-professionals for decades, the term frailty was attributed to the concept of a geriatric syndrome much later [3]. Since then it has attracted wide-spread scientific interest amongst researchers and clinicians, even reaching popular print media [4]. How can these two entities then be interrelated and what conclusions should be drawn?

This textbook focuses on sarcopenia and most of the relevant aspects are detailed in other chapters. This chapter tries to delineate the interplay of sarcopenia and the frailty syndrome, to put them into perspective with other clinical entities such as cachexia, in order to strengthen the view in the current partly semantic debate of all these terms. This will hopefully help in the future to better focus on specificities of these different clinical pictures to foster research and development of (specific) therapeutic strategies.

SARCOPENIA

Definition of sarcopenia (see also Chapter 6)

Sarcopenia has emerged as a core concept to understand function and by that independence in older age. As muscle mass accounts for about 40% of body mass, its decline with age is not just a part of senescence, but also an important research field to understand the causes of decline, considering that muscle is replaced by other tissue types, especially fat mass. After the age of 50 years, about 1-2% of muscle mass is lost per year [5]. Thus, a

Sarcopenia, First Edition. Edited by Alfonso J. Cruz-Jentoft and John E. Morley.
© 2012 John Wiley & Sons, Ltd. Published 2012 by John Wiley & Sons, Ltd.

continuous loss of muscle mass with aging is observed in different populations [6,7]. This loss of muscle mass is more pronounced in men than in women, the former showing a higher absolute muscle mass in earlier years, but a steeper decline in later adulthood and old age. A correlation between loss of muscle mass and loss of muscle strength has also been established. The decrease of muscle strength is approximately 20% to 40% when adults around 20 years of age are compared to individuals around age 70 and may increase to above 50% when compared to individuals in their 90s [8,9]. In addition, muscle strength is lost even faster with age [10], indicating that muscle mass is only partially responsible for strength and functionality in old age.

Sarcopenia is present when there is a less-than-expected muscle mass in an individual of a specified age, gender and race. Using the definition of Janssen [11], the prevalence for class II sarcopenia – two standard deviations below that of young adults – above age 80 was calculated at 7% for men and 11% for women in the United States. This prevalence compared to the one described for frailty for the same age-group (see below), indicates that sarcopenia can only partly describe the full picture of the frailty syndrome in many older persons.

Nevertheless, large scale studies focusing on the functional consequences of sarcopenia are rare. For example, in the nursing home environment, where sarcopenia allegedly shows a regular high prevalence, not a single study has been undertaken to date that applied the classical definition of sarcopenia as muscle mass. Moreover, the vast majority of older persons living in nursing homes are frail.

Another shortcoming of the definitions introduced by Baumgartner [2] and Janssen [11] is that they solely rely on the measurement of muscle mass and lack a functional component. Newer definitions either add up gait speed [12] or gait speed or muscle strength [13]. Such additional factors indeed make sense for the diagnosis of sarcopenia, as its diagnosis is a major cause of frailty and disability in older persons [14,15].

Sarcopenia beyond muscle mass loss and locomotion

Even though the focus of sarcopenia research has mainly concentrated on locomotion (e.g. gait speed, falls), muscle tissue is abundant and important in other body tissues. Loss of muscle mass in these organs also hampers functionality in affected persons. As muscle mass loss is a general phenomenon of aging, its loss beyond a certain threshold renders a person more vulnerable to different health outcomes (see below for frailty). Cardiac output, respiratory capacity, glucose homeostasis and insulin sensitivity, amino acid supply, as well as drug bioavailability and tolerance (due to changes in body composition) are such factors. As for frailty, sarcopenia may aggravate other diseases as well as their prognosis by negatively influencing their progress. Such diseases include congestive heart failure, chronic obstructive lung disease, diabetes mellitus, chronic kidney disease, diabetes mellitus, and even stroke and dementia.

It is still a challenge inasmuch as these different frequent diseases – often being part of multimorbidity in older persons – are not just accompanied by sarcopenia, but altogether may cluster in more defined entities with different progression rates. If such clusters can be found, they may theoretically finally lead to distinct therapeutic approaches, as is the actual tendency in cachexia research (see Chapter 10).

DEFINITION OF FRAILTY

The frailty concept

The concept of frailty has attracted increasing interest since well-based approaches to define it have been more widely acknowledged. Frailty may now be regarded as a geriatric syndrome of decreased reserve and resistance to stressors, resulting from cumulative declines across multiple physiologic systems, causing vulnerability to adverse health outcomes including falls, hospitalization, institutionalization and mortality (16). This could imply that a common underlying biological process is responsible for its development. Concepts focusing on inflammatory processes, hormonal changes and body composition follow this hypothesis.

The frailty syndrome is a multidimensional entity which comprises of physical, psychological and sociological components. To date most research has clearly been performed on the physical and disease-related aspects of frailty, while the other two areas are still predominantly unexplored. Frailty may be seen as a continuum stretching from early stages that cannot be identified clinically under the circumstances of everyday life and only become obvious when the individual faces external stressors, to late stages of full-blown frailty that are easily recognized as they interfere with daily routine activities and come close to a state of disability [17]. According to most experts, frailty does not exist in the absence of chronic disease. If no chronic comorbidity is present when frailty is diagnosed, subclinical or undiagnosed disease might therefore be present [16].

Nevertheless, some characteristics of frailty apply for normal aging, such as decreased physiologic reserve, decreased organ function, decreased functional reserve and loss of complexity [18]. According to some authors, it might therefore not be possible to distinguish frailty unambiguously from advanced stages of the aging process. This will also depend on the measures that are used to diagnose frailty as pointed out below.

Grip strength – strongly correlated with sarcopenia – is also a predictor of falls, physical disability and the frailty syndrome [19]. The strong correlation of gait speed as a functional parameter in the lower extremities with functionality per se and even mortality has therefore also found its way into the description of frailty [20,21].

As the term frailty was first described in the field of neonatology, one may ask why it is now so prominent in geriatric medicine. It cannot just be a metaphor for the demographic shift and the challenge of aging societies. No, frailty means in both contexts the inability of an organism to cope with stressors, especially with regard to functionality. Here there is a link to sarcopenia, as muscle mass is one of the tissues mainly affected, as is also true for pre-term babies.

Diagnosing frailty

The diagnostic tool for practical assessment of frailty should be well defined and graded to different severities of the syndrome. On a theoretical basis, a diagnosis of frailty will be reasonable when the general condition of an individual deteriorates in such a way that he or she faces an increased risk of developing illness and death.

Table 11.1 Criteria for the phenotypic definition of frailty developed by Fried et al. [3]

• Weight loss:	> 5 kg/a
• Exhaustion:	depression scale CES-D (2 points)
• Weakness:	grip strength (lowest 20%)
• Gait speed:	5 m (slowest 20%)
• Low physical activity:	kcal/week (lowest 20%)
Diagnosis of frailty:	3 or more criteria met
Diagnosis of pre-frailty:	1-2 criteria met

The two most widely utilized approaches are the phenotypic definition of frailty developed by Fried and co-workers based on data from the Cardiovascular Health Survey [3] and the Frailty Index developed by Rockwood and co-workers [22].

The Fried definition proposes five items (Table 11.1): weight loss, exhaustion, weakness, slow walking speed and low levels of physical activity [3]. Frailty is diagnosed when at least three criteria are met. An individual is said to be pre-frail when one or two of these criteria are present.

Based on the results of several recent studies, the criterion weight loss may be regarded as one-dimensional, as high BMI-values above 30 kg/m^2 are also associated with a loss of functionality, which may be an expression of being frail. Furthermore, weight loss thresholds given in the Fried criteria may be too high for the European population, as shown in a study on community-dwelling older persons [23]. This is corroborated by the fact that in most trials using the Fried criteria, small adaptations of the original definition have been utilized [24]. Nevertheless, the good applicability of the frailty assessment by the Fried criteria could be demonstrated even in a general practitioner setting.

For the calculation of the Frailty Index by Rockwood, it is necessary to count a number of pre-specified deficits that are present in an individual [25]. In the most extensive study Rockwood and co-workers have published, 70 deficits were used for the evaluation (Table 11.2). These included active diseases, ability to perform activities of daily living and physical signs from clinical and neurological examinations. The presence of each deficit scored one point. Theoretically, but not practically, a maximum score of 70 was possible. The Frailty Index is calculated by the sum of scores of present deficits divided by 70. The highest number of deficits the authors found in any setting was 47 [25].

Both measures of frailty have recently been shown to be associated with incident disability and mortality in community-dwelling people and nursing home inhabitants [25,26]. Nevertheless, the clinical applicability of these two measures has to be regarded differently. While the Fried criteria concentrate on the physical aspects of frailty and are more easy and quick to work with, the Frailty Index by Rockwood incorporates a more diverse spectrum of information on the elderly individual and therefore requires a more elaborate work-up. Both measures use criteria that are familiar to the clinician and are closely linked to functionality, thereby showing links to sarcopenia.

The relationship between frailty and a wide spectrum of clinical diseases, such as coronary heart disease [27], Parkinson's disease [28], stroke [29], Alzheimer's disease [30], venous thromboembolism [31] and esophagitis [32] has been explored by different research groups. This underlines the growing interest of clinical researchers in this geriatric syndrome.

Table 11.2   List of variables used for the 70-item Frailty Index by Rockwood et al. (22)

Changes in everyday activities	Mood problems	Others
Head and neck problems	Feeling sad, blue, depressed	Seizures, generalised
Poor muscle tone in neck	History of depressed mood	Syncope, blackouts
Bradicinesia, facial	Depression	Headache
Bradicinesia, limbs	(clinical impression)	Cerebrovascular problems
Problems getting dressed	Sleeping changes	History of stroke
Problems with bathing	Restlessness	History of diabetes mellitus
Problems carrying out	Memory changes	Arterial hypertension
personal grooming	Short-term memory	Peripheral pulses
Urinary incontinence	impairment	Myocardial infarction
Toileting problems	Long-term memory	Arrhythmia
Poor muscle bulk	impairment	Congestive heart failure
Rectal problems	Changes in general mental	Lung problems
Gastrointestinal problems	functioning	Respiratory problems
Problems cooking	Onset of cognitive symptoms	History of thyroid disease
History of Parkinson's disease	Clouding or delirium	Thyroid problems
Problems going out alone	Paranoid features	Malignant disease
Impaired mobility	History relevant to	Breast problems
Musculoskeletal problems	cognitive impairment or loss	Abdominal problems
Tired all the time	Family history relevant to	Presence of snout reflex
Abnormal muscle tone in limbs	cognitive impairment or loss	Palmomental reflex
Impaired limb coordination	Impaired vibration	Cardiac problems
Impaired coordination, trunk	Tremor at rest	Other medical history
Poor standing posture	Postural tremor	
Irregular gait pattern	Intention tremor	
Skin problems	Suck reflex	
	Family history of	
	neuro-degenerative disease	
	Falls	

Pathophysiology of frailty

Several pathophysiological processes are related to the development of frailty [18]. A predominant role has been attributed to inflammatory mechanisms. Increased levels of CRP and proinflammatory cytokines are associated with the presence of frailty [33–35]. Especially increased IL-6 levels have repeatedly been observed, with a close association with an increased risk for being frail.

A series of studies have concentrated on the relationship between nutrition and frailty. It was shown that frailty is significantly associated with a daily energy intake below 21 kcal / kg bodyweight as well as a low protein intake [36]. Data from the InCHIANTI study have proved a statistically significant association between frailty and low vitamin E levels [37]. From the Women's Health and Aging Studies we know that pre-frail and frail individuals have a higher prevalence of being deficient in vitamin B12, vitamin D and alpha-tocopherol than non-frail individuals [38]. The simultaneous prevalence of more than one vitamin deficiency is also significantly higher in pre-frail and frail individuals.

The current understanding of the involvement of the above mentioned multiple factors in the pathogenesis of frailty is summarized in Figure 11.1. It also shows that sarcopenia plays a central role in this concept.

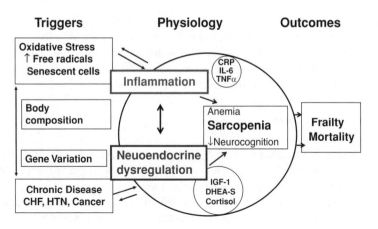

Figure 11.1 Modal pathway to adverse outcomes in the elderly - Adapted after Walston J 2007 (personal communication).

Pathophysiological overlaps between sarcopenia and frailty

Pathophysiological overlaps between sarcopenia and frailty are important. With regard to grading sarcopenia, attempts have been made to parallel classification of the frailty syndrome. Whereas the Fried criteria grade subjects as non-frail, prefrail and frail, the European Working Group on Sarcopenia in Older People (EWGSOP) consensus definition of sarcopenia, using three parameters (low muscle mass, low muscle strength, and low physical performance), also proposes a staging system that includes three levels: presarcopenia, sarcopenia and severe sarcopenia [13]. The presarcopenia stage is determined by a low muscle mass with preserved muscle strength (grip strength) and normal physical performance (gait speed). The sarcopenia stage is defined as low muscle mass and either diminished grip strength or gait speed, whereas severe sarcopenia adds up all three factors. The factors contributing to sarcopenia as detailed in the recent article by Cederholm et al. [39], interplay with the frailty syndrome, as detailed below.

Senescence

Different hormonal axes show significant changes during aging. The growth hormone, insulin like growth factor-1 (IGF-1), but also sex hormones including testosterone, estrogens and the pro-hormone dehydroepiandrosterone sulphate all decrease with age. Some of them have been used in an attempt to counteract the sarcopenia process. Nevertheless, studies using single hormonal replacements have been disappointing. Present concepts favour a multiple hormonal deregulation leading to frailty [40]. Thus, the absolute burden of several anabolic hormonal deficiencies partly predicts sarcopenia and frailty, suggesting a generalized endocrine deficiency [41].

Starvation

Anorexia is frequent in older persons, both in those showing signs of sarcopenia and/or frailty. A correlation between anorexia, subsequent weight loss and the frailty syndrome has therefore been put forward [42]. Using anthropometric measurements (e.g. triceps skinfold thickness) a correlation can be found between the degree of frailty, inflammatory parameters such as C-reactive protein, and also with the anorectic hormone leptin [43]. As anorexia often leads to protein-energy malnutrition – being a major cause for sarcopenia – a further interlink between sarcopenia and frailty can be found.

Inflammatory processes

Inflammatory signals that are part of the 'inflamm-aging' concept [44,45] – also related to nutrition – are associated with muscle wasting (sarcopenia, cachexia), which then may lead to frailty and functional decline. Most studies have focused on interleukin 6 (IL-6) and tumour necrosis factor alpha (TNF-alpha). In addition, the monocyte/macrophage-derived immune activation marker neopterin is (independent of IL-6) correlated with frailty [46]. This indicates that monocyte/macrophage-mediated immune activation is also part of the frailty syndrome.

Studies have demonstrated an independent association of proinflammatory cytokines such as tumour necrosis factor alpha and interleukin 1 and 6 with lower muscle strength, lower physical performance and a higher risk of disability in sarcopenic persons [47]. In a frail population, typical age-related diseases are more often seen. In addition to a pro-inflammatory state being correlated with the degree of frailty, different chronic diseases such as chronic cardiovascular and kidney diseases, but also anaemia and depressive states, are often combined in sarcopenic and frail older adults [48].

When considering that a diet rich in anti-oxidant can counteract oxidative stress – both from internal and external sources – and by that inflammatory processes such as sarcopenia and frailty, it may well be that such processes not only reduce the risk of becoming frail as part of functional decline, but also for other components of the frailty syndrome [49]. Such a correlation has indeed been described in elderly community-dwelling persons for different markers of the redox balance [50], including reduced oxidized gluthatione (GSSG) levels. Moreover, increased levels of tumour necrosis alpha and malonaldehyde and 4-hydroxy-2,3-nonrenal protein plasma adducts have been found [51]. A genetic basis for such alterations has been described at a mitochondrial level [52].

Endocrine alterations

Besides different endocrine axes, growth hormone has received special attention as being a strong anabolic hormone, its plasma levels decreasing in the normal aging process as does muscle mass. A correlation between growth hormone and the IGF-1 axis with skeletal muscle mass loss has indeed been described [53]. The replacement of low growth hormone levels to counteract the sarcopenic process and frailty has been disappointing to date, but its use is still being debated, especially as part of a more orchestrated intervention including several anabolic substances [54].

Vitamin D

Low vitamin D levels are clearly related to functional muscle strength loss and falls as an indirect sign of sarcopenia [55–57]. The correlation of a low vitamin D status as a single parameter for frailty risk has also been described. Nevertheless, even though lower vitamin D levels in community-dwelling older men are independently correlated with frailty, they do not predict further progression in the following years [58]. Similar findings are described for women, where low vitamin D levels are also associated with an increased risk of incident frailty or death during follow-up [59]. These findings have been nevertheless challenged by others, as such correlation could only be found in men [60]. In summary, low vitamin D levels as a single biomarker only modestly predict progression of frailty, but vitamin D deficiency at a serum concentration <15 ng mL as a punctual measurement is linked to an approximately 4-fold increase in the odds of frailty [61]. Finally, a further link between vitamin D status, inflammatory load and the 6-minute walk has been described in frail elderly persons with heart failure [62].

Insulin resistance

Not only insulin resistance predicts frailty, but diabetes mellitus also accelerates the loss of muscle strength [63]. The frailty status is correlated with altered glucose-insulin dynamics in older women with undiagnosed non-insulin dependent diabetes mellitus. Specifically, glucose and insulin responses are exaggerated and prolonged in frail versus non-frail and pre-frail women [64]. This is corroborated by findings that insulin resistance is not only correlated to frailty, but also to gait speed, indicating a link to sarcopenia and frailty [65]. Frailty in association with insulin resistance and glucose metabolism may also depend on increased abdominal fat, linking frailty to sarcopenic obesity [66]. A high waist circumference, even among underweight older adults, may be an additional target of intervention to counteract frailty [67].

FUTURE CHALLENGES

Sarcopenic obesity

Changes in body composition, especially a relative and absolute increase in fat mass, may be seen as another important aspect in the pathogenesis of frailty. In this context, it has recently been shown by data from the Cardiovascular Health Study, that frail individuals are characterized by higher weight, more central obesity, higher insulin resistance and a higher probability for the metabolic syndrome [68].

Obesity is defined as an increased body mass index (BMI). Despite this, BMI does not say anything about body composition. As an example, fluid retention due to heart failure increases body weight and thus BMI, without improving a state of malnutrition. An increased BMI is correlated to self-reported low mobility, but not to reduced balance [69]. To overcome these limitations, we explored in data sets from all continents whether calf circumference as a parameter to measure muscle mass could substitute the BMI when this parameter is missing. Indeed, when screening for nutritional status, BMI can be replaced by calf-circumference [70], indirectly correlating body weight with body composition.

This means that obesity can very well be related to sarcopenia, functional decline and the frailty syndrome. This interrelationship is well described for both research and treatment strategies in an aging and more and more obese society [71] and is substantiated in Chapter 13.

Cachexia and sarcopenia

Protein-energy malnutrition (PEM) was first described as a severe clinical problem in the 1980s and 1990s with a fast increasing understanding of its pathophysiological background. Mounting research to tackle this problem came out of oncology, where cancer-associated PEM was strongly related to inflammatory processes. A semantically good example of this period is the description of the tumour necrosis factor alpha. Even more important, it was and is still well-known that this high inflammatory load renders nutritional treatment rather disappointing [72,73]. Cachexia was then defined as disease-related loss of body cell mass, not necessarily linked with concurrent weight loss. In contrast, conditions with weight loss irrespective of the effects on body composition are termed wasting disorders, and the involuntary age-associated non disease-related – e.g. age-specific – muscle loss was called sarcopenia. This has now changed regarding the diagnosis of sarcopenia; the finding of a reduced age-adjusted muscle mass has to be combined with a functional parameter (gait speed or handgrip strength) to be diagnosed as sarcopenia [12,13,39].

In the consensus paper of Evans and colleagues [74], three out of five of the classification items of the Fried frailty criteria were used for the diagnosis of frailty (weight loss, fatigue and decreased muscle strength). The question now arises if sarcopenia, frailty and even cachexia share common pathways and clinical presentations. As sarcopenia is always part of cachexia but not vice versa, one can argue differently on the interplay of these three clinical entities:

- Frailty is an umbrella syndrome, under which both sarcopenia and cachexia can be covered.
- Sarcopenia and frailty are brothers and sisters, and cachexia is an outburst of the two in high inflammatory states.
- Sarcopenia is one of the phenotypes of frailty, cachexia another, and also quite different ones, such as psychological and social failure to cope with internal and external stressors.

If the last feature may fit best, this has implications for the diagnosis and especially for the treatment of frailty. The specificity of the different pathophysiological origins of frailty still needs to be tackled separately. This means that research and drug/treatment developments for frailty have to concentrate on the specific predominant backgrounds. Sarcopenia may well need different therapeutic approaches than cachexia. This is substantiated by the fact that nutritional intervention is successful for sarcopenia and frailty, but much less for cachexia. Such a concept can also help to critically analyze present therapeutic strategies involving nutritional interventions and physical activity programs, which may well differ in their goals and success.

With regard to cancer cachexia, an interesting crosslink to both frailty and sarcopenia has recently been published [75]. The diagnostic criterion of cachexia is additional weight loss in individuals who already show signs of a diminished BMI (<20kg/m2) or reduced skeletal muscle mass (sarcopenia). Assessments for clinical classification and management should include the following domains: anorexia or reduced food intake, catabolic drive, muscle mass and strength, functional and psychological impairment. The items muscle mass, muscle strength and functional impairment depict the overlap to sarcopenia, as these parameters are an integral part of the sarcopenia definition.

Strictly speaking, one can summarize that the definition of cachexia by Evans and colleagues uses different items of the frailty definition, whereas the one by Fearon and co-workers for cancer cachexia uses the sarcopenia definition, in addition demanding a weight loss or a BMI <20 kg/m2. The latter two items are not part of the sarcopenia definition and therefore indicate that weight loss or a low BMI adds up to sarcopenia to a state of cancer cachexia. The reasons for this weight loss may indeed be quite diverse, one of them being the inflammatory load. It is hoped that biomarkers of inflammation will be better defined and thresholds found, as this may influence therapeutic strategies.

CONCLUSIONS

Sarcopenia, as with many other geriatric phenomena, involves a number of underlying causes and mechanisms. Factors involved are not just intrinsic changes within the muscle tissue itself, but also neuronal, humoral, and lifestyle factors. Inadequate protein intake and physical inactivity may accelerate sarcopenia.

Sarcopenia may be regarded as a non-specific clinical sign that can be an age-associated phenomenon, but may also be caused by a multitude of clinical conditions that are independent of the aging process. Sarcopenia is a fundamental component of frailty, but may be seen as too one-dimensional, as the general condition of the elderly individual is determined by a complex interplay of multiple factors that may in several instances be overlooked by the diagnosis of sarcopenia alone.

Although many open questions still remain, frailty has nevertheless already created an immense interest among clinicians, one main reason being that the frailty concept is more clinically oriented than the concept of sarcopenia. Whilst the tools to measure frailty are still not perfect, they are at least clinically applicable within a routine setting. The frailty concept corresponds more directly to the needs of clinicians in defining patient groups that might suffer from complications of therapeutic interventions (operative, pharmacological) being considered for the treatment of age-associated comorbidities like cancer or coronary heart disease.

Basic researchers are asked to cooperate with their clinical colleagues to elucidate the true nature of frailty and to improve medical therapy in this important field of care for the elderly.

REFERENCES

1. Rosenberg IH. Sarcopenia: origins and clinical relevance. J Nutr 1997; 127(5 Suppl):990S–991S.
2. Baumgartner R, Koehler KM, Gallagher D, Romero L, Heymsfield SB, Ross RR, Garry PJ, Lindeman RD. Epidemiology of sarcopenia among the elderly in New Mexico. Am J Epidemiol 1998;147:755–763.
3. Fried L, Tangen CM, Walston J et al. Frailty in older adults: evidence for a phenotype. J Gerontol A Biol Sci Med Sci 2001;56:M146–M156.
4. Kolata G. Old but not frail: a matter of heart and head. The New York Times. October 5, 2006:A1.

5. Frontera WR, Hughes VA, Fielding R et al. Aging of skeletal muscle: a 12-yr longitudinal study. J Appl Physiol 2000;88:1321–1326).

6. Doherty TJ. Invited review: Aging and sarcopenia. J Appl Physiol 2003;95(4):1717–1727.

7. Iannuzi-Sucich M, Prestwood KM, Kenny AM. Prevalence of sarcopenia and predictors of skeletal muscle mass in healthy older men and women. J Gerontol Biol Sci Med Sci 2002;57:M772–M777.

8. Baumgartner R.N., Waters L.W., 2006. Sarcopenia and sarcopenic-obesity, in: Pathy M.S., Sinclair A.J., Morley J.E. (Eds.), Principles and practice of geriatric medicine. John Wiley & Sons Ltd., Chichester, pp. 909–933.

9. Goodpaster B, Won Park S, Harris TB, Kritchevsky SB, Nevitt M, Schwartz AV, Simonsick EM, Tylavsky FA, Visser M, Newman AN. THe loss of skeletal muslce strength, mass, and quality in older adults: The Health, Aging and Body Composition Study. J Gerontol Biol Sci Med Sci 2006;61A:1059–1064.

10. Ferrucci L, Guralnik JM, Buchner D et al. Departures of linearity tin the relationship between measures of muscular strength and physical performance of the lower extremities.: the Women's Health and Aging Study. J Gerontol A Biol Sci Med Sci 2007;52:M275–M285.

11. Janssen I, Heymsfield SB, Ross Robert. Low relative skeletal muscle mass (sarcopenia) in older persons is associated with functional impairment and physical disability. J Am Geriatr Soc 2002;50:889–896.

12. Muscaritoli M, Anker SD, Argıles J, et al. Consensus definition of sarcopenia, cachexia and pre-cachexia: Joint document elaborated by Special Interest Groups (SIG) "cachexia-anorexia in chronic wasting diseases" and "nutrition in geriatrics". Clin Nutr 2010;29; 154–159.

13. Cruz-Jentoft AJ, Baeyens JP, Bauer JM, Boirie Y, Cederholm T, Landi F, Martin FC, Michel JP, Rolland Y, Schneider SM, Topinkova E, Vandewoude M, Zamboni M (2010) Sarcopenia: European consensus on definition and diagnosis: Report of the European Working Group on Sarcopenia in Older People. Age Ageing 39:412–423.

14. Morley JE, Kim MJ, Haren MT, Kevorkian R, Banks WA. Frailty and the aging male. Aging Male 2005;8:135–140.

15. Abellan van Kan G, Rolland YM, Morley JE, Vellas B. Frailty: toward a clinical definition. J Am Med dir Assoc 2008;9:71–71.

16. Bergman H, Ferrucci L, Guralnik J, Hogan DB, Hummel S, Karunananthan S, Wolfson C. Frailty: an emerging research and clinical paradigm - issues and controversies. J Gerontol A Biol Sci Med Sci 2007;62(7):731–737.

17. Whitson HE, Purser JL, Cohen HJ. Frailty thy name is . . . Phrailty? J Gerontol A Biol Sci Med Sci 2007;62(7):728–730.

18. Strandberg T, Pitkälä K. Frailty in elderly people. Lancet 2007;369:1328–1329.

19. Xue QL, Walston JD, Fried LP, Beamer BA. Prediction of risk of falling, physical disability, and frailty by rate of decline in grip strength: the women's health and aging study. Arch Intern Med 2011;171:1119–1121.

20. Cesari M, Pahor M, Lauretani F, Zamboni M, Bandinelli S, Bernabei R, Guralnik JM, Ferrucci L. Skeletal muscle and mortality from the InCHIANTI Study. J Gerontol A Biol Sci Med Sci 2009;64:377–384.

21. Studenski S, Perera S, Patel K, Rosano C, Kaulkner K, Inzitari M, Brach J, Chandler J, Cawthon J, Cawthon P, Connor EB, Nevitt M, Visser M, Kritchevsky S, Badinelli S, Harris T, Newman AB, Cauley J, Ferrucci L, Guralnik J. Gait speed and survival in older adults. JAMA 2011;305:50–58.

22. Rockwood K, Song X, MacKnight C, Bergman H, Hogan DB, McDowell I, Mitnitski A. A global clinical measure of fitness and frailty in elderly people. CMAJ 2005;173(5):489–495.

23. Drey M, Wehr H, Wehr G, Uter W, Lang F, Rupprecht R, Sieber CC, Bauer JM. The frailty syndrome in general practitioner care: a pilot study. Z Gerontol Ger 2011;44:48–54.

24. Drey M, Pfeifer K, Sieber CC, Bauer JM. The Fried frailty criteria as inclusion criteria for a randomized controlled trial: personal experience and literature review. Gerontology 2011;57:11–18).

25. Rockwood K, Abeysundera MJ, Mitnitski A. How should we grade frailty in nursing home patients? J Am Med Dir Assoc 2007;8(9):595–603.

26. Rockwood K, Andrew M, Mitnitski A. A comparison of two approaches to measuring frailty in elderly people. J Gerontol A Biol Sci Med Sci 2007;62(7):738–743.

27. Purser JL, Kuchibhatla MN, Fillenbaum GG, Harding T, Peterson ED, Alexander KP. Identifying frailty in hospitalized older adults with significant coronary artery disease. J Am Geriatr Soc 2006;54(11):1674–1681.

28. Ahmed NN, Sherman SJ, Vanwyck D. Frailty in Parkinson's disease and its clinical implications. Parkinsonism Relat Disord. 2007 Nov 7 [Epub ahead of print]

29. Ertel KA, Glymour MM, Glass TA, Berkman LF. Frailty modifies effectiveness of psychosocial intervention in recovery from stroke. Clin Rehabil. 2007 Jun; 21(6):511–522.

30. Buchman AS, Boyle PA, Wilson RS, Tang Y, Bennett DA. Frailty is associated with incident Alzheimer's disease and cognitive decline in the elderly. Psychosom Med. 2007 Jun;69(5):483–489.

31. Folsom AR, Boland LL, Cushman M, Heckbert SR, Rosamond WD, Walston JD. Frailty and risk of venous thromboembolism in older adults. J Gerontol A Biol Sci Med Sci. 2007 Jan;62(1):79–82.

32. Cardin F, Minicuci N, Siviero P, Bertolio S, Gasparini G, Inelmen EM, Terranova O. Esophagitis in frail elderly people. J Clin Gastroenterol. 2007 Mar;41(3):257–263.

33. Leng SX, Xue QL, Tian J, Walston JD, Fried LP. Inflammation and frailty in older women. J Am Geriatr Soc 2007;55(6):864–871.

34. Hubbard RE, O'Mahony MS, Calver BL, Woodhouse KW. Nutrition, Inflammation, and Leptin Levels in Aging and Frailty. J Am Geriatr Soc 2007.

35. Walston J, McBurnie MA, Newman A, Tracy RP, Kop WJ, Hirsch CH, Gottdiener J, Fried LP. Frailty and activation of the inflammation and coagulation systems with and without clinical comorbidities: results from the Cardiovascular Health Study. Arch Intern Med 2002;162(20):2333–2341.

36. Bartali B, Frongillo EA, Bandinelli S, Lauretani F, Semba RD, Fried LP, Ferrucci L. Low nutrient intake is an essential component of frailty in older persons. J Gerontol Med Sci 2006;61A:589–593.

37. Ble A, Cherubini A, Volpato S, Bartali B, Walston JD, Windham BG, Bandinelli S, Lauretani F, Guralnik JM, Ferrucci L. Lower plasma vitamin E levels are associated with the frailty syndrome: the InCHIANTI study. J Gerontol A Biol Sci Med Sci 2006;61(3):278–283.

38. Michelon E, Blaum C, Semba RD, Xue Q, Ricks MO, Fried LP. Vitamin and Carotenoid status in older women: Associations with the frailty syndrome. J Gerontol Med Sci 2006;61A: 600–607.

39. Cederholm TE, Bauer JM, Boirie Y et al. Towards a definition of sarcopenia. Clin Geriatr Med 2011;27:341–353.

40. Maggio M, Cattabiani C, Lauretani F, Ferrucci L, Luci M, Valenti G, Ceda G. The concept of multiple hormonal dysregulation. Acta Biomed 2010;81(Suppl 1):19–29.

41. Cappola AR, Xue QL, Fried LP. Multiple hormonal deficiencies in anabolic hormones are found in frail older women: the Women's Health and Aging studies. J Gerontol A Biol Sci Med Sci 2009;64:243–248.

42. Morley JE. Anorexia, weight loss, and frailty. J Am Med Dir Assoc 2010;11:225–228.

43. Hubbard RE, O'Mahony MS, Calver BL, Woodhouse KW. Nutrition, inflammation, and leptin levels in aging and frailty. J Am Geriatr Soc 2008;56:279–284.

44. Salvioli S, Capri M, Valensin S, Tieri P, Monti D, Ottaviani E, Franceschi C. Inflamm-aging, cytokines and aging: state of the art, new hypotheses on the role of mitochondria and new perspectives from systemic biology. Curr Pharm Des 2006;12:3161–3171.

45. Biagi E, Nylund L, Candela M, Ostan R, Bucci L, Pini E, Nikkila J, Monti D, Satokari R, Franceschi C, Brigidi P, de Vos W. Through ageing, and beyond: gut microbiota and inflammatory status in seniors and centenarians. PLoS One 2010;5(5):310667.

46. Leng SX, Tian X, Matteini A, Li H, Hughes J, Jain A, Walston JD, Fedarko NS. IL6-independent association of elevated serum neopterin levels with prevalent frailty in community-dwelling older adults. Age Ageing 2011;40:475–481.

47. Pahor M, Manini T, Cesari M. Sarcopenia: clnical evaluation, biological markers and other evaluation tools. J Nutr Health Aging 2009;13:724–728.

48. Chang SS, Weiss CO, Xue QL, Fried LP. Association between inflammatory-related disease burden and frailty: results from the women's Health and Aging Studies (WHAS) I and II. Arch Gerontol Geriatr 2012;54:9–15.

49. Semba RD, Ferrucci L, Sun K, Walston J, Varadhan R, guralnik JM, Fried JP. Oxidative stress and severe walking disability among older women. Am J Med 2007;120:1084–1089.

50. Espinoza SE, Guo H, Fedarko N, DeZern A, fried LP, Xue QL, Leng S, Beamer B, Walston JD. Glutathione peroxidise enzyme activity in aging. J Gerontol A Biol Sci Med Sci 2008;63:505–509.

51. Serviddio G, Romano AD, Greco A, Rollo T, Bellanti F, Altomare E, Vendemiale G. Frailty syndrome is associated with altered circulating redox balance and increased markers of oxidative stress. Int J Immunpathol Pharmacol 2009;22:819–827.

52. Moore AZ, Biggs ML, Matteini A, O'Connor A, McGuire S, Beamer BA, Fallin MD, Fried LP, Walston J, Chakravarti A, Arking DE. Polymorphisms in the mitochondrial DNA control region and frailty in older adults. PLoS One 2010;5:e11069.

53. Perrini S, Laviola L, Carreira MC, Cignarelli A, Natalicchio A. Giorgino F. The GH/IGF1 axis and signalling pathways in the muscle and bone: mechanisms underlying age-related skeletal muscle wasting and osteoporosis. J Endocrinol 2010;205:201–210.

54. von Haehling S, Morley JE, Anker SD. An overview of sarcopenia: facts and numbers on prevalence and clinical impact. J Cachexia Sarcopenia Muscle 2010;1:129–133.

55. Bischoff-Ferrari HA, Shao A, Dawson-Hughes B, Hathcock J, Giovannucci E, Willett WC. Benefit-risk assessment of vitamin D supplementation. Osteoporos Int 2010;21:1121–1132.

56. Bischoff-Ferari HA, Dawson-Hughes B, Staehelin HB, Oray JE, Stuck AE, Theiler R, Wong JB, Egli A, Kiel DP, Henschkowski J. Fall prevention with supplemental and active forms of vitamin D: a meta-analysis of randomised controlled trials. BMJ 2009;339:b3692.

57. Pramyothin P, Techasurungkul S, Lin J, Wang H, Shah A, Ross PD, Puapong R, Wasnich RD. Vitamin D status and falls, frailty, and fractures among postmenopausal Japanese women living in Hawai. Osteoporos Int 2009;20:1955–1962).

58. Ensrud KE, Blackwell TL, Cauley JA, Cummings SR, Barrett-Connor E, Dam TT, Hoffman AR, Shikany JM, Lane NE, Stefanick ML, Orwoll ES, Cawthon PM: Osteoporotic Fractures in Men Study Group. J Am Geriatr Soc 2011;59:101–106.

59. Ensrud KE, Ewing SK, Fredman L, Hochberg MC, Cauley JA, Cummings SR, Yaffe K, Cawthon PM: Study of Osteoporotic Fractures Research Group. Circulating 25-hydroxyvitamin D levels and frailty status in older women. J Clin Endocrinol Metab 2010;95:5266–5273.

60. Shardell M, Hicks GE, Miller RR, Kritchevsky S, Andersen D, Bandunelli S, Cherubini A, Ferrucci L. Association of low vitamin D levels with the frailty syndrome in men and women. J Gerontol A Biol Sci Med Sci 2009;64:69–75.

61. Wilhelm-Leen ER, Hall YN, Deboer IH, Chertow GM. Vitamin D deficiency and frailty in older Americans. J Intern Med 2010;268:171–180.

62. Boxer RS, Dauser DA, Walsh SJ, Hager WD, Kenny AM. The association between vitamin D and inflammation with the 6-minute walk and frailty in patients with heart failure. J Am Geriatr Soc 2008;56:454–461.

63. Chen LK, Chen YM, Lin MH, Peng LN, Hwang SJ. Care of elderly patients with diabetes mellitus: a focus on frailty. Ageing Res Rev 2010;Suppl 1:S18-S22.

64. Kalyani RR, Varadhan R, Weiss CO, Fried LP, Cappola AR. Frailty status and altered glucose-insulin dynamics. J Gerontol A Biol Sci Med Sci 2011;(Epub ahead of print).

65. Kuo CK, Lin LY, Yu YH, Wu KH, Kuo HK. Inverse association between insulin resistance and gait speed in nondiabetic older men: results from the U.S. National Health and Nutrition Examination survey (NHANES) 1999-2002. BMC Geriatr 2009;9:49.

66. Goulet ED, Hassaine A, Dionne IJ, Gaudreau P, Khalil A, Fulop T, Shatenstein B, Tessier D, Morais JA. Frailty in the elderly is associated with insulin resistance of glucose metabolism in the postabsorptive state only in the presence of increased abdominal fat. Exp Gerontol 2009;44:740–744.

67. Hubbard RE, Lang IA, Llewellyn DJ, Rockwood K. Frailty, body mass index, and abdominal obesity in older people. J Gerontol A Biol Sci Med Sci 2010;65:377–381.

68. Barzilay JI, Blaum C, Moore T, Xue QL, Hirsch CH, Walston JD, Fried LP. Insulin resistance and inflammation as precursors of frailty: the Cardiovascular Health Study. Arch Intern Med 2007;167(7):635–641.

69. Hergenroeder AL, Wert DM, Hile ES, Studenski SA, Brach JS. Association of body mass index with self-report and performance-based measures of balance and mobility. Phys Ther 2011;91:1223–1234.

70. Kaiser M, Bauer JM, Ramsch C, Uter W, Guigoz Y, Cederholm T, Thomas DR, Anthony P, Charlton KE, Maggio M, Tsai AC, Grathwohl D, Vellas B, Sieber CC. MNA-International Group. J Nutr Health Aging 2009;13:782–788.

71. Zamboni M, Mazzali G, Fantin F, Rossi A, Di fFrancesco V. Sarcopenic obesity: a new category of obesity in the elderly. Nutr Metab Cardiovasc Dis 2008;18:388–395.

72. Cederholm T, Hellström K. Reversibility of protein-energy malnutrition in a group of chronically ill elderly out-patients. Clin Nutr 1995;14:81–87.

73. Creutzberg EC, Schols AM, Welinh-Scheepers CA et al. Characterization of non-response to high caloric oral nutritional therapy in depleted patients with chronic obstructive pulmonary disease. Am J Respir Crit Care Med 2000;161:745–752.

74. Evans WJ, Morley JE, Argiles J, Bales C, Baracos V, Guttridge D, Jatoi A, Kalantar-Zadeh K, Lochs H, Mantovani G, Marks D, Mitch WE, Muscaritoli M, Najand A, Ponikowski P, Rossi Fanelli F, Schambelan M, Schols A, Schuster M, Thomas DR, Wolfe R, Anker SD. Cachexia: a new definition. Clin Nutr 2008;27:793–799.

75. Fearon K, Strasser F, Anker SD, Bosaeus I, Bruera E, Fainsinger RL, Jatoi A, Loprinzi C, MacDonald N, Mantovani G, Davis M, Muscaritoli M, Ottery F, Radbruch L, Ravasco P, Walsh D, Wilcock A, Kaasa S, Baracos VE. Definition and classification of cancer cachexia: an international consensus. Lancet Oncol 2011;12:489–495.

CHAPTER 12

Sarcopenia, Osteoporosis and Fractures

Tommy Cederholm

Clinical Nutrition and Metabolism, Department of Public Health and Caring Sciences, Uppsala University, Sweden; Department of Geriatric Medicine, Uppsala University Hospital, Sweden

THE MUSCULO-SKELETAL LOCOMOTOR SYSTEM – ROLE FOR FALL AND FRACTURE PREVENTION

Locomotion is a major denominator of independent living, primarily provided by the combined action of muscles, joints and bones, i.e. the musculo-skeletal organ system. The prevention of falls depends on axial stability and the capacity to correct for imbalance, sway and trips, which is determined by the combined neuromuscular fitness. Fractures as a consequence of a fall, like hip fractures, are prevented by strong bones and by soft tissue cushioning and impact absorption. Moreover, skeletal fitness is of underrated importance for fracture prevention. Thus, apart from independence and mobility sarcopenia, i.e. the loss of muscle mass associated with increasing age, has to be recognized also for fracture prevention in the old population.

Two main features of sarcopenia are loss of fast-twitch type II fibres and loss of motorneurons. These losses are both important factors involved in the onset of a fall. The trip that precedes the fall is counteracted by a quick, strong and well-coordinated corrective action that requires fast and strong muscle action and well innervated muscle fibres. Thus, the capacity to counteract a trip is markedly reduced by sarcopenia. All features of sarcopenia that are related to lower limb dysfunction, e.g. reduced chair-rising capacity and reduced gait speed are acknowledged risk factors for hip fracture.

This chapter will deal with the common features of sarcopenia and osteoporosis, like shared mechanistic pathways, similarities in definition, and treatment alternatives with simultaneous effects on osteoporosis and sarcopenia.

Sarcopenia, First Edition. Edited by Alfonso J. Cruz-Jentoft and John E. Morley.
© 2012 John Wiley & Sons, Ltd. Published 2012 by John Wiley & Sons, Ltd.

COMMON MUSCLE AND SKELETAL CATABOLIC PROCESSES DURING AGEING AND DISEASE

Modelling and re-modelling of bone and muscle

The mechanisms for growth and catabolism of the two tissues differ greatly, whereas the anabolic and catabolic signals show many resemblances. Genetic traits are the major denominators of muscle, skeletal and body size. Still the continuous remodeling of the two tissues is under a number of modifiable influences.

Bone

Bone mass is built during adolescence, and peak mass is reached early in adulthood. The skeleton is gradually broken down from early middle-age with an average loss of ~1% of the skeletal bone per year. Thus, osteoporosis and its sequelae, i.e. fragility fractures of the hip, vertebra and wrist, are disorders confined to old adults. Bone remodeling is regulated by the concerted action of *osteoblasts* (growth) and *osteoclasts* (break-down). Throughout life there is a shifting balance between osteoblast production of new bone matrix, its mineralization and osteoclast bone reabsorption. Between 5 and 10% of the skeleton is exchanged annually. The skeleton comprises trabecular (20%) and cortical (80%) bone.

Major determinants for bone anabolism and maintenance are good nutrition and loading, especially early in life. Good nutrition from a bone perspective is a sufficient intake of calcium and proteins, together with adequate serum levels of vitamin D. The latter is provided mainly by sun exposure, but also by intake of vitamin D rich food like fat fish and fortified dairy products. Vitamin D acts in concert with parathyroid hormone for calcium absorption in the gut and also for calcium deposition, i.e. mineralization of the bone. The mechanical load provided by the muscle attachment to the skeleton contributes to the bone strength. Thus, prolonged resting as well as reduced muscle strength may result in reduced bone fitness.

Muscle

Growth of muscle mass depends on the synthesis of the myofibrillar contractile proteins actin and myosin. Myofibrillar protein synthesis is under the regulation of protein availability and is enhanced by external loading, i.e. exercise, and further enhanced by endocrine signals, like androgens, estrogens (in women), vitamin D and certain cytokines. In response to resistance exercise insulin-like growth factor-I (IGF-I) is elevated and stimulates skeletal muscle growth.

Satellite cell dysfunction is an emerging field for improved molecular understanding of the development of sarcopenia [1]. Satellite cells are myogenic stem cells that merge with myocytes and differentiate to new muscle fibres in order to facilitate growth, maintenance and repair of damaged skeletal muscle tissue. Satellite cells are located on the outer surface of the muscle fibre and are usually dormant. Especially when muscle fibres are damaged, for example from resistance training overload, the satellite cells become activated. Activated cells proliferate and are drawn to the damaged muscle site to fuse with the existing muscle fibre. The satellite cell nucleus helps to regenerate the muscle fibre. Thus, muscle repair or growth by satellite cell action does not result in more fibres, but increase the size and number of contractile proteins within the muscle fibre. Since slow-twitch type I fibres are used to much larger extents in daily life, these cells have many more satellite cells attached to them than the fast-twitch type II fibres. Myostatin D is a recently described molecule that inhibits the generation of satellite cells [2].

Hormonal and inflammatory pathogenesis for sarcopenia and osteoporosis

Ageing per se, chronic disease, reduced physical activity, insufficient energy, protein and nutrient intake, insufficient sun exposure are some examples of conditions that together have added detrimental effects on both muscle and skeletal integrity.

Bone

Osteoblasts are under positive influence by the gonadal hormones estrogen and testosterone, as well as of other anabolic hormones like IGF-I, dehydroepiandrostendione (DHEA) and growth hormone (GH). During ageing the production of gonadal hormones is reduced. The female menopause is caused by the fairly abrupt cease of estrogen production, whereas the reduction of testosterone production in men, i.e. andropause, is more gradual. When the trophic actions on osteoblast activities are reduced, the relative impact of osteoclast bone resorption increases. Not only gonadal hormone production is reduced by ageing, but also that of other anabolic hormones like GH, DHEA and IGF-1, further paving the way for bone catabolism. Cortisol, i.e. the steroid hormone produced in the adrenal cortex, is a stress hormone which initiates and support protein catabolism both in the muscle and bone. Thus, the use of glucocorticoids for the treatment of a number of illnesses of inflammatory character, not uncommonly occurring at old age, is not only related to the development of osteoporosis but also to sarcopenia.

Inflammatory cytokines like interleukin(IL)-1, IL-6 and tumor necrosis factor-alpha (TNF-a) are partly regulated by anabolic hormones. Ageing per se, but also reduced gonadal hormone levels is responsible for the increase of catabolic cytokine production seen during ageing, a condition that has been denominated "inflammaging" [3]. It is well established from observational studies that inflammatory diseases like rheumatoid arthritis or Crohn's disease are associated with reduced BMD and osteoporosis. Although the inflammatory pathways for increased bone resorption are not fully understood, the active and crucial role for the receptor activator of NF-kB ligand (RANKL), a member of the TNF cytokine family, is recently described for the differentiation of osteoclast precursors into activated osteoclasts [4]. Cathepsin K is a protease with specific action on collagen, recently acknowledged to contribute to bone resorption [4].

Muscle

Protein synthesis in the muscle fibres are under similar endocrine and inflammatory influence as the osteoblasts and osteoclasts of the bone. Oestrogen deficiency has a stronger effect on bone than on muscle, which is obvious from the observation that osteoporosis is more pronounced than sarcopenia in women, whereas the contrary is imminent for men with a more pronounced sarcopenic than osteoporotic trajectory. Insulin resistance which is often observed in ageing and partly due to 'inflammaging' contributes to muscle wasting [5]. Obesity and myosteatosis are additional causes of insulin resistance at old age. Intramyocellular lipidaccumulation, i.e. the fat infiltration of aging muscles, may impair skeletal muscle insulin signalling not only for glucose but also for amino acid utilization [6]. While muscle mass decreases during aging, the relative and sometimes also the absolute amount of fat mass increases. This condition has been called sarcopenic obesity, which is a transition of body composition that fuels a vicious cycle of insulin resistance and further loss of muscle mass. Satellite cells also have the capacity to become adipocytes and are consequently also involved in the development of myosteatosis [1].

Systemic inflammation, i.e. elevated activity of TNF-alpha, IL-6 and IL-1, leads to muscle protein breakdown. Although disease is the major cause of inflammation in older age, also aging itself by 'inflammaging' is linked to muscle catabolism. The search for the molecular basis of inflammation-triggered muscle atrophy has rendered the discovery of up-regulated genes of E3 ubiquitin ligases MuRF1 and Atrogin-1 which are both involved in the activation of *the ubiquitin-proteasome system* and the muscle fibre actin and myosin proteolysis [7]. The muscle protein breakdown caused by the activated ubiquitin-proteasome system provide the inflammatory metabolism with amino acids like alanine for gluconeogenesis in the liver and glutamine for DNA synthesis and for gut energy expenditure.

In contrast to disease-triggered muscle wasting being dominated by protein breakdown, senescence-related muscle atrophy is suggested to be mainly an effect of reduced protein synthesis especially in response to feeding [8]. The molecular basis of such perturbed signalling pathways involves the action of the mammalian target of rapamycin (mTOR) kinase which is recognized as a key regulator of cell growth by initiating gene transcription and protein translation. mTOR is a sensor of nutritional status, and may play a role as a potential target of amino acid induced protein synthesis [7].

SIMILARITIES AND DIFFERENCES IN DEFINING OSTEOPOROSIS AND SARCOPENIA

Definitions of osteoporosis and sarcopenia

Osteoporosis

The severity of bone loss is categorized in relation to the mean peak bone mineral density (BMD) in the healthy young individual. The World Health Organization [9] defines osteoporosis as a BMD of >2.5 standard deviations (SD) below the mean BMD of healthy young subjects in the same population, i.e. a T-score < -2.5 SDs. Osteopenia is a corresponding T-score of -1 SD to -2.5 SD, whereas normal BMD is a T-score of ± 1 SD [9]. Dual energy X-ray absorptiometry (DXA) is the dominating technique to measure and monitor BMD. The spine and hip are the preferred sites for measurements. Single X-ray absorptiometry (SXA) of the wrist and Quantitative Ultra Sound (QUS) are alternative techniques. The quality or strength of the bone is determined by its mineralization and by its macro- as well as micro-architecture. BMD is the hallmark for the assessment of bone quality, and is suggested to account for ~70% of the bone strength [10].

The reliability of biochemical markers of osteoblast (e.g. osteocalcin) as well as of osteo-clast (e.g. C-terminal cross-linking telopeptide of type I collagen CTX) activity improves continuously as diagnostic tools, but they are still seldom used in clinical practice.

Osteoporosis is classified as primary in post-menopausal women or at old age, and as secondary when diseases, e.g. rheumatoid arthritis, or pharmacological treatment, e.g. glucocorticoids are the major triggering events.

Sarcopenia

The majority of epidemiological studies on prevalence of sarcopenia have used mus-cle mass-based definitions, in line with that suggested for osteoporosis. Thus, a value >2 SD below the mean of a young reference population has been defined as sarcopenia [11]. Accumulating data have indicated that muscle mass is not linearly related to muscle function. Longitudinal observational studies, for example the Health ABC Study, have shown that indices of function are better predictors of adverse outcomes than muscle mass [12]. Piling evidence confirms that muscle function, as assessed for example by gait speed, is a strong predictivor of survival [13]. Therefore, the definition of sarcopenia has recently been re-assessed. The European Society for Clinical Nutrition and Metabolism (ESPEN) stated 2010 that:

> 'sarcopenia is a condition characterized by loss of muscle mass and muscle strength. Although sarcopenia is primarily a disease of the elderly, its development may be associated with conditions that are not exclusively seen in older persons, like disuse, malnutrition and cachexia. Like osteopenia, it can also be seen in younger patients such as those with inflammatory diseases. The loss of muscle mass and muscle strength caused by such conditions is usually functionally less relevant in younger individuals, as their muscle mass and muscle strength is higher before it is affected by these conditions' [14].

Several international working-groups have recently suggested definitions that in major respects overlap [15–17]. For example, The European Working Group on Sarcopenia in Older People (EWGSOP), endorsed by ESPEN, EUGMS, IAGG(ER) and IANA, stated that 'Sarcopenia is a syndrome characterized by progressive loss of muscle mass and strength with a risk of adverse outcomes' [15]. The diagnosis was suggested to be based on the combined presence of a low muscle mass, i.e. more than 2 SDs below the mean measured in young adults, and gait speed ≤0.8 m/s in a 4 m walk test.

Like with osteoporosis, sarcopenia is suggested to be classified as primary when old age is the only obvious cause for muscle wasting, and secondary sarcopenia if disease, inactivity or insufficient nutrition are the major underlying causes [15].

Case-finding procedures

Osteoporosis

BMD gives a good estimation of fracture susceptibility, but the assessment requires access to a DXA machine. Such access varies and it is valuable to use methods for case-finding that are based on clinical assessment. There are several clinical signs implying the presence of osteoporosis in the old subject, for example; >5 cm loss of height, weight below 50 kg, thoracic and neck kyfosis and tooth loss [18]. Recently, in order to evaluate fracture risk on clinical signs The Fracture Risk Assessment Tool (FRAX®️ tool) has been developed by WHO (www.shef.ac.uk/FRAX) . The tool is based on the compilation of 11 individual risk factors, i.e. age, sex, weight, height, previous fracture, parent fractured hip, current smoking, glucocorticoids, rheumatoid arthritis, secondary osteoporosis and alcohol consumption. Femoral neck BMD may be added, but is not necessary. The calculation gives a 10-year probability of a major osteoporotic fracture (clinical spine, forearm, hip or shoulder fracture). The FRAX®️ model has been developed from population-based cohorts from Europe, North America, Asia and Australia.

Sarcopenia

Like for osteoporosis, case-finding of sarcopenia is facilitated by clinical assessment. Thus, to identify subjects with sarcopenia the European Working Group on Sarcopenia in Older People (EWGSOP) suggested an algorithm based on gait speed measurement as the easiest and most reliable way to begin sarcopenia screening in practice [15]. A cut-off point of less than 0.8(-1.0) m/s identifies risk for sarcopenia. If this criterion is fulfilled it is suggested that a DXA is performed. If gait speed would exceed the cut-off value, but the suspicion of sarcopenia remains, it is advised to test the hand grip strength. If low, body composition measurement is suggested.

The accessibility to DXA machines varies by countries and hospitals. For clinical use bioelectrical impedance analysis is acknowledged by some, more reluctantly by others. A major point to consider is that the technique to measure body composition should comply with the technique that was used in the reference population in order to define cut-off values.

THE DEVASTATING EFFECTS OF CONCURRENT SARCOPENIA AND OSTEOPOROSIS

The combined effect of sarcopenia and osteoporosis, i.e. 'the hazardous duet' [19], is a devastating threat to the old adult, especially if frail. The sarcopenic propensity for falls may in the end result in an osteoporotic hip fracture. This single event may reduce life expectancy by up to two years [20], corresponding to an excess mortality of 20–25% in the first year after the fracture. One-year mortality after a hip fracture is estimated to 10–15%. Moreover, morbidity is increased and mobility is reduced, leading to increased expected time spent in nursing homes by up to a year [20]. Nine out of ten hip fractures occur in adults >65 years of age and 80% strikes women. The remaining life time risk of a 50-year-old woman sustaining a fragility fracture is 50%, with about one in five being struck by a hip fracture. Life expectancy in affluent societies has increased from around 50 to 80 years during the last century. Linked to this process is the observation that the population aged >65 years grows faster, i.e. 1.9% annually, than any other age group (1.2%). From this it is easy to deduct that fragility fractures will soon or have already reached epidemic levels. The annual rate of hip fractures is estimated to increase world-wide from 1.7 million in 1990 to 6.3 million fractures in 2050 [21].

Hip fractures entail heavy economic burdens on the society, i.e. direct medical costs for fracture care alone represent a greater burden than costs for stroke, breast cancer, diabetes or chronic lung disease [22]. Health economic projections on the societal costs for sarcopenia are not as abundant. However, Janssen et al. used large US cohorts of elderly people and calculated the cost generated by sarcopenia related disability to an astonishing 18.5 billion USD, corresponding to about 1.5% of the total health care expenditures for the corresponding year [23]. The on-going demographic changes in society will increase the societal burdens of sarcopenia and osteoporosis-related illness substantially.

THE CONCERTED PREVENTION AND TREATMENT OF SARCOPENIA AND OSTEOPOROSIS

The best approach to meet the challenge of sarcopenia and osteoporosis in an ageing society is to identify the modifiable factors and focus on measures of primary, secondary and tertiary prevention. Primary prevention of osteoporosis aims at maximizing peak bone mass during adolescence, and to reduce bone loss during middle ages and in early menopause. Conversely, treatment of sarcopenia will markedly reduce societal care burden. The muscle organ system of the aged individual is more plastic and prone for growth and improved function than the skeleton. Nevertheless, both tissues benefit from many common measures. The prevention and treatment of sarcopenia is usually also positive for bone strength, whereas treatment for osteoporosis does not always have corresponding effects on muscles. For example, treatments of osteoporosis with bisphosphonates or raloxifene (a selective estrogen receptor modifier) have so far not displayed positive effects on muscle.

Although genetic factors play a major role for peak bone mass and that the peak is usually determined before the age of 30 years, BMD and bone strength may be influenced later in life. For example, vitamin D from sun exposure, energy and protein intake, and strength training will improve bone strength even in senescence.

Vitamin D and calcium

Osteoporosis

Calcium and vitamin D are crucial nutrients for the bone and usually gain the focus when nutritional measures are discussed. Dairy products and fish are rich in calcium, e.g. a glass of milk contains ~300 mg calcium. Milk products are estimated to provide about 80% of the daily calcium intake. Oily fish is also rich in vitamin D, as is liver, while dairy products are often fortified with vitamin D. National Food Administrations in general advocate a daily food intake of 7.5–10 ug (i.e. 300–400 IU) vitamin D and 800–1200 mg of calcium. In the very old (>80 years old) and in institutionalized elderly people supplementation with 1200 mg calcium and 20 µg (800 IU) vitamin D daily is advocated by most regulatory bodies in several countries. Whether younger postmenopausal women with manifest or with increased risk of osteoporosis should also receive calcium and vitamin D supplementation is today controversial, although such treatment is advocated by many. The most recent Cochrane meta-analysis update 2009 included 45 trials and concluded that 'frail older people confined to institutions may sustain fewer hip fractures if given vitamin D with calcium. Vitamin D alone is unlikely to prevent fracture'. [24] The major vitamin D action for bone is to facilitate gut absorption of calcium. To prevent secondary hyperparathyroidism and subsequent bone resorption circulating vitamin D should not be <50 nmol/l.

Sarcopenia

It is suggested that vitamin D has important roles in muscles as well [25], although the exact mechanisms for such actions are not yet defined. Vitamin D receptors are abundant on muscle fibre membranes, and in vivo models show that exposure to vitamin D triggers muscle protein synthesis [26]. Increased risk of falls is observed with low vitamin D status, and recent meta-analyses indicate that vitamin D treatment reduces the risk of falls [27]. In 2010 the American Institute of Medicine, however, settled that the evidence status at that moment did not permit other indications for vitamin D and calcium treatment than fracture prevention [28].

Nutrient, energy and protein balance

Osteoporosis

Fruit and vegetables contain anti-oxidants and phytoestrogenes, both with potentially beneficial effects on bone health. Although no human intervention studies on fruit and vegetables intake for bone health have been performed it is safe to follow the general recommendation of five servings or 500 g fruit and vegetables/day.

Oily fish contains *n-3 fatty acids* (FA) and these are shown experimentally to have positive effects on BMD. Epidemiologic studies show somewhat conflicting results. For example, longitudinal observations from the Framingham Osteoporosis Study indicated that fish consumption may protect against bone loss in women [29]. Meanwhile cross-sectional data from the large Women's Health Initiative suggest that saturated fat intake may increase hip fracture risk [30]. The evidence status for the moment does not allow for strong recommendations on fat intake according to bone health.

Low body mass index show a strong positive correlation to osteoporosis and fracture risk. For the elderly a sufficient energy intake is needed to avoid weight loss and underweight, i.e. a BMI >22 kg/m² is desirable. Consequently, for thin elderly patients supplementation with energy and protein is recommended, especially for those who are at risk or already have sustained a hip fracture [31].

There is still some controversial evidence on the relation between *protein* and bone health [32], since low and high protein intakes are both suggested to be associated with osteoporosis. According to ecological observations the highest prevalence of fractures is found in countries with the highest protein consumption. It has been suggested that high protein intakes, i.e. >~2 g protein/kg body weight, are associated with increased urinary calcium excretion [33], but the current belief is that this is explained by increased intestinal calcium absorption rather than by increased bone resorption [34]. On the other hand several epidemiological studies show positive associations between protein intake and BMD. For example, again the Framingham data display augmented bone loss with low protein intake;

i.e. persons in the lowest quartile of protein intake had after four years lost 4 % of BMD as compared to 1 % among those in the highest quartile of protein intake [35]. Protein intake below 1 g protein/kg body weight is linked to decreased intestinal calcium absorption and secondary hyperparathyroidism [36]. It appears that an intake of protein between 1–1.5 g/kg body weight is safe and probably optimal for bone health [37]. Thin patients that have sustained a hip fracture increase IGF-I serum concentrations and preserves their BMD by ingesting a protein enriched liquid supplementation [38].

Sarcopenia

Protein is the crucial macronutrient for muscle anabolism, and vitamin D (see above) and n-3 FAs may play as important roles for muscle growth as they do for skeletal anabolism.

About ten years ago there was a great research interest in n-3 FA treatment for cancer cachexia since reports had implicated possible protection against muscle wasting [39]. In 2003 a large RCT in pancreatic cancer patients failed to confirm such effects when intention-to-treat analyses were performed, whereas post-hoc tests clearly indicated positive effects on preserved lean body mass by high serum concentrations of n-3 FAs [40]. Recently a new interest on this potentially effective treatment has arisen, e.g. there are indications that the intake of n-3 FAs is associated with phosphorylation of mTOR, i.e. the key regulator of protein synthesis [41].

Traditional nitrogen balance studies indicate that whole body balance between resorption and excretion of nitrogen is achieved in healthy subjects by an intake of 0.8 g *protein*/kg body weight and day. This long established recommendation has been repeatedly questioned, especially for the old and for ill catabolic patients. Strict intake of 0.8 g protein/kg body weight resulted in urinary nitrogen excretion and radiologic decrease in thigh-muscle cross-sectional area [42]. It is suggested that the old subject has an anabolic resistance to amino acids, justifying an increased intake. It is also shown that the gut and liver retention of amino acids absorbed in the gut is larger for old than for young subjects. Thus less amino acids enter the systemic circulation and become available for the muscle. As described elsewhere in this book intense research is currently performed to resolve the question if protein supplementation in itself or targeted amino acid treatment, like that of leucin has the capacity to increase muscle protein synthesis and increase muscle function [43].

Exercise

The cheapest and most effective measure to counteract both sarcopenia and osteoporosis is exercise.

Bone

The plasticity of the skeleton cannot compare with that of the muscle, still there is compelling evidence that resistance training may improve BMD even in old adults with established osteoporosis. The most recent Cochrane update from 2011 [44] compiles 43 RCTs and concludes that there is a small but possibly important effect of exercise on BMD. A prerequisite for such effects is the unlimited access to calcium, vitamin D and protein. Osteogenic exercise is suggested to be composed by dynamic-not static modules, strain that exceeds a threshold, brief and intermittent bouts of exercise, and by exposure of unusual loading to the bone [45]. Desensitizing is suggested to be crucial, i.e. the training sessions have to actively use rest periods for maximal effect. Interestingly, the mechanosensing apparatus appears to be confined to the osteocytes, i.e. the most abundant cell in the skeleton [46].

Muscle

Sarcopenia is commonly very responsive to progressive resistance training, especially in the old subject. Improvements of strength up to 200% are not unusual, whereas the corresponding increase in muscle mass usually does not exceed 10% in the old adult. The recent Cochrane up-date in 2009 compiling altogether 121 RCTs concludes that resistance training confers 'modest improvement in gait speed', 'moderate-large effect for getting out of chair' and 'large effect on muscle strength' [47]. Exercise and resistance training for the treatment of sarcopenia is described in detail elsewhere in this book.

There is traditionally a pronounced respect or fear of causing injuries by imposing true resistance training for the weak frail sarcopenic old adult. On the contrary, the careful introduction of such activities holds the promise to provide the old frail sarcopenic adult with new vitality and a more independent lifestyle.

CONCLUDING REMARKS

The hazardous duet of osteoporosis and sarcopenia, i.e. the age-related degeneration of the musculo-skeletal system, leading to reduced mobility, risk for falls and subsequent fractures, holds many pathogenic and treatment features in common. Daily physical training combining endurance and resistance exercises, daily outdoor activities providing sun exposure, daily sufficient intake of proteins, e.g. of dairy products, meat, fish, egg, legumes like peas and beans, as well as of antioxidant and phytoestrogene rich fruit and vegetable intake will provide a life-style that will improve muscle fitness, reduce the risk of falls and reduce the fragility fracture risk in the old adult.

REFERENCES

1. Thornell LE. (2010) Sarcopenic obesity: satellite cells in the aging muscle. Curr Opin Clin Nutr Metab Care 14,22–27.
2. Huang Z, Chen X, Chen D. (2011) Myostatin: a novel insight into its role in metabolism, signal pathways, and expression regulation. Cell Signal 23,1441–1446.
3. Franceschi C, Capri M, Monti D et al. (2007) Inflammaging and anti-inflammaging: a systemic perspective on aging and longevity emerged from studies in humans. Mech Ageing Dev 128,92–105.
4. Rachner TD, Khosla S, Hofbauer LC. (2011) Osteoporosis: now and the future. Lancet 377,1276–1287.

5. Guillet C, Boirie Y (2005). Insulin resistance: a contributing factor to age-related muscle mass loss? Diabetes Metab 31, Spec No 2:5S20–5S26.

6. Guillet C, Delcourt I, Rance M et al. (2009) Changes in basal and insulin and amino acid response of whole body and skeletal muscle proteins in obese men. J Clin Endocrinol Metab 94,3044–3050.

7. Glass, DJ. (2010) Signalling pathways perturbing muscle mass. Curr Opin Clin Nutr Metab 13,225–220.

8. Short KR, Nair KS. (2000) The effect of age on protein metabolism. Curr Opin Clin Nutr Metab 3,39–44.

9. World Health Organization. (1994) Assessment of fracture risk and its application to screening for post-menopausal osteoporosis. Geneva, Switzerland: World Health Organization. WHO Technical Report Series 843.

10. Faulkner KG. (2000) Bone matters: are density increases necessary to reduce fracture risk? J Bone Miner Res 15,183–187.

11. Baumgartner RN, Koehler KM, Gallagher D et al. (1998) Epidemiology of sarcopenia among the elderly in New Mexico. Am J Epidemiol 147,755–763.

12. Newman AB, Kupelian V, Visser M et al. (2006) Strength, but not muscle mass, is associated with mortality in the health, aging and body composition study cohort. J Gerontol A Biol Sci Med Sci 61,72–77.

13. Studenski S, Perera S, Patel K et al. (2011) Gait speed and survival in older adults. JAMA 305,50–58.

14. Muscaritoli M, Anker SD, Argiles J et al. (2010) Consensus definition of sarcopenia, cachexia and pre-cachexia: Joint document elaborated by Special Interest Groups (SIG) "cachexia-anorexia in chronic wasting diseases" and "nutrition in geriatrics". Clin Nutr 29,154–159.

15. Cruz-Jentoft A, Baeyens JP, Bauer J et al. (2010) Sarcopenia: European consensus on definition and diagnosis. Age Ageing 39,412–423.

16. Fielding RA, Vellas B, Evans WJ et al. (2011) Sarcopenia: an undiagnosed condition in older adults. Current consensus definition: prevalence, etiology, and consequences. International working group on sarcopenia. J Am Med Dir Assoc 12,249–256.

17. Morley JE, Abbatecola AM, Argiles JM et al. (2011) Sarcopenia with Limited Mobility: An International Consensus. J Am Med Dir Assoc 12,403–409.

18. Wilkins CH, Birge SJ. (2005) Prevention of osteoporosis. Am J Med 118,1190–1195.

19. Crepaldi G, Maggi S. (2005) Sarcopenia and osteoporosis: A hazardous duet. J Endocrinol Invest 28(10 Suppl), 66–68.

20. Braithwaite RS, Col NF, Wong J. (2003) Estimating hip fracture morbidity, mortality and costs. J Am Ger Soc 51,364–370.

21. Prentice A. Diet, nutrition and the prevention of osteoporosis. (2004) Public Health Nutr 7,227–243.

22. Becker DJ, Kilgore ML, Morrisey MA. (2010) The societal burden of osteoporosis. Curr Rheumatol Rep 12,186–191.

23. Janssen I, Shepard DS, Katzmarzyk PT, Roubenoff R. (2004) The healthcare costs of sarcopenia in the United States. J Am Geriatr Soc 52,80–85.

24. Avenell A, Gillespie WJ, Gillespie LD, O'Connell D. (2009) Vitamin D and Vitamin D analogues for preventing fractures associated with involutional and post-menopausal osteoporosis. Cochrane Database Syst Rev CD000227.

25. Dirks-Naylor AJ, Lennon-Edwards S. (2011) The effects of vitamin D on skeletal muscle function and cellular signaling. J Steroid Biochem Mol Biol 125(3–5), 159–168.

26. Ceglia L, da Silva Morais M, Park LK et al. (2010) Multi-step immunofluorescent analysis of vitamin D receptor loci and myosin heavy chain isoforms in human skeletal muscle. J Mol Histol 41(2–3), 137–42.

27. Bischoff-Ferrari HA, Dawson-Hughes B, Staehlen HB et al. (2009) Fall prevention with supplemental and active forms of vitamin D: a meta-analysis of randomised controlled trials. Br Med J 339,b3692

28. Institute of Medicine. (2010) Dietary Reference Intakes for Calcium and Vitamin D. www.iom.edu

29. Farina EK, Kiel DP, Roubenoff R et al. (2011) Protectiv effects of fish intake and interactive effects of long-chain polyunsaturated fatty acid intakes on hip bone mineral density in older adults: the Framingham Osteoporosis Study. Am J Clin Nutr 93,1142–1151.

30. Orchard TS, Cauley JA, Frank GC et al. (2010) Fatty acid consumption and risk of fracture in the Women's Health Initiative. Am J Clin Nutr 92,1452–1460.

31. Avenell A, Handoll HHG. (2010) Nutritional supplementation for hip fracture aftercare in older people. Cochrane Database Syst Rev CD001880.

32. Barzel US, Massey LK. (1998) Excess dietary protein can adversely affect bone. J Nutr 128,1051–1053.

33. Kerstetter JE, O'Brien KO, Insogna KL. (2003) Dietary protein, calcium metabolism, and skeletal homeostasis revisited. Am J Clin Nutr 78(3 Suppl), 584S–592S.

34. Kerstetter JE, O'Brien KO, Caseria DM et al. (2005) The impact of dietary protein on calcium absorption and kinetic measures of bone turnover in women. J Clin Endocrinol Metab 90,26–31.

35. Hannan MT, Tucker KL, Dawson-Hughes B et al. (2000) Effect of dietary protein on bone loss in elderly men and women: The Framingham Osteoporosis Study. J Bone Mineral Res 15,2504–2512.

36. Kerstetter J, O'Brien KO, Insogna KL. (2003) Low protein intake: the impact on calcium and bone homeostasis in humans. J Nutr 133,855S-61S.

37. Gaffney-Stomberg E, Insogna KL, Rodriguez NR, Kerstetter JE. (2009) Increasing dietary protein requirements in elderly people for optimal muscle and bone health. J Am Ger Soc 57,1073–1079.

38. Schurch MA, Rizzoli R, Slosman D et al. (1998) Protein supplements increase serum insulin like growth factor-I levels and attenuate proximal femur bone loss in patients with hip fracture. Ann Intern Med 128,801–809.

39. Wigmore SJ, Barber MD, Ross JA et al. (2000) Effect of oral eicosapentaenoic acid on weight loss in patients with pancreatic cancer. Nutr Cancer 36,177–184.

40. Fearon KC, Von Meyenfeldt MF, Moses AG et al. (2003) Effect of a protein and energy dense N-3 fatty acid enriched oral supplement on loss of weight and lean tissue in cancer cachexia: a randomised double blind trial. Gut 52,1479–1486.

41. Smith GI, Atherton P, Reeds DN et al. (2011) Dietary omega-3 fatty acid supplementation increases the rate of muscle protein synthesis in older adults: a randomized controlled trial. Am J Clin Nutr 93,402–412.

42. Campbell WW, Trappe TA, Wolfe RR, Evans WJ. (2001) The recommended dietary allowance for protein may not be adequate for older people to maintain skeletal muscle. J Gerontol A Biol Sci Med Sci 56,M373–80.

43. Rieu I, Balage M, Sornet C et al. (2006) Leucine supplementation improves muscle protein synthesis in elderly men independently of hyperaminoacidaemia. J Physiol 575,305–315.

44. Howe TE, Shea B, Dawson LJ et al. (2011) Exercise for preventing and treating osteoporosis in postmenopausal women. Cochrane Database Syst Rev 7,CD000333.

45. Borer KT. (2005) Physical activity in the prevention and amelioration of osteoporosis in women: interaction of mechanical, hormonal and dietary factors. Sports Med 35,779–830.

46. Turner CH, Warden SJ, Bellido T et al. (2009) Mechanobiology of the skeleton. Sci Signal 2,pt3.

47. Liu CJ, Latham NK. (2009) Progressive resistance strength training for improving physical function in older adults. Cochrane Database Syst Rev CD002759.

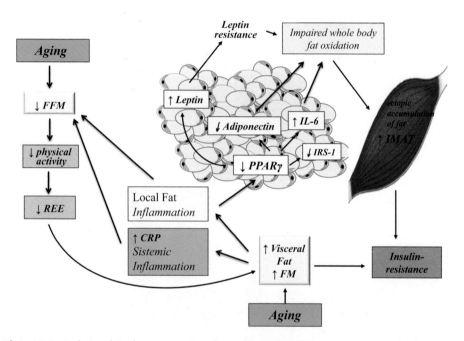

Plate 13.1 Relationships between aging, fat and muscle inflammation. FFM = fat free mass, FM = fat mass, REE = resting energy expenditure, CRP = C reactive protein, IMAT = intermuscular adipose tissue, IRS-1 = insulin receptor substrate-1, IL-6 = interleukine-6, PPAR-γ = peroxisome proliferator-activated receptor gamma.

Sarcopenia, First Edition. Edited by Alfonso J. Cruz-Jentoft and John E. Morley.
© 2012 John Wiley & Sons, Ltd. Published 2012 by John Wiley & Sons, Ltd.

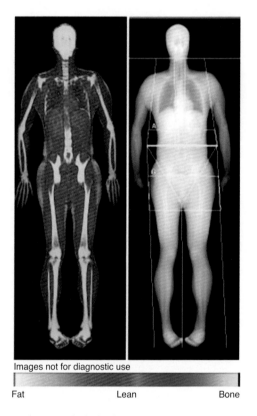

Images not for diagnostic use

Fat   Lean   Bone

Plate 14.1 Patient image from a whole body composition measurement made by a Hologic Discovery a DXA scanner.

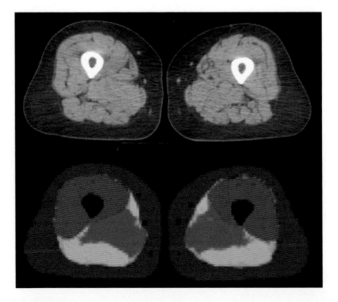

Plate 14.2 Mid thigh CT scans and segmentation of muscle groups using analytic software. Top row: CT scans of mid thigh. Bottom row: Segmentation of main muscle groups, including quadriceps (purple), adductors (grey), hamstrings (yellow) and Sartorius (off white). Red and green pixels are subcutaneous and intermuscular fat respectively.

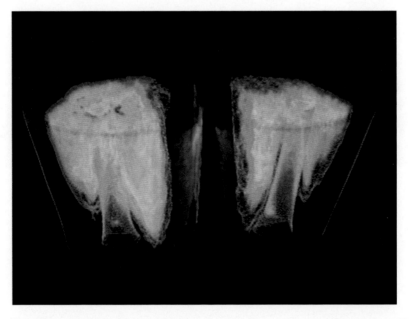

Plate 14.4 Three dimensional reconstruction fan image from the mid-thigh from a PET/CT acquisition using 11C-L-Methyl Methionine (11C-MET) to estimate protein synthesis rate of skeletal muscle. Colored pixels represent uptake of 11C-MET and transparent greyscale represents the delination of the thigh anatomy. This image was obtained of a female subject one hour after completion of unilateral leg resistance exercise of the right leg (left leg on the image). Note increased uptake in exercised leg.

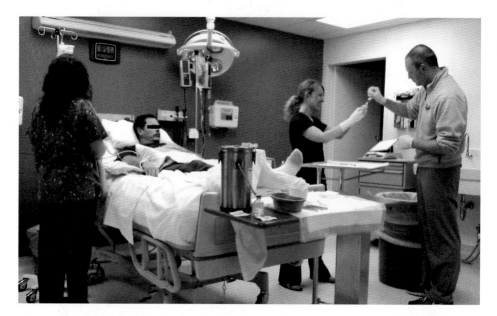

Plate 19.4 Stable isotope methodology can provide a direct assessment of muscle protein anabolism in healthy and clinical populations.

CHAPTER 13

Sarcopenic Obesity

Mauro Zamboni, Andrea P. Rossi and Elena Zoico

Department of Medicine, Geriatric Division, University of Verona, Verona, Italy

INTRODUCTION

The aging of the world population together with the epidemic of obesity, raises serious concern for health care systems in developed countries. The prevalence of obesity in old people has dramatically increased in recent years: in the United States represents nearly 30% in men and in women aged 60 years and over, with an increase also in extreme degrees of obesity [1]. Spain and Italy showed similar patterns in studies carried out between 2006 and 2011 [2,3].

Normal aging itself is associated with a progressive increase in fat mass, which normally peaks at about age 65 years in men and later in women [4]. Body fat distribution also changes with age, with visceral abdominal fat increase, and subcutaneous abdominal fat decrease [5]. Moreover aging is also associated with ectopic fat deposition within non-adipose tissue such as the skeletal and cardiac muscle, liver and pancreas [6,7]. Age related changes in fat deposition occur even without significant changes in body mass index (BMI) or body weight. In the meantime, age associated loss of muscle mass and strength occurs even in relatively weight stable healthy individuals [8].

HOW TO DEFINE SARCOPENIC OBESITY

Years ago, Baumgartner introduced the term of Sarcopenic-Obesity (SO), a condition in which older adults experience both a low muscle mass and a high fat mass [9]. Age-related body composition changes, i.e. muscle mass decline and fat mass increase, in particular when coupled with weight gain, are responsible for this condition [10].

The prevalence of SO in epidemiological studies depends on the definition used (Table 13.1). The definition of SO necessarily should combine those of sarcopenia and obesity. A common definition of sarcopenia and SO was proposed by Baumgartner et al. [10]; SO was defined by concurrence of sarcopenia and high amount of fat mass (i.e.

Sarcopenia, First Edition. Edited by Alfonso J. Cruz-Jentoft and John E. Morley.
© 2012 John Wiley & Sons, Ltd. Published 2012 by John Wiley & Sons, Ltd.

Table 13.1   Different Sarcopenic Obesity definitions and prevalence

Study	Definition of Sarcopenic Obesity	n	Mean age (SD)	Prevalence
New Mexico Aging Process Study	• Sarcopenia: skeletal muscle mass $-2SD$ below mean of young population or <7.26 kg/m^2 in men and <5.45 kg/m^2 in women • Obesity: percentage body fat greater than median or $>27\%$ in men and $>38\%$ in women	831	60 and over	M: 4.4% W: 3.0%
NHANES III	• Sarcopenia: two lower quartiles of muscle mass (<9.12 kg/m^2 in men and <6.53 kg/m^2 in women) • Obesity: two higher quintiles of fat mass ($>37.2\%$ in men and $>40.0\%$ in women)	2982	M: 76.3 (1.7) W: 77.3 (2.2)	M: 9.6% W: 7.4%
Verona, Italy	• Sarcopenia: two lower quintiles of muscle mass (<5.7 kg/m^2 in women) • Obesity: two higher quintiles of fat mass ($>42.9\%$ in women)	167	W: 71.7 (2.4)	W:12.4%
Baltimora Longitudinal Study on Aging	• Impaired strength: lower gender-specifics tertile of handgrip strength (<33kg for men and <20kg for women) • Obesity BMI ≥ 30 kg/m^2	1026	75.8 (7.1)	M: 3.5% W: 6.6%
InCHIANTI, Italy	• Impaired strength: lower gender-specifics tertile of handgrip strength (<32 kg for men and <18 kg for women) • Obesity BMI ≥ 30 kg/m^2	856	74.3 (6.9)	M: 6.3% W: 8.7%
Longitudinal Aging Study Amsterdam	• Impaired strength: lower gender-specifics tertile of handgrip strength (<33 kg for men and <20 kg for women) • Obesity BMI ≥ 30 kg/m^2	1189	75.8 (7.2)	M: 5.1% W: 8.9%
EXERNET Study, Spain	• Sarcopenia: two lower quintiles of muscle mass (<8.61 kg/m^2 in men and <6.19 kg/m^2 in women) • Obesity: two higher quintiles of fat mass ($>30.3\%$ in men and $>40.9\%$ in women)	3176	M: 72.4 (5.5) W: 72.1 (5.2)	M: 17.7% W: 14.0%
Health 2000 Survey, Finland	• Impaired strength: lower gender-specifics tertile of handgrip strength (<322 N for men and <176 N for women) • Obesity BMI ≥ 30 kg/m^2	1413	75.8 (7.1)	M: 6.1% W: 11.0%

percentage of body fat greater than 27% in men and 38% in women or high values of BMI). Sarcopenia was defined by dividing appendicular skeletal muscle mass, as assessed by dual energy X-ray absorptiometry (DXA), by height squared (ASM/h^2), thus obtaining a relative skeletal muscle index. Individuals were defined as having class I sarcopenia when ASM/h^2 was within -1 and -2 standard deviations (SD) of the sex-specific mean of a young reference group, and sarcopenia class II when ASM/h^2 was below -2 SD of the sex specific mean of a young reference group. However, almost 15% of men and women enrolled in the New Mexico Elder Health Survey were considered to be sarcopenic obese when using this definition [9].

Actually, Newman et al. [10] observed that the prevalence of sarcopenia among overweight and obese elderly subjects differed significantly depending on the method used to define sarcopenia. They used two criteria to define sarcopenia: appendicular lean mass (aLM) relative to height squared and aLM relative to height and total fat mass computed from the residuals of the linear regression used to model the relationship between aLM on height and fat mass; a positive residual was indicative of a relatively muscular individual, whereas a negative value indicative of relatively sarcopenic individual [10]. The 20th percentile of the distribution of residuals was used in both cases as the cut-off point for sarcopenia. However, 8.9% of overweight men and 7.1% of overweight women were classified as sarcopenic using the Baumgartner definition of sarcopenia, while 15.4% of overweight men and 21.7% of overweight women were classified as sarcopenic using the method of residuals. Interestingly, none of the subjects with a BMI >30 kg/m^2 was classified as sarcopenic using aLM/h^2, while 11.5% of men and 14.4% of obese women were defined as being sarcopenic using the method of residuals. These findings clearly show that since obese individuals tend to increase amount of fat together with that of fat free mass, even if in an unbalanced way [11], they may have an apparently 'normal' absolute quantity of muscle mass, and they would not appear to be sarcopenic even if their muscle mass is inadequate for their size. As a consequence, higher BMI could mask the presence of sarcopenia, and the definition proposed by Baumgartner et al. [9] may underestimate sarcopenia in overweight and obese subjects, thus leading to an underestimation of SO.

An alternative definition of SO was subsequently suggested by Davison et al. [12], who defined sarcopenic-obese individuals as those in the upper two quintiles of body fat and in the lower three of muscle mass. In a sample of 1391 men and 1526 women aged 70 years and older, they reported a prevalence of SO of 9.6% and 7.4%, respectively. By using a definition of SO in line with that of Davison et al. [12] we also observed a similar prevalence of SO in 167 women aged 67 to 78 years [13].

All the above mentioned SO definitions raise some concern, some related to sarcopenia definition and some others to obesity definition.

Limits related to the definition of sarcopenia:

1. When using a definition of sarcopenia based on the amount of muscle mass, quality of muscle, in terms of fat infiltration (the so called myosteatosis) or fibrosis, is not taken into account (Figure 13.1). It has been documented that the amount of triglycerides in muscle increases with both ageing and obesity [14,15]: mid-thigh low-density lean tissue, a surrogate of muscle fat infiltration, as evaluated by computed tomography, has been observed to be directly associated with age and adiposity [16]. Further, it must be noted that both DXA and BIA, the body composition methods usually recommended for definition of sarcopenia, are not able to recognize neither myosteatosis nor myofibrosis [11].

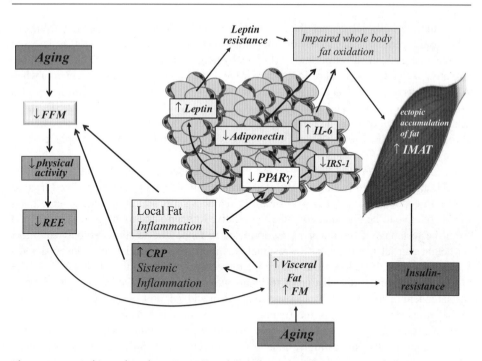

Figure 13.1 Relationships between aging, fat and muscle inflammation. FFM = fat free mass, FM = fat mass, REE = resting energy expenditure, CRP = C reactive protein, IMAT = intermuscular adipose tissue, IRS-1 = insulin receptor substrate-1, IL-6 = interleukine-6, PPAR-γ = peroxisome proliferator-activated receptor gamma. (*A full color version of this figure appears in the color plate section.*)

2. Muscle function in terms of strength and performance is even not taken into account. This raises great concern because it is known that both muscle strength and performance decline more than muscle mass with aging. This concept has been extensively considered by the European Working Group on Sarcopenia in Older People [17], who developed a practical clinical definition of sarcopenia that recommends the presence of both low muscle mass and low muscle function (strength or performance) for the diagnosis of sarcopenia. In line with these recommendations are also recent statements from the International Sarcopenia Consensus Conference Working Group Meeting [18].

Quality of muscle, as evaluated by the ratio between muscle quantity and muscle strength, should be taken into account in particular in obese people. Villareal et al. [19] compared obese elderly subjects, non-obese frail subjects, and normal weight, non-frail subjects and observed that, although obese elderly subjects had higher absolute muscle mass, when compared to the other two groups they showed the poorest muscle quality, as expressed as force per unit of cross-sectional muscle area. They also had reductions in their functional status, aerobic capacity, strength, balance and walking speed in which they were comparable to the group of frail non-obese elders.

It has also been observed that subjects with poor muscle strength were approximately two times more likely to be obese compared to those with normal strength when adjusted for age, gender and body weight [20].

Interestingly, a significantly higher decline in muscle quality, as expressed as force per unit of cross-sectional muscle area, was observed in subjects with diabetes compared with those without in the Health ABC Body Composition Study [21].

Therefore, defining of sarcopenia just based on low muscle mass is likely sub-optimal.

The term Dynapenic Obesity has been coined to define subjects with both high fat mass and low muscle strength [22]. Measurements of both muscle strength and physical performance should be carried out in subjects with overweight and obesity and should be taken carefully into consideration.

Limits related to the definition of Overweight and Obesity:

1. Overweight is defined as BMI ranging between 25 and 30 kg/m^2 and obesity as BMI $\geq$ 30 kg/m^2 [23]. However, there is still debate about the most appropriate indices and cut-off for overweight and obesity in the elderly [24]. Further, as with aging, an increase in abdominal fat and in particular in visceral abdominal fat can be observed, even without changes in BMI, the use of indices of fat distribution may be more representative than those of fat mass degree [24]. Thus, measurements of abdominal circumferences, widely considered good surrogate of fat distribution and in particular of visceral abdominal adipose tissue, may be more adequate than BMI.

   The ratio between ASM/h, as evaluated by DXA, and visceral abdominal adipose tissue, as evaluated by computed tomography, has been recently suggested as a tool for SO definition [25].

2. It should also be noted that obesity in the elderly is not just characterized by visceral abdominal fat increase, but also by ectopic fat deposition (in muscle, liver, pancreas and heart) as well as by subcutaneous fat decline (in some areas of the body).

Theoretically, all these aspects should be taken into account in the definition of SO (Figure 13.2).

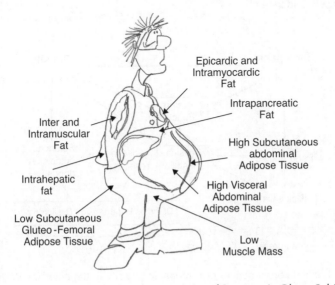

Figure 13.2   Body composition characteristics of Sarcopenic Obese Subjects.

PATHOGENESIS OF SO

The age-related reduction in muscle mass and the increase in fat mass seem to be strictly related to each other from a pathogenic point of view (Figure 13.3).

It is possible to hypothesize that the age-related decrease in muscle mass and strength may lead to reduced physical activity. A reduction in muscle mass and physical activity reduces total energy expenditure and may lead to weight gain [26].

Moreover obesity has been associated with a state of subacute low-grade inflammation, resulting from the secretion of many adipokines that may contribute to the progression of sarcopenia, acting both at a local and at a systemic level. In fact it has been hypothesized that several adipokines, such as TNF-alpha, IL-6 and leptin which are known to influence insulin resistance, energy metabolism and growth hormone secretion, may lead to progressive loss of muscle mass and further increase in fat mass. Schrager et al. [27] demonstrated that the degree and distribution of adiposity can directly affect inflammation and the development and progression of sarcopenia. In the InCHIANTI Study SO was associated with elevated levels of IL-6, CRP, IL-1 receptor antagonist, and soluble IL-6 receptor even after multiple adjustments [27].

An increase in total and central adiposity may lead to sarcopenia, not only decreasing muscle mass quantity but also profoundly affecting muscle quality. From a physiopatho-logical point of view, the main predictors of muscle quality appear to be the degree of Myosteatosis (MS) and Myofibrosis (MF). In fact aging of skeletal muscle is associated with an impairment in muscle quality characterized by an increase in fibrous connective tissue [28], and a reduction in muscle regenerative potential [28], resulting in a progressive replacement of muscle by fibrous connective and adipose tissue.

MS has been observed to be directly and strongly associated with metabolic abnormal-ities, poorer strength and scores on performance tests, as well as with incident mobility disability [20,29]. The mechanisms by which an increase in total body adiposity may lead to an increase in MS and all its unfavorable metabolic and functional consequences, are still not precisely understood.

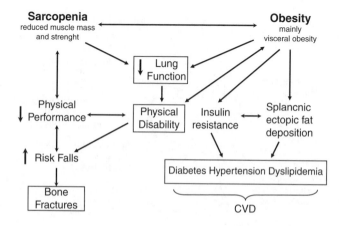

Figure 13.3   Clinical consequences of Sarcopenic Obesity in the elderly. CVD = cardiovas-cular disease.

In a group of healthy overweight and obese elderly men, we recently observed that MS increases with age and adiposity and is associated with the degree of insulin resistance as well as to serum leptin levels [30]. A high serum level of leptin, a marker of leptin resistance, may lead to lower fatty acid oxidation in muscle and consequently to ectopic fat deposition and insulin resistance [31]. In turn this down-regulation of lipid oxidation may lead to an accumulation of lipid metabolites interfering with insulin signaling. In the Health ABC Study population, the degree of thigh intermuscular fat was significantly associated with higher levels of inflammatory markers [32]. We recently found that IL-6 gene expression in subcutaneous adipose tissue near the muscle was positively related to the degree of MS possibly suggesting a prevalent role of tissue inflammation rather than of systemic inflammation [30]. Moreover in our study hs-CRP was negatively related to PPARγ gene expression in SAT, with a consequent down-regulation of adiponectin and up-regulation of IL-6 production in adipose tissue and finally ectopic fat accumulation [30].

MF has not been yet the object of extensive studies even though functional consequences of MF are relevant. MF is associated with a decrease in muscle strength, elasticity and blood supply of muscle fibers, further increasing muscle atrophy [33]. Sections from muscles of mice at different ages showed accumulation of collagen with age, similar to those of myo-dystrophic mice, even though to a lesser extent [28]. Muscle stem cells from aged mice tend to convert more to a fibrogenic lineage compared to cells from young muscles [34]. The pathways involved in this impaired muscle regeneration and enhanced fibrotic response are still incompletely known. Preliminary observations in a small sample of healthy elderly men undergoing elective vertebral surgery seem to show that not only the degree of MS but also the degree of MF were associated with a pattern of increased adiposity, with central fat distribution and a worse metabolic profile (unpublished observations). Elderly sarcopenic subjects with a worse muscle quality hystologically determined presented significantly higher values of BMI, waist circumference and FM (unpublished observations).

CLINICAL IMPLICATIONS OF SO

Functional limitation and disability

Obesity is a risk factor for poor health, reduced functional capacity and quality of life in older persons [24,25]. Analogously, low muscle strength has proven to be a predictor of functional capacity, institutionalization and mortality [17,18]. Thus, it is intuitive that having high levels of fat mass together with low muscle mass may lead to more functional limitations and disability.

Some evidence indicates that when obesity and muscle impairment co-exist they act synergistically on the risk of developing multiple health related outcomes.

For instance, in a cross-sectional study, participants of the New Mexico Aging Process Study cohort, [9] the odds ratios for disability in sarcopenic, obese, and sarcopenic-obese groups, relative to the group of seniors with a normal body composition, were 2.07, 2.33, and 4.12, respectively.

A more recent study by Rolland et al. [35] reinforced these findings by showing that compared with women with a healthy body composition, those with SO had a 2.60 higher odds of having difficulty climbing stairs, 2.35 higher odds of having difficulty going down stairs, and 1.54 higher odds of having moving difficulties.

Baumgartner et al. [36], in an eight-year follow-up of the New Mexico Aging Process Study [36], showed that subjects with SO at baseline were two or three times more likely to develop instrumental disability than lean sarcopenic or non-sarcopenic obese subjects.

Some studies evaluated the joint effect of obesity and poor muscle strength. Increased fat mass percentage and decreased muscle strength in the Finnish Health 2000 Survey was shown to be associated with higher prevalence of walking limitation compared to those with only high fat percentage or low muscle strength [37].

In a cross-sectional study of 2039 men and women aged 55 years and older, where leg extension strength was measured with a dynamometer, 12% of the non dynapenic and non obese group had walking disability, compared with 18% of those with obesity alone, 24% of those with dynapenia, and 36% of those with dynapenic obesity [22]. Interestingly, they [22] observed that dynapenyc obese subjects had a walking speed of approximately 0.14 m/s than the non dynapenic and non obese subjects determining a difference of 2.8 seconds every 20 meters distance.

A study published in 2010 of 904 men and women aged 67–84 years reported that combining handgrip strength and fat mass is the best predictor of a low physical function score, compared with any other body composition and strength marker [38].

When combined, these findings show that dynapenia and obesity have independent, additive and negative effects on physical function.

Pulmonary disease and SO

Obesity has been shown to be associated with worse pulmonary function [24]. Just a few studies evaluated the joint effects of both sarcopenia and SO on pulmonary function. In a longitudinal study involving 77 elderly men and women with BMI ranging from 19.8 to 37 Kg/m^2 evaluated over a seven-year follow-up period, suggesting that the age related combination of FFM loss and fat gain may have additive negative effects on pulmonary function [39].

In a recent longitudinal study it has been shown that not only fat mass increase, but also intermuscular fat infiltration, associated with SO, is negatively related with lung function decline in the elderly, suggesting that age-associated changes in muscle quality, may also in part contribute to worsening pulmonary function among older adults [40].

Taken together, these findings show that SO should be associated with worse pulmonary function. As fat and in particularly abdominal fat are much more deleterious for lung function in a lying position than in a standing position (as obviously evaluated in the above mentioned studies), the negative impact of SO on lung function in the elderly in clinical practice should be even more relevant.

Cardiovascular and metabolic consequences of SO

Association between obesity, metabolic alterations and cardiovascular diseases has been observed even in older ages [23,24]. Some evidence shows association between sarcopenia, both defined as low muscle mass or low muscle strength, and metabolic alterations, in particular diabetes [20].

Only a few studies evaluated the association between SO and metabolic alterations and their findings are not conclusive.

In the cross sectional analysis of the New Mexico Aging Process Study [36], subjects with SO did not show higher incidence of congestive heart disease and hip fracture. Despite the fact that type 2 diabetes was more frequent in SO subjects, the incidence of type 2 diabetes was not affected by the SO status.

Aubertin-Leheudre et al. [41] in a small study sample of postmenopausal women did not observe any difference in cardiovascular and metabolic risk factor profile between obese old women with a normal muscle mass and those with SO.

A longitudinal follow-up study of over 3000 older adults reported that the combination of low muscle mass and abdominal obesity was not associated with an increased risk for the development of cardiovascular disease over an eight-year follow-up period [42].

Recently, association between SO, evaluated as ASM to visceral abdominal fat ratio, metabolic syndrome and arterial stiffness has been observed in 526 apparently healthy adults enrolled in the Korean Sarcopenic Obesity Study, an ongoing prospective observational cohort study [25]. By multiple logistic regression analysis, the odds ratio for metabolic syndrome was 5.43 higher in subjects with SO [25]. These findings seem to suggest that if fat distribution is taken into account in the definition of SO, its association with metabolic syndrome and vascular damage may reach evidence.

It is tempting to speculate that if ectopic fat deposition, besides fat distribution and BMI, could be considered in the SO definition, its association with metabolic alterations could be even more evident. Several studies in fact show strong association between ectopic fat depots and insulin resistance and metabolic risk [6–8].

Mortality risk associated with obesity coupled with poor strength has been evaluated [43] in a 30-years prospective study in initially healthy men. They observed that overweight persons in the lowest grip strength tertile had 1.39 times higher mortality risk compared to normal weight persons in the highest grip strength tertile.

Increased mortality related to SO is an important finding and may help to clarify some un-answered questions about the relation between obesity in old age and mortality [44].

Treatment

Debate has been raised in the past about the hazard of obesity in the elderly and thus about the need for its treatment. However, since SO is associated with poor outcomes, its treatment should be considered. It must be kept in mind that weight loss is usually associated with decline in fat mass, as well as decline in fat free mass and bone [44]. However, it seems crucial that any treatment of SO should reduce fat mass, in particular abdominal fat mass with maintenance of muscle mass function and improvement in its quality.

Some evidence shows that improvement of muscle quality after weight loss as well as of its function may be obtained if physical exercise is combined with dietary counseling and if a weight loss goal is moderate, ranging from 5 to 10% of initial body weight.

Villareal et al. showed that six months weight loss treatment aimed to be no more than 1.5% per week combined with exercise training three times per week (with each session lasting 90 min) ameliorates function and frailty in obese older subjects [45]. We observed that a moderate weight loss (nearly 5%) in a group of elderly women determines a significant improvement in insulin resistance, fat distribution and more importantly of muscle lipid infiltration, with just a small decrease in appendicular lean tissue [46].

No clinical study specifically addressed the topic of SO treatment.

Some recommendations should be considered:

1. Careful clinical examination is mandatory before starting any treatment with weight trajectories examined in each subject as well as usual food intake. It is also important to remember that many chronic conditions of old age may be associated with a wasting period that signals transition to a more severe phase of the disease.
2. Energy restriction must be moderate (with a maximum energy deficit of 500 kcal/day) [23] and a very low hypo-energetic diet should be avoided.
3. Weight loss goal should range between 5 to 10%.
4. Diet should be enriched in high biological value protein (at least 1.2 g/kg/day) and supplementation with leucine-enriched amino-acid essential mixture should be considered.
5. Dietary treatment should be combined with short-term resistance training and aerobic exercise.
6. Supplementation with Vitamin D and calcium is mandatory.

CONCLUSION

With aging, loss of muscle mass and gain in fat seem to be linked each other and contribute, in the presence of positive energy balance, to the development of SO.

Identification of elderly subjects with SO could help to identify a group of subjects with particularly high health risk, and the concept of SO may help to clarify the relation between obesity, morbidity and mortality in the elderly.

Recently, great effort has been done to improve sarcopenia definition in order to get it carried out in the clinical assessment of elderly people. However, similar effort seems to be mandatory also for SO definition.

REFERENCES

1. Ogden CL, Carroll MD, Curtin LR et al. (2006) Prevalence of overweight and obesity in the United States, 1999-2004. JAMA 295, 1549–1555.
2. Micciolo R, Di Francesco V, Fantin F et al. (2010) Prevalence of overweight and obesity in Italy (2001-2008): is there a rising obesity epidemic? Ann Epidemiol 20, 258–264.
3. Gomez-Cabello A, Pedrero-Chamizo R, Olivares PR et al. (2011) Prevalence of overweight and obesity in non-istitutionalized people aged 65 or over from Spain: the elderly EXERNET multi-centre study. Obes Rev 12, 583–592.
4. Prentice AM, Jebb SA. (2001) Beyond body mass index. Obes Rev 2, 141–147.
5. Zamboni M, Armellini F, Harris T et al. (1997) Effects of age on body fat distribution and cardiovascular risk factors in women. Am J Clin Nutr 66, 111–115.
6. Unger RH. (2003) Minireview: weapons of lean body destruction: the role of ectopic lipids in the metabolic syndrome. Endocrinolgy 144, 5159–5165.
7. Rossi AP, Fantin F, Zamboni GA et al. (2011) Predictors of ectopic fat accumulation in liver and pancreas in obese men and women. Obesity 19, 1747–1754.
8. Gallagher D, Ruts E, Visser M et al. (2000) Sarcopenia and weight stability mask in elderly men and women. 279, E366–375.
9. Baumgartner RN. (2000) Body composition in healthy aging. Ann N Y Acad Sci 904, 437–448.

10. Newman AB, Lee JS, Visser M et al. (2005) Weight change and the conservation of lean mass in old age: the Health, Aging and Body Composition Study. Am J Clin Nutr 82, 872–878.

11. Gallagher D, DeLegge M. (2011) Body composition (Sarcopenia) in obese patients: implication for care in the intensive care unit. J Parenter Enter Nutr 35, 21S–8S.

12. Davison KK, Ford ES, Cogswell ME et al. (2002) Percentage of body fat and body mass index are associated with mobility limitations in people aged 70 and older from NHANES III. J Am Geriatr Soc 50, 1802–1809.

13. Zoico E, Di Francesco V, Guralnik JM et al. (2004) Physical disability and muscular strength in relation to obesity and different body composition indexes in a sample of healthy elderly women. Int J Obes 28, 234–241.

14. Cree MG, Newcomer BR, Katsanos CS et al. (2004) Intramuscular and liver triglycerides are increased in the elderly. J Clin Endocrinol Metab 89, 3864–3871.

15. Song MY, Ruts E, Kim J et al. (2004) Sarcopenia and increased adipose tissue infiltration of muscle in elderly African American women. Am J Clin Nutr 79, 874–880.

16. Goodpaster BH, Carlson CL, Visser M et al. (2001) Attenuation of skeletal muscle and strength in the elderly: The Health ABC Study. J Appl Physiol 90, 2157–2165.

17. Cruz-Jentoft AJ, Baeyens JP, Bauer JM et al. (2010) Sarcopenia: European consensus on definition and diagnosis. Age and Ageing 39, 412–423.

18. Fielding RA, Vellas B, Evans WJ et al. (2011) Sarcopenia: an undiagnosed condition in older adults. Current consensus definition: prevalence, etiology, and consequences. International working group on Sarcopenia. J Am Med Dir Assoc 12, 249–256.

19. Villareal DT, Banks M, Siener C et al. (2004) Physical frailty and body composition in obese elderly men and women. Obes Res 12, 91–96.

20. Stenholm S, Harris TB, Rantanen T et al. (2010) Sarcopenic obesity-definition, etiology and consequences. Curr Opin Clin Nutr Metab Care 11, 693–700.

21. Park SW, Goodpaster BH, Strotmeyer ES et al. (2007) Accelerated loss of skeletal muscle strength in older adults with type 2 diabetes: the Health, aging and body composition study. Diabetes Care 30, 1507–1512.

22. Bouchard SR, Janssen J. (2010) Dynapenic-Obesity and Physical Function in older adults. J Gerontol Med Sci 1, 71–77.

23. Villareal DT, Apovian CM, Kushner RF et al. (2005) American Society for Nutrition and NAASO, The Obesity Society. Obesity in older adults: technical review and position statement of the American Society for Nutrition and NAASO, The Obesity Society. Am J Clin Nutr 82, 923–934.

24. Zamboni M, Mazzali G, Zoico E et al. (2005) Health consequences of obesity in the elderly: a review of four unresolved questions. Int J Obes; 29, 1011–1029.

25. Lim KI, Yang SJ, Kim TN et al. (2010) The association between the ratio of visceral fat of thigh muscle area and metabolic syndrome: the Korean sarcopenic obesity study (KSOS). Clinical Endocrinology 73, 588–594.

26. Nair KS. (2005) Aging muscle. Am J Clin Nutr 81, 953–963.

27. Schrager MA, Metter EJ, Simonsick E et al. (2007) Sarcopenic obesity and inflammation in the InCHIANTI study. J Appl Physiol 102, 919–925.

28. Goldspink G, Fernandes K, Williams PE et al. (1994) Age-related changes in collagen gene expression in the muscles of mdx dystrophic and normal mice. Neuromuscul Disord 4, 183–191.

29. Goodpaster BH, Thaete FL, Kelley DE. (2000) Thigh adipose tissue distribution is associated with insulin resistance in obesity and type 2 diabetes mellitus. Am J Clin Nutr 71, 885–892.

30. Zoico E, Rossi A, Di Francesco V et al. (2010) Adipose tissue infiltration in skeletal muscle of healthy elderly men: relationship with body composition, insulin resistance, and inflammation at the sistemic and tissue level. J Gerontol Med Sci 3, 295–299.

31. Unger RH. (2005) Longevity, lipotoxicity and leptin: the adipocyte defense against feasting and famine. Biochimie 87, 57–64.

32. Beasley LE, Koster A, Newman AB et al. (2009) The Health ABC Study. Inflammation and race and gender differences in computerized tomography-measured adipose depots. Obesity 17, 1062–1069.

33. Huard J, Li Y, Fu FH. (2002) Muscle injuries and repair: current trends in research. J Bone Joint Surg Am 84, 822–832.

34. Brack AS, Conboy MJ, Roy S et al. (2007) Increased Wnt signaling during aging alters muscle stem cell fate and increases fibrosis. Science 317, 807–810.

35. Rolland Y, Lauwers-Cances V, Cristini C et al. (2009) Difficulties with physical function associated with obesity, sarcopenia, and sarcopenic-obesity in community-dwelling elderly women: the EPIDOS study. Am J Clin Nutr 89, 1895–1900.

36. Baumgartner RN, Wayne SJ, Waters DL et al. (2004) Sarcopenic obesity predicts instrumental activities of daily living disability in the elderly. Obes Res 12, 1995–2004.

37. Stenholm S, Rantanen T, Heliövaara M et al. (2008) The mediating role of C-reactive protein and handgrip strength between obesity and walking limitation. J Am Geriatr Soc 56, 462–469.

38. Choquette S, Bouchard DR, Doyon CY et al. (2010) Relative strength as a determinant of mobility in elders 67–84 years of age. A nuage study: nutrition as a determinant of successful aging. J Nutr Health Aging 14, 190–195.

39. Rossi A, Fantin F, Di Francesco V, et al. (2008) Body composition and pulmonary function in the elderly: a 7-year longitudinal study. Int J Obes 32, 1423–1430.

40. Rossi AP, Watson NL, Newman AB et al. (2011) Effects of body composition and adipose tissue distribution on respiratory function in elderly men and women: the health, aging and body composition study. J Gerontol A Biol Sci Med Sci 66, 801–808.

41. Aubertin-Leheudre M, Lord C, Goulet EDB et al. (2006) Effect of sarcopenia on cardiovascular disease risk factors in obese postmenopausal women. Obesity 14, 2277–2283.

42. Stephen WC, Janssen I. (2009) Sarcopenic-obesity and cardiovascular disease risk in the elderly. J Nutr Health Aging 13, 460–466.

43. Rantanen T, Guralnik JM, Foley D et al. (1999) Midlife hand grip strength as a predictor of old age disability. JAMA 281, 558–560.

44. Zamboni M, Mazzali G, Fantin F et al. (2008) Sarcopenic obesity: a new category of obesity in the elderly. Nutr Metab Cardiovasc Dis 18, 388–395.

45. Villareal DT, Banks M, Sinacore DR et al. (2006) Effect of weight loss and exercise on frailty in obese older adults. Arch Intern Med 166, 860–866.

46. Mazzali G, Di Francesco V, Zoico E et al. (2006) Interrelations between fat distribution, muscle lipid content, adipocytokines, and insulin resistance: effect of moderate weight loss in older women. Am J Clin Nutr 84, 1193–1199.

CHAPTER 14

Imaging of Skeletal Muscle

Thomas F. Lang
University of California, San Francisco, San Francisco, USA

INTRODUCTION

Modern definitions of sarcopenia describe it as the loss of physical function secondary to loss of muscle quantity. The quantity of muscle may be assessed using DXA, CT or MRI. DXA is a two-dimensional measurement which assesses the masses of lean, fat and osseous components in the body. CT and MRI are three-dimensional modalities that can assess muscle cross-sectional area or volume, depending on whether the acquisition techniques involve single section or volumetric imaging. In addition to muscle mass, CT, MRI and MRS can be employed to assess the composition of skeletal muscle, in particular the extent of adipose infiltration of skeletal muscle tissue and the distribution of the adipose content between and within specific muscle groups, as well as the partition of intramuscular triglyceride between adipoctyes, and the skeletal muscle fibers themselves. MRS and PET may be utilized to study the metabolic activity of skeletal muscle tissue, including production of ATP/ADP as well as glucose and amino acid metabolism.

DUAL X-RAY ABSORPTIOMETRY

Dual x-ray absorptiometry (DXA) is an accurate, clinically available method of assessing body composition at any anatomic site [1]. Originally developed to assess bone mineral density (BMD), DXA was introduced in the late 1980s and has become the mainstay of osteoporosis diagnosis and clinical evaluation worldwide. In the DXA concept, x-rays with a bimodal energy spectrum, obtained either by rare-earth filtration [2] of an x-ray tube, or rapid switching of kVp [3], are passed through the body. The DXA scanner has a detector system which measures the attenuation of the 'high' and 'low' energy x-rays by the object being scanned, determining the difference in attenuation of the two x-ray energies. With this technique, bone can readily be differentiated from soft tissue on the basis of this attenuation difference. By relating these measurements to calibration standards, it is possible to measure the mass of bone in grams at each point or pixel of the projectional image. An areal bone density in g/cm^2 is obtained by determining a region of interest, such as the lumbar, spine or the femoral neck, and dividing the total mass in g summed across all the pixels in the region by the region's area in cm^2. Starting in the early 1990s, prospective studies have documented the association of areal BMD with incident osteoporotic fracture and have documented therapy responses to anti-resorptives and other osteoporosis medications [4]. DXA has been widely adopted in the clinical setting due to its low cost, high reliability and a radiation dose which is close to daily background radiation and much smaller than that received during a transatlantic flight.

In those regions of the image that have no bone, it is possible to use the differential x-ray absorption measurement described above to separate lean from fat tissue. This composition measurement is used both to correct BMD values for the variability introduced by the adipose content of soft tissue which overlies bone, as well as to generate quantitative image maps of the composition of soft tissue [1,5]. For correction of BMD measurements, the ratio of adipose/lean tissue adjacent to the bone is extrapolated to the region directly above the bone, where only the total mass of soft tissue has been quantified. Applying this ratio to the soft tissue mass allows for the estimation of adipose, lean and bone tissue mass in skeletal regions. When this three compartment estimate is joined to the adipose and lean tissue measurements from the non-bone regions, a full three compartment body composition estimate can be made. Body composition measurements require a whole body scan. Analytic software is then used to partition the bone, adipose and lean content into anatomic segments, including the trunk, pelvis limbs etc (Figure 14.1). Generally, the precision for body composition measurements by commercial scanners is quite good, with values of roughly 1% for bone content and 2–3% for lean and adipose content. The algorithms to accomplish these partitions, the precision, and the sources of error vary between DXA manufacturers, and the reader is referred to technical papers that describe this approach, along with its strengths and limitations [1,5–10].

Constant hydration is an assumption common to all DXA body composition measurements [11]. DXA systems assume that the hydration of fat free mass is constant at 73%, although there is a small amount of normal variation in this property which does not appear to introduce clinically significant errors into the measurement. However, pathologic over- or under-hydration can introduce errors into the percentage fat estimates. Clinically, such conditions can be caused by excessive water retention or edema. DXA software enables one to determine bone mineral and soft-tissue composition in different regions of the body.

DXA body composition measurements have been widely employed to track the changes in lean and fat mass associated with sarcopenia [12–18]. In the limbs, the lean tissue mass is employed as a surrogate for muscle mass, and these appendicular mass measurements have been employed in early attempts to establish the definition and prevalence of sarcopenia, to track the loss of skeletal muscle with age, and to estimate the association of low skeletal muscle mass with prevalent and incident functional impairments, with falls and with sarcopenia-related skeletal conditions such as osteoporosis and skeletal fracture. However, as shown in the following sections, an estimate of skeletal muscle mass alone is of limited value in understanding the relationship between the status of skeletal muscle tissue and the functional impairments associated with sarcopenia [19]. Other image-based techniques can be used to combine a mass estimate with measures of tissue composition and metabolism which greatly improve the detail in the clinical portrait of sarcopenia.

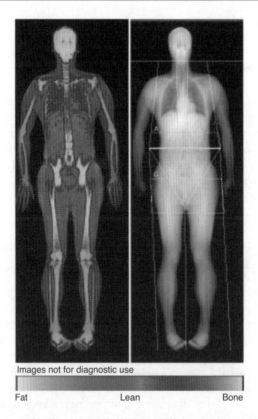

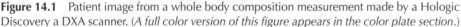

Figure 14.1 Patient image from a whole body composition measurement made by a Hologic Discovery a DXA scanner. (*A full color version of this figure appears in the color plate section.*)

COMPUTED TOMOGRAPHY (CT)

CT is a three-dimensional x-ray absorptiometric measurement which provides the distribution of linear attenuation coefficient in thin cross-sections of tissue [20]. In the transverse plane, the object being scanned is contained within a fan of x-rays defined between the individual elements of the detector array and the x-ray source. The detector array consists of multiple rows of detectors, which depending on the model of CT scanner, typically ranges from 16 to 256 rows that extend in the direction of the table axis. Modern CT scanners are typically based on 'helical' acquisitions, where the detector array and x-ray tube rotate while the table continuously translates the subject along the z-axis [21]. At distinct intervals (typically 360 per gantry rotation), the attenuation of the x-ray beams between the x-ray spot and the individual x-ray detectors is measured by the system. This attenuation measurement is the logarithm of the measured intensity of the x-ray beam with the subject in place to the intensity measured in air. The rotation of the x-ray tube and detector thus acquire a helix of data around the subject and interpolative techniques which employ data from the multiple rows of detector arrays are employed to fill in the gaps between the arms of the helices and generate a fully cylindrical volume of encasing the subject. The volume of data is reconstructed into cross sections of varying thickness, ranging from 0.5 mm to 10 mm depending on the specific clinical imaging requirements. These cross-sections are sampled into square matrices of picture elements, or 'pixels'. Because the image represents a slice of tissue, the picture elements have a thickness, and thus are volume elements, or 'voxels'. The dimensions of the voxels may be adjusted depending on the size of the organ being imaged. Depending on the type of scanner, the voxel dimensions range from the μM level to roughly 1 mm 'in plane' and up to several mm in slice thickness. In the resulting CT image, the voxel values map to linear attenuation coefficient, a measure of density and electron density of the tissue. Because these linear attenuation coefficients depend on the effective x-ray energy (which varies between CT scanner models and different kVp settings of the same scanner), a simple scale, known as the Hounsfield scale, is used to standardize them. The gray-scale value of each voxel is represented as a Hounsfield Unit, which is defined as the difference of the linear attenuation coefficient of a given voxel from that of water, divided by the linear attenuation coefficient of water. The HU scale is a linear scale in which air has a value of -1000, water 0, muscle 30, with bone typically ranging from 300 to 3000 units.

The value of the Hounsfield unit for a given tissue type depends on several technical factors. First, if the sizes of the structures in the tissue are smaller than the dimensions of the voxel, the HU value is subject to partial volume averaging, in which the HU value is the average HU of the constituent tissues of the voxel, weighted by their volume fractions. For example, a 0.78mm x 0.78mm x10mm voxel of trabecular bone is a mixture of bone, collagen, cellular marrow and fatty marrow, and HU is the volume-weighted average of these four constituents. Beam hardening is a second source of variation in HU. In a CT image, the result of this is that for the same tissue, attenuation coefficients at the outside of the patient are systematically higher than those in the interior. Although manufacturers of CT equipment have implemented beam-hardening corrections, the efficacy of these corrections varies between manufacturers and between technical settings on different machines.

CT imaging may be employed to quantify bulk characteristics of muscle and body composition that are highly related to muscle strength and to overall functional ability in the elderly. In particular, CT imaging is widely used to study muscle and fat in epidemiologic studies of body composition. Typically, acquisitions have included single cross sections at the L1/2 or L4/5 intervertebral space to image body fat or volumetric measurements obtained in the abdomen and in the thigh, usually relating to the midthigh or to a bony landmark [22–28]. As shown in Figure 14.2, the key variables quantified include the total muscle CSA of the midthigh, the CSA values of the quadriceps and hamstrings, the total CSA of subcutaneous fat, and the attenuation coefficients of the total thigh muscle and the hamstrings and quadriceps separately. The CSA values of the total thigh muscle and quadriceps muscle are positively associated with increasing knee extensor strength.

The CSA declines with age, as does the muscle strength, and is smaller in females than in males [22–24]. Another property of great interest to the study of sarcopenia is the mean attenuation coefficient, which is computed within all of the muscle regions after a threshold is applied to exclude depots of fat embedded within each muscle group. In elderly subjects, the mean attenuation coefficient, when calculated in this manner, has been shown histologically to correspond to fat accumulation within and between the muscle cells. The increasing fat infiltration into the muscle with aging may be an important, if not central, aspect of sarcopenia [22–24,29]. Lower values of the mean thigh muscle attenuation coefficient correspond to increasing fattiness of muscle tissue. Decreasing thigh muscle attenuation is correlated to decreasing muscle strength, a relationship which

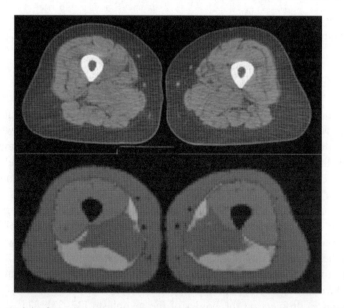

Figure 14.2 Mid thigh CT scans and segmentation of muscle groups using analytic software. Top row: CT scans of mid thigh. Bottom row: Segmentation of main muscle groups, including quadriceps (purple), adductors (grey), hamstrings (yellow) and Sartorius (off white). Red and green pixels are subcutaneous and intermuscular fat respectively. (*A full color version of this figure appears in the color plate section.*)

is independent of the muscle CSA and the total amount of adipose tissue in the thigh. Measures of CSA and muscle attenuation assessed at multiple skeletal sites are associated with indices of functional capacity in elderly adults, including chair stand and leg strength measurements which have been shown to be strongly predictive of falls [26–28]. Several studies based on the Health, Aging, and Body Composition Study, a large NIH-funded population study, have related measures of body composition derived by CT to indices of functional ability and quality of life in the independently living elderly. Visser et al. examined the relationship between measures of thigh composition and lower-extremity performance (LEP), assessed by two timed tests: a series of five chair stands without use of arms and a 6-m walk [28]. Reduced thigh CSA was associated with poorer LEP, as was reduced thigh muscle attenuation coefficient, even after the adjustment for muscle area. The attenuation coefficient of thigh muscle is not only related to current physical performance but is also related to incident functional decline. Analyzing longitudinal data from the Health ABC study, Visser et al. observed that low baseline values of thigh muscle attenuation predicted incident mobility limitation, defined as inability to walk one-quarter mile or climb ten steps [27]. These data on mobility limitations are consistent with later studies that examined association of muscle attenuation with incident fracture. Lang et al. showed that reduced attenuation of the thigh muscle was associated with incident hip fracture [30], and Schafer et al. showed that reduced thigh muscle attenuation was associated with clinical fractures in elderly subjects with diabetes [31]. Reduced thigh muscle attenuation coefficient is also associated with increased insulin resistance and the presence of metabolic syndrome in the elderly. Diabetes and other weight-related health conditions are associated with poor vision, musculoskeletal pain, and other conditions which are themselves indicators of increased fall risk [22].

MAGNETIC RESONANCE IMAGING

MRI is an imaging technique that is based on using radio waves to excite protons in the presence of an external magnetic field. The resonance frequency at which protons maximally absorb the radioenergy is based on their local chemical environment. Because musculoskeletal tissues are rich in proton-containing molecules such as muscle proteins and lipids, MRI is an inherently powerful tool at depicting the anatomy of muscle tissues, particularly in the delineation of lean and adipose components of muscles. While some investigators have used 3D MRI acquisitions to determine lean tissue and intermuscular fat volumes in a range of applications, the true advantage of MRI is the ability to obtain spectroscopic data that can probe in vivo the ATP-generating functions within skeletal muscle and the storage of important nutrients such as lipid and glycogen.

Proton magnetic resonance spectroscopy (1H-MRS) is a technique that can differentiate lipids stored within adipocytes (extramyocellular lipid, EMCL) from intramyocellular lipid (IMCL) stored as droplets on the border of the myoplasm [32–35]. This differentiation is based on the variance in resonance frequency between protons contained in relatively cylindrical deposits of EMCL in adipocytes and protons contained in IMCL deposits which are spherical in shape. These resonances show up as different peaks on the proton spectrum of skeletal muscle (Figure 14.3). Probing IMCL is of clinical importance because IMCL stores represent lipid which borders mitochondria and which represent an energy supply of free fatty acids for oxidation. IMCL intensity determined by 1H-MRS has been found to correlate with insulin resistance and obesity. The risk of insulin resistance is known to increase with age, and aging skeletal muscle is characterized by decreasing oxidative capacity that may lead to increased IMCL. MRS may also be used to detect resonances of 31P and 13C nuclei contained in ATP, ADP inorganic phosphate, glycogen, and other chemical forms in skeletal muscle estimate the intracellular pH, as well as the free concentrations of ADP and $Mg2+$ ions. These measurements allow the technique to be used to estimate rates of ATP synthesis under ischemic (glycogenolytic) conditions or aerobic (oxidative) conditions. Other applications in skeletal muscle studies include estimates of the oxidative capacity of skeletal muscle, as well as the proton efflux and buffer capacity, which provide insight into the recovery of skeletal muscle from exercise. The wide chemical shift of the 13C resonance allows 13C-MRS to assess the relative abundances of a wide range of molecules related to glycogen synthesis and glycogenolysis. Using the natural abundance (1.1%) of 13C, it is possible to detect resonances of 13C in glycogen and triglyceride. This allows for estimates of glycogen turnover in skeletal muscle and for studies of insulin resistance and type 2 diabetes. By administration of 13C glucose, it is possible to enrich 13C, allowing for more advanced determinations, such as examining glycogen synthesis rate and quantifying organelle and mitochondrial activity during the TCA cycle cells, shedding important light on muscle metabolism. 31PMRS can be used to directly analyze relative abundances of 31P contained in compounds of interest to energetics of skeletal muscle, including ATP, inorganic phosphate, and phosphocreatine [32,36–40].

Other physiologic measurements that can be obtained with MRI include fiber microstructure, blood flow and ion fluxes. Diffusion-weighted tensor imaging (DTI) was developed to

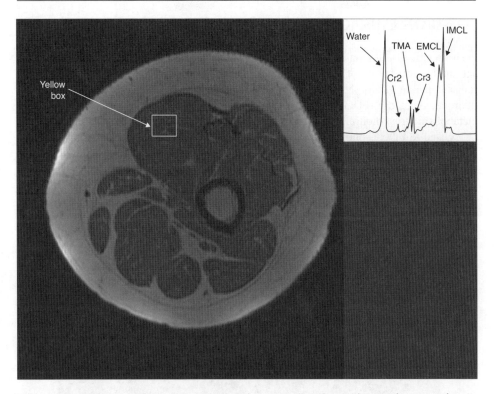

Figure 14.3 MRI image of distal femur at left showing yellow box indicating location of spectroscopic acquisition of the quadriceps muscle. Proton spectroscopy studies may be used to assess the relative amounts of intra and extramyocellular lipid. At right, a proton spectrum corresponding to the soleus muscle shows 1H resonances associated with creatinine (CR2 and CR3), water, extramyocellular lipid (EMCL), intramyocellular lipid (IMCL) and trimethylamines (TMA).

study the microstructural ordering of the white matter tracts of the central nervous system. DTI images are based on the anisotropy of the diffusion of water and tissues that have distinctly ordered microstructures, such as the white matter of the brain, display anisotropic diffusion properties. Recently, improved clinical scanners and acquisition methods have permitted this approach to be extended to the study of skeletal muscles. Studies have examined the potential application to fiber tracking to measure fiber length, cross-sectional area and pennation angles [41–45]. Arterial Spin Labelling (ASL) and Blood Oxygen Level Dependent (BOLD) imaging can be used to study blood flow in skeletal muscle. ASL imaging provides a signal which is proportional to perfusion [46–49], whereas the signal in BOLD imaging depends on a combination of microvascular density, blood flow and volume and rate of oxygen extraction [50–55]. ASL has been employed to study changes in perfusion during and after exercise, and BOLD imaging has been applied to study impaired blood flow in degenerative muscle disorders. 23Na imaging has been applied to study disorders of muscle associated with impairment of ion channel function [56]. In this application, increases in the 23Na signal intensity are associated with muscle membrane depolarization in muscle myotonia and paramyotonia, indicating that MRI imaging can be used to image cellular changes in muscle function.

POSITRON EMISSION TOMOGRAPHY

Positron emission tomography (PET) is an imaging technique which is employed to image the biodistribution of a compound of interest labeled with a positron-emitting atom, for example an 18F or 11C. The most commonly employed PET imaging agent is 18F-fluorodeoxyglucose (FDG), a glucose analog which is widely employed to study glucose metabolism across multiple tissue types. 18FFDG penetrates the cell membrane and is phosphorylated to FDG-6-phosphate and is no longer metabolized and thus is trapped within the cell. It builds up in the cell in proportion to the rate of glucose transport across the cell membrane and also in relation to the activities of hexokinase and glucose-6-phospotase within the cell. In skeletal muscle, FDG imaging has been employed to study glucose utilization. When used in conjunction with compartmental modeling, this approach has been employed to dissect the rate of glucose utilization in terms of the components of cell membrane transport and phosphorylative activity in insulin resistance associated with both obesity and diabetes [57,58]. 11C-acetate imaging has been employed to measure perfusion and oxygen utilization of skeletal muscle tissue [59]. Another application of PET which is relevant to skeletal muscle is the use of 11C-methyl-methionine to estimate the rate of protein synthesis (Figure 14.4). This agent accumulates in skeletal muscle as 11C-labeled protein, and the use of this methylated agent has advantages over radiolabeled leucine in

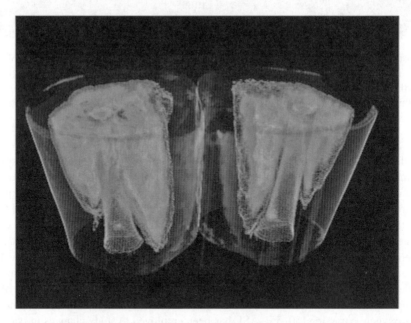

Figure 14.4   Three dimensional reconstruction fan image from the mid-thigh from a PET/CT acquisition using 11C-L-Methyl Methionine (11C-MET) to estimate protein synthesis rate of skeletal muscle. Colored pixels represent uptake of 11C-MET and transparent greyscale represents the delination of the thigh anatomy. This image was obtained of a female subject one hour after completion of unilateral leg resistance exercise of the right leg (left leg on the image). Note increased uptake in exercised leg. (*A full color version of this figure appears in the color plate section.*)

that the latter accumulates in the blood as 11Clabeled CO_2. Fischmann and others have validated this technique against skeletal muscle biopsy and have used it to outline the rate of skeletal muscle protein synthesis in healthy young volunteers [60].

CONCLUSION

In summary, imaging can be used to derive skeletal muscle tissue properties of relevance to aging and sarcopenia. While DXA may be used to characterize skeletal muscle mass at appendicular sites, three dimensional techniques such as CT, MRI and PET allow direct characterization of skeletal muscle tissue at multiple anatomic sites, including both central and peripheral anatomy. These characterizations not only include muscle mass, a parameter which is clinically important but which has limited value to predict deleterious outcomes of sarcopenia, but also muscle metabolism measures which may have the potential to improve our ability to predict outcomes and to better understand the mechanisms underlying clinical interventions. The advent of multi-modality imaging such as PET/CT and PET/MRI, allow for the ability to improve our mapping of functional measures to anatomy, as well as to spatially correlate multiple metabolic measures of skeletal muscle.

REFERENCES

1. Chun KJ. Bone densitometry. Semin Nucl Med 2011;41:220–228.
2. Mazess RB, Collick B, Trempe J, Barden H, Hanson J. Performance evaluation of a dual energy x-ray bone densitometer. Calcif Tissue Int 1989;44:228–232.
3. Stein JA, Lazewatsky JL, Hochberg AM. Dual energy x-ray bone densitometer incorporating an internal reference system. Radiology 1987;165(P):313.
4. Black D, Cummings S, Karpf D, Cauley Jea. Randomised trial of effect of alendronate on risk of fracture in women with existing vertebral fractures. The Lancet 1996; 348.
5. Andreoli A, Scalzo G, Masala S, Tarantino U, Guglielmi G. Body composition assessment by dual-energy X-ray absorptiometry (DXA). Radiol Med 2009;114:286–300.
6. Blake GM, Fogelman I. Technical principles of dual energy x-ray absorptiometry. Semin Nucl Med 1997;27:210–228.
7. DeVita MV, Stall SH. Dual-energy X-ray absorptiometry: a review. J Ren Nutr 1999;9:178–181.
8. Lohman TG, Harris M, Teixeira PJ, Weiss L. Assessing body composition and changes in body composition. Another look at dual-energy X-ray absorptiometry. Ann N Y Acad Sci 2000;904:45–54.
9. Pietrobelli A, Formica C, Wang Z, Heymsfield SB. Dual-energy X-ray absorptiometry body composition model: review of physical concepts. Am J Physiol 1996;271:E941–51.
10. Albanese CV, Diessel E, Genant HK. Clinical applications of body composition measurements using DXA. J Clin Densitom 2003;6:75–85.
11. Pietrobelli A, Wang Z, Formica C, Heymsfield SB. Dual-energy X-ray absorptiometry: fat estimation errors due to variation in soft tissue hydration. Am J Physiol 1998;274:E808–16.
12. Abellan van Kan G. Epidemiology and consequences of sarcopenia. J Nutr Health Aging 2009;13:708–712.
13. Abellan van Kan G, Andre E, Bischoff Ferrari HA, et al. Carla Task Force on Sarcopenia: propositions for clinical trials. J Nutr Health Aging 2009;13:700–707.

14. Aubertin-Leheudre M, Lord C, Labonte M, Khalil A, Dionne IJ. Relationship between sarcopenia and fracture risks in obese postmenopausal women. J Women Aging 2008;20:297–308.

15. Di Monaco M, Vallero F, Di Monaco R, Tappero R. Prevalence of sarcopenia and its association with osteoporosis in 313 older women following a hip fracture. Arch Gerontol Geriatr 2011;52:71–74.

16. Frisoli A, Jr., Chaves PH, Ingham SJ, Fried LP. Severe osteopenia and osteoporosis, sarcopenia, and frailty status in community-dwelling older women: results from the Women's Health and Aging Study (WHAS) II. Bone 2011;48:952–957.

17. Kenny AM, Dawson L, Kleppinger A, Iannuzzi-Sucich M, Judge JO. Prevalence of sarcopenia and predictors of skeletal muscle mass in nonobese women who are long-term users of estrogen-replacement therapy. J Gerontol A Biol Sci Med Sci 2003;58:M436–40.

18. Walsh MC, Hunter GR, Livingstone MB. Sarcopenia in premenopausal and postmenopausal women with osteopenia, osteoporosis and normal bone mineral density. Osteoporos Int 2006;17:61–67.

19. Woods JL, Iuliano-Burns S, King SJ, Strauss BJ, Walker KZ. Poor physical function in elderly women in low-level aged care is related to muscle strength rather than to measures of sarcopenia. Clin Interv Aging 2011;6:67–76.

20. Hsieh J. Computed tomography. Bellingham, WA: SPIE Optical Engineering Press; 2002.

21. Multidetector-row computed tomography scanning and contrast protocols. Springer, 2005. (Accessed at http://www.myilibrary.com?id=31271.)

22. Goodpaster BH, Brown NF. Skeletal muscle lipid and its association with insulin resistance: what is the role for exercise? Exerc Sport Sci Rev 2005;33:150–154.

23. Goodpaster BH, Kelley DE, Thaete FL, He J, Ross R. Skeletal muscle attenuation determined by computed tomography is associated with skeletal muscle lipid content. J Appl Physiol 2000;89:104–110.

24. Goodpaster BH, Park SW, Harris TB, et al. The loss of skeletal muscle strength, mass, and quality in older adults: the health, aging and body composition study. J Gerontol A Biol Sci Med Sci 2006;61:1059–1064.

25. Taaffe DR, Henwood TR, Nalls MA, Walker DG, Lang TF, Harris TB. Alterations in Muscle Attenuation following Detraining and Retraining in Resistance-Trained Older Adults. Gerontology 2008.

26. Visser M, Deeg DJ, Lips P, Harris TB, Bouter LM. Skeletal muscle mass and muscle strength in relation to lower-extremity performance in older men and women. J Am Geriatr Soc 2000;48:381–386.

27. Visser M, Goodpaster BH, Kritchevsky SB, et al. Muscle mass, muscle strength, and muscle fat infiltration as predictors of incident mobility limitations in well-functioning older persons. J Gerontol A Biol Sci Med Sci 2005;60:324–333.

28. Visser M, Kritchevsky S, Goodpaster B, et al. Leg muscle mass and composition in relation to lower extremity performance in men and women aged 70–79: The Health Aging and Body Composition Study. J Amer Ger Society 2002;50:897–905.

29. Goodpaster BH, Carlson CL, Visser M, et al. Attenuation of skeletal muscle and strength in the elderly: The Health ABC Study. J Appl Physiol 2001;90:2157–2165.

30. Lang T, Cauley JA, Tylavsky F, Bauer D, Cummings S, Harris TB. Computed tomographic measurements of thigh muscle cross-sectional area and attenuation coefficient predict hip fracture: the health, aging, and body composition study. J Bone Miner Res 2010;25:513–519.

31. Schafer AL, Vittinghoff E, Lang TF, et al. Fat infiltration of muscle, diabetes, and clinical fracture risk in older adults. J Clin Endocrinol Metab 2010;95:E368–72.

32. Boesch C. Musculoskeletal spectroscopy. J Magn Reson Imaging 2007;25:321–338.

33. Machann J, Stefan N, Schick F. (1)H MR spectroscopy of skeletal muscle, liver and bone marrow. Eur J Radiol 2008;67:275–284.

34. Torriani M. Measuring muscle lipids with 1H-MR spectroscopy. Skeletal Radiol 2007;36:607–608.

35. Weis J, Johansson L, Ortiz-Nieto F, Ahlstrom H. Assessment of lipids in skeletal muscle by high-resolution spectroscopic imaging using fat as the internal standard: comparison with water referenced spectroscopy. Magn Reson Med 2008;59:1259–1265.

36. Bendahan D, Mattei JP, Guis S, Kozak-Ribbens G, Cozzone PJ. [Non-invasive investigation of muscle function using 31P magnetic resonance spectroscopy and 1H MR imaging]. Rev Neurol (Paris) 2006;162:467–484.

37. Brosseau OE, Mahdjoub R, Seurin MJ, Thiriet P, Gozal D, Briguet A. Kinetics of anaerobic metabolism in human skeletal muscle: influence of repetitive high-intensity exercise on sedentary dominant and non-dominant forearm. A 31P NMR study. Biochimie 2003;85:885–890.

38. Lanza IR, Wigmore DM, Befroy DE, Kent-Braun JA. In vivo ATP production during free-flow and ischaemic muscle contractions in humans. J Physiol 2006;577:353–367.

39. Mairiang E, Hanpanich P, Sriboonlue P. In vivo 31P-MRS assessment of muscle-pH, cytolsolic-[Mg2+] and phosphorylation potential after supplementing hypokaliuric renal stone patients with potassium and magnesium salts. Magn Reson Imaging 2004;22:715–719.

40. Taylor JH, Beilman GJ, Conroy MJ, et al. Tissue energetics as measured by nuclear magnetic resonance spectroscopy during hemorrhagic shock. Shock 2004;21:58–64.

41. Levin DI, Gilles B, Madler B, Pai DK. Extracting skeletal muscle fiber fields from noisy diffusion tensor data. Med Image Anal 2011;15:340–353.

42. Englund EK, Elder CP, Xu Q, Ding Z, Damon BM. Combined diffusion and strain tensor MRI reveals a heterogeneous, planar pattern of strain development during isometric muscle contraction. Am J Physiol Regul Integr Comp Physiol 2011;300:R1079–90.

43. Sinha S, Sinha U. Reproducibility analysis of diffusion tensor indices and fiber architecture of human calf muscles in vivo at 1.5 Tesla in neutral and plantarflexed ankle positions at rest. J Magn Reson Imaging 2011;34:107–119.

44. Sinha U, Sinha S, Hodgson JA, Edgerton RV. Human soleus muscle architecture at different ankle joint angles from magnetic resonance diffusion tensor imaging. J Appl Physiol 2011;110:807–819.

45. Virtanen SM, Lindroos MM, Majamaa K, Nuutila P, Borra RJ, Parkkola R. Voxelwise analysis of diffusion tensor imaging and structural MR imaging in patients with the m.3243A>G mutation in mitochondrial DNA. AJNR Am J Neuroradiol 2011;32:522–526.

46. Wu WC, Mohler E, 3rd, Ratcliffe SJ, Wehrli FW, Detre JA, Floyd TF. Skeletal muscle microvascular flow in progressive peripheral artery disease: assessment with continuous arterial spin-labeling perfusion magnetic resonance imaging. J Am Coll Cardiol 2009;53:2372–2377.

47. Frouin F, Duteil S, Lesage D, Carlier PG, Herment A, Leroy-Willig A. An automated image-processing strategy to analyze dynamic arterial spin labeling perfusion studies. Application to human skeletal muscle under stress. Magn Reson Imaging 2006;24:941–951.

48. Raynaud JS, Duteil S, Vaughan JT, et al. Determination of skeletal muscle perfusion using arterial spin labeling NMRI: validation by comparison with venous occlusion plethysmography. Magn Reson Med 2001;46:305–311.

49. Frank LR, Wong EC, Haseler LJ, Buxton RB. Dynamic imaging of perfusion in human skeletal muscle during exercise with arterial spin labeling. Magn Reson Med 1999;42:258–267.

50. Towse TF, Slade JM, Ambrose JA, DeLano MC, Meyer RA. Quantitative analysis of the post-contractile blood-oxygenation-level-dependent (BOLD) effect in skeletal muscle. J Appl Physiol 2011;111:27–39.

51. Sanchez OA, Copenhaver EA, Elder CP, Damon BM. Absence of a significant extravascular contribution to the skeletal muscle BOLD effect at 3 T. Magn Reson Med 2010;64:527–535.

52. Bulte DP, Alfonsi J, Bells S, Noseworthy MD. Vasomodulation of skeletal muscle BOLD signal. J Magn Reson Imaging 2006;24:886–890.

53. Duteil S, Wary C, Raynaud JS, et al. Influence of vascular filling and perfusion on BOLD contrast during reactive hyperemia in human skeletal muscle. Magn Reson Med 2006;55:450–454.

54. Meyer RA, Towse TF, Reid RW, Jayaraman RC, Wiseman RW, McCully KK. BOLD MRI mapping of transient hyperemia in skeletal muscle after single contractions. NMR Biomed 2004;17:392–398.

55. Noseworthy MD, Bulte DP, Alfonsi J. BOLD magnetic resonance imaging of skeletal muscle. Semin Musculoskelet Radiol 2003;7:307–315.

56. Chang G, Wang L, Schweitzer ME, Regatte RR. 3D 23Na MRI of human skeletal muscle at 7 Tesla: initial experience. Eur Radiol 2010;20:2039–2046.

57. Bertoldo A, Pencek RR, Azuma K, et al. Interactions between delivery, transport, and phosphorylation of glucose in governing uptake into human skeletal muscle. Diabetes 2006;55:3028–3037.

58. Bertoldo A, Price J, Mathis C, et al. Quantitative assessment of glucose transport in human skeletal muscle: dynamic positron emission tomography imaging of [O-methyl-11C]3-O-methyl-D-glucose. J Clin Endocrinol Metab 2005;90:1752–1759.

59. Croteau E, Lavallee E, Labbe SM, et al. Image-derived input function in dynamic human PET/CT: methodology and validation with 11C-acetate and 18F-fluorothioheptadecanoic acid in muscle and 18F-fluorodeoxyglucose in brain. Eur J Nucl Med Mol Imaging 2010;37:1539–1550.

60. Fischman AJ, Yu YM, Livni E, et al. Muscle protein synthesis by positron-emission tomography with L-[methyl-11C]methionine in adult humans. Proc Natl Acad Sci U S A 1998;95:12793–12798.

CHAPTER 15

Measurements of Muscle Mass, Equations and Cut-off Points

Marjolein Visser

*Department of Health Sciences, Faculty of Earth and Life Sciences,
VU University Amsterdam, The Netherlands; and
Department of Epidemiology and Biostatistics, VU University Medical Center,
Amsterdam, The Netherlands*

Laura Schaap

*Department of Epidemiology and Biostatistics, VU University Medical Center,
Amsterdam, The Netherlands*

INTRODUCTION

This chapter will describe different methods that can be used to measure or estimate muscle mass. Furthermore, several sarcopenia cut-off points based on these methods will be discussed. In the first paragraph, the estimation of muscle mass by anthropometric methods such as arm and calf circumference will be explained as well as prediction equations based on anthropometric measures to predict appendicular skeletal muscle mass (ASMM). Second, the bioelectrical impedance method will be described including the currently available muscle mass prediction equations. Then, the use of dual-energy x-ray absorptiometry (DXA) will be described and finally the use of the imaging techniques computed tomography (CT) and magnetic resonance imaging (MRI). The focus of this chapter will be on the single assessment of muscle mass rather than on multiple muscle mass assessments, because a single measurement of muscle mass is more clinically feasible. Advantages and disadvantages of each method and of the developed sarcopenia cut-off points, when available, will be discussed.

Sarcopenia, First Edition. Edited by Alfonso J. Cruz-Jentoft and John E. Morley.
© 2012 John Wiley & Sons, Ltd. Published 2012 by John Wiley & Sons, Ltd.

ANTHROPOMETRY – METHOD DESCRIPTION

Efforts have been made in examining the use of anthropometric measurements to estimate muscle size and to define sarcopenia. Assessment of a single anthropometric measurement as well as combination of anthropometric measurements have been used as indicators of skeletal muscle mass or have been used to predict skeletal muscle mass. A potential advantage of this approach is the greater feasibility of simple anthropometric measures in clinical practice although these measurements will provide a less precise estimate of the amount of muscle mass and the inter-observer variability of the measurement may be large.

Anthropometric measurements at the mid-upper arm have been frequently used as indicators of muscle mass. The following standard formulae [1] are being used: *Arm muscle circumference (cm) = arm circumference – (π*triceps skinfold thickness)* and *Arm muscle cross-sectional area (cm^2) = (arm circumference – (π*triceps skinfold thickness))^2/4*π*. The latter formula assumes that the arm and muscle within it are circular and that the skinfold thickness represents the average thickness between skin and muscle. Skinfold thickness is relatively more important in calculating muscle cross-sectional area in obese individuals. In young adults the latter equation was shown to overestimate arm muscle area as assessed by computed tomography by 20–25%. This was due to the assumption of a circular mid-arm muscle compartment and due to inclusion of mid-arm cross-sectional bone area [1].

Arm circumference and arm muscle area have been related to total body muscle mass as determined by urinary creatinine excretion method, showing a rather low explained variance of 52% and 38% in younger persons [2]. This low explained variance, together with the large standard error of estimation (2.91 kg and 3.29 kg), shows their limited use to assess muscle mass. In a sample of 617 Chinese persons aged 69–82 years, arm circumference and arm muscle area were correlated with arm lean mass as assessed by DXA in older men (r = 0.60 and r = 0.61 [3]). In older women, these correlations were much lower; r = 0.28 and r = 0.39. Other studies also confirm that single anthropometric measurements at the arm are insufficiently correlated with ASMM as determined by DXA [4].

The correlation between calf circumference and ASMM from DXA is generally stronger as compared to the correlation between arm circumference and ASMM [4]. This was confirmed in a sample of 158 older men from the Longitudinal Aging Study Amsterdam (Table 15.1). However, in women the correlations of arm circumference and calf circumference with ASMM were similar (Table 15.1). In both men and women the correlation between body weight and ASMM was highest; r = 0.62 in men and r = 0.69 in women. In 1,458 French women aged 70 years the correlation between different anthropometric measurements and ASMM from DXA was examined [5]. Of the anthropometric measures, including waist circumference, hip circumference, calf circumference and grip strength, the calf circumference was most strongly associated with ASMM (r = 0.63, 95% CI 0.60-0.66). Similar as in the Longitudinal Aging Study Amsterdam, body weight was more strongly associated with ASMM (r = 0.83, 95% CI 0.71-0.76) than any other anthropometric parameter.

Another approach to estimate skeletal muscle mass from anthropometry is to perform multiple circumference measurements across a body segment to estimate the total muscle volume in that segment. The estimated muscle volume is then validated against muscle volume based on multiple magnetic resonance imaging scans (MRI) [6,7]. Muscle volume of the thigh segment, based on three estimates of muscle area across the thigh, was 40% (SD 21) higher as compared to MRI. For the calf segment the overestimation was 18%

Table 15.1   Correlation between individual anthropometric parameters and appendicular skeletal muscle mass (ASMM) from dual-energy x-ray absorptiometry in 303 men and women aged 68–90 years from the Longitudinal Aging Study Amsterdam

	Men	Women
Characteristics (mean (SD))		
Age (y)	76.5 (5.9)	76.2 (6.2)
Body height (cm)	174 (7)	161 (6)
Body weight (kg)	79.5 (11.8)	69.7 (12.0)
Body mass index (kg/m²)	26.0 (3.4)	26.7 (4.7)
Mid-upper arm circumference (cm)	29.6 (2.8)	30.0 (3.8)
Calf circumference (cm)	36.4 (2.7)	35.8 (3.1)
Waist circumference (cm)	100.2 (10.6)	92.4 (11.6)
Hip circumference (cm)	101.7 (6.3)	104.0 (9.5)
ASMM (kg)	22.1 (2.7)	14.9 (2.3)
Pearson correlation coefficients* with ASMM		
Height (cm)	0.59	0.53
Body weight (kg)	0.76	0.69
Body mass index (kg/m²)	0.54	0.45
Mid-upper arm circumference (cm)	0.58	0.49
Calf circumference (cm)	0.66	0.45
Waist circumference (cm)	0.54	0.51
Hip circumference (cm)	0.59	0.53

*All p-values < 0.0001.

(SD 14) [6,7]. These studies show the limited use of multiple anthropometric measurements to estimate segmental muscle volume.

Apart from single anthropometric indicators of muscle mass, prediction equations based on a set of different anthropometric measurements have been developed and cross-validated. Cadaver studies showed that total body skeletal muscle mass could be predicted based on equations including at least six different anthropometric measurements [8,9]. The percentage of variance in total body skeletal muscle explained by the anthropometric variables was 96–97% but the standard error of estimation was substantial (1.49–1.53 kg). More recently, Baumgartner et al. developed and validated a prediction equation to predict ASMM from DXA using three anthropometric measurements, grip strength and sex [10]. This equation was developed in a random sample of the New Mexico Elder Health Survey, including 199 older men and women and was used to propose the first cut-off points to define sarcopenia. The following equation was developed in 149 persons: *ASMM (kg) = (0.2487*body weight) + (0.0483*body height) − (0.1584*hip circumference) + (0.0732*grip strength) + (2.5843*sex) + 5.8828* (explained variance 91%, standard error of estimation 1.58 kg). The validity of this equation was then tested in the other 50 persons of the sample. Predicted muscle mass was highly correlated with measured muscle mass: the explained variance was 86% with a standard error of estimation of 1.72 kg. It should be noted that individual prediction errors in the total sample ranged from +4.2 kg to −5.1 kg, and that in 17% of the sample the prediction error was larger than 2 kg. In 2003, Rolland and others also developed a prediction equation to estimate ASMM as assessed by DXA in a large sample of French women aged 70 and older (5). The following equation was developed: *ASMM (kg) = (0.31*calf circumference (cm)) + (0.05*waist circumference (cm)) + (0.08*hip circumference (cm)) + (0.02*grip strength (kPa)) − (0.16*body mass* *index (kg/m²)) − 5.1.* The reported explained variance was 48%, which is rather low, and the standard error of estimation was not reported. These two studies suggest that predicted appendicular skeletal muscle mass based on a set of anthropometric variables, combined with a grip strength assessment, should always be interpreted very carefully, especially when this is done on an individual level.

ANTHROPOMETRY – CUT-OFF POINTS IN SARCOPENIA RESEARCH

Anthropometric measures of muscle mass in older persons have been related to different health outcomes in observational studies. Most of these studies have used mortality as an outcome but some studies investigating functional status are available. These studies may provide some insight into a potential cut-off point for sarcopenia.

A study among 357 older Italian men and women showed that persons in the lowest tertile of arm muscle circumference (<21.1 cm in men and <19.2 cm in women) had a poorer four-year survival compared to those with high arm muscle circumference [11]. A lower arm muscle area (lowest tertile <23.5 cm²) was associated with two-year mortality risk in 957 Japanese frail older persons [12]. An arm muscle area of <21.4 cm² (men) and <21.6 cm² (women), corresponding with the lowest quartile, was also associated with an almost two-fold higher risk of death during a four-year follow-up among 1376 community-dwelling men and women aged 70 years and older living in Australia [13]. Follow-up data from the same study, the Australian Longitudinal Study of Ageing, showed that these cut-off points were also predictive of eight-year mortality [14] while no significant associations were observed for body mass index. A study among 219 geriatric patients also confirmed the strong association between lower arm muscle area and 4.5 year mortality risk [15]. Recent findings from the Longitudinal Aging Study Amsterdam showed, after excluding (ex)smokers, cancer patients and persons with obstructive lung disease, an inversely, J-shaped association between upper-arm circumference and 15-year mortality in both older men and women [16]. Based on the dose-response plots, the mortality risk already started to increase at values below 30 cm. These studies consistently show that a smaller arm circumference, arm muscle circumference and arm muscle area are related to an increased mortality risk in older men and women. However, none of the studies specifically developed a cutoff value below which this risk was increased. Therefore, no consistent cutoff value can be established as a criterion for the presence of sarcopenia based on anthropometric measurements at the arm.

Studies have also investigated the association between arm anthropometric measurements and functional decline in older persons. In a cross-sectional study among 357 older Italian men and women persons those in the lowest tertile of arm muscle circumference (<21.1 cm in men and <19.2 cm in women) showed a poorer functional performance and poorer grip strength compared to those with high arm muscle circumference (>23.4 cm and >21.3 cm) [11]. A recent prospective study among 543 community-dwelling, frail Japanese older persons showed that a single measurement of arm circumference or arm muscle area was not an indicator of future decline in activities of daily living scores during a two-year follow-up [17]. However, a decline in arm circumference equal or greater than 1.6 cm was associated with a decline in activities of daily living scores, although cause and effect cannot clearly be distinguished.

Rolland et al. [5] examined the potential use of the calf circumference as an indicator of sarcopenia. Using receiver operating characteristic curves, the optimal cut-off point for calf circumference to determine sarcopenia was investigated among 1458 older French women [5]. Sarcopenia was defined based on DXA measurements using the cut-off point of Baumgartner et al. which was based on a young sample from the Rosetta Study [10]. A calf circumference value cut-off point of 32 cm was optimal based on the combination of sensitivity and specificity, however, the authors decided to set the cut-off point at 31 cm to maximize specificity without reducing the sensitivity too much. Women with a calf circumference below 31 cm were 2.5 times more likely to have activity of daily living disabilities and were two- to three-fold more likely to have physical function difficulties. A low calf circumference was not associated with fall history of the previous six months. Although the calf circumference cut-off point resulted in a good specificity (91.4%), its sensitivity was rather low (44.3%). These results again show the limited usefulness of anthropometric measurements to assess sarcopenia.

BIOELECTRICAL IMPEDANCE – METHOD DESCRIPTION

Bioelectrical impedance analysis (BIA) is a relatively simple, quick and non-invasive method for estimating body water and fat free mass. The use of BIA in studies of body composition has grown rapidly over the past two decades. Fat free mass (FFM) as predicted by BIA has traditionally been used as a surrogate measure of skeletal muscle in the absence of better instruments. FFM however, not only consists of skeletal muscle mass ($\sim 51\%$ [18]), but also includes other organs, bone and water of which the latter can show great variation.

BIA is based on the principle that lean body mass, which consists largely of ions in a water solution, conducts electricity far better than fat tissue. Therefore, the resistance of the body to an electrical current is inversely related to the lean body mass. The two main determinants of impedance, resistance and reactance, respond differently at any given frequency to intracellular and extracellular fluids. The reciprocal of the impedance is proportional to total body water for a current frequency ≥ 50 kHz or, to extracellular fluid, for frequencies below 5 kHz. Impedance values are then converted into values specific for total body water or extracellular fluid and then into fat-free mass by means of prediction equations that are population specific. Prediction of lean mass can be improved by accounting for sex as well as height and weight. Most BIA measurements are made at a single frequency (50 kHz), while some instruments can make measurements at multiple frequencies. The BIA method is very simple in practice. Electrodes (either two or four) are attached to a person's extremities (usually wrist and ankle) (Figure 15.1). A weak radio frequency signal is applied to the electrodes, and the impedance is measured. Usually several measurements are made, but the whole procedure takes less than a minute. Because the BIA method is simple, quick, safe and non invasive, it is potentially useful in clinical practise.

Many researchers have investigated the applicability of BIA prediction equations in various populations. BIA results have been shown to be confounded by fluid retention, as found in patients with COPD [19]. Hydrostatic disturbances, peripheral oedema and the use of diuretic medication may affect the validity of BIA measurements in older age groups [20]. As shown by Visser et al. [21] and Deurenberg et al. [22], BIA measurements are effected by an increase in extracellular fluid in skeletal muscle of older persons. Therefore, Pietrobelli et al. [23] explored BIA prediction equations for appendicular skeletal muscle mass at increasing electrical frequencies in 49 healthy men and women by using

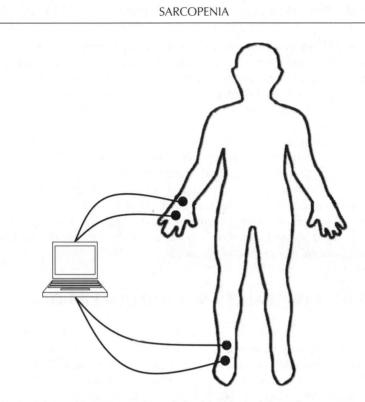

Figure 15.1   Schematic representation of the bioelectrical impedance measurement. Two electrodes are placed on the hand and foot.

segmental BIA (measurement of the arms and legs). The hypothesis of this study was that appendicular skeletal muscle mass prediction equations would no longer include age as an independent predictor at frequencies greater than 50 kHz (which is the standard used electrical frequency). It was shown however, that age was a significant predictor in the prediction equation at all frequencies under study, suggesting other age-related changes in the skeletal muscle besides fluid increase that influence BIA measurement in older persons. In this study it was also found that the prediction equation for appendicular skeletal muscle mass improved at higher frequencies, which implies that multiple frequency BIA systems may offer an advantage over the conventional 50 kHz BIA method when evaluating muscle mass. However, this has yet to be confirmed by other studies.

Unfortunately, BIA methods that have been validated for the prediction of fat-free mass in young individuals have been found to be inadequate when used in older populations [20]. Visser et al. [21] found that existing prediction equations for BIA that were based on young and middle-aged subjects overestimated lean mass and underestimated the percentage of body fat in an older (aged 60–87 years) population. Other studies have suggested that the errors in BIA equations are not related to age, but to the specific populations under study [24,25]. In contrast, Genton et al. [26] compared four equations specific for BIA analysis in older persons and found only the equations derived by Kyle et al. [27] to accurately predict fat-free mass in a group of persons with an age range of 65–94 years. The BIA equations developed by Deurenberg et al. [28] (age range 60–83 years), Roubenoff et al. [24] (average

age 78) were not found to be valid by Dey et al. [29]. In conclusion, when determining body composition in older persons, one should keep in mind that BIA equations are subject to errors, either due to age-related changes in hydration or population specific characteristics. Therefore, BIA equations should be validated in the population in which they are to be applied, which of course hampers the use of BIA as a fast and simple method [30] and its use in clinical practice.

BIOELECTRICAL IMPEDANCE – CUT-OFF POINTS IN SARCOPENIA RESEARCH

In the past 15 years, BIA prediction equations have been developed to estimate total or appendicular muscle mass. In general, equation models include height squared, the BIA resistance, sex and age as independent predictors of muscle mass. Janssen et al. developed a prediction equation for estimating whole body skeletal muscle [31]. Whole body skeletal muscle mass, determined by magnetic resonance imaging, was compared with BIA measurements in a multiethnic sample of 388 men and women, aged 18–86 years, at two different laboratories. Within each laboratory, equations of skeletal muscle mass were developed using the impedance measured with BIA, body height squared, sex and age in the Caucasian subsample. Second, both equations were cross validated and pooled to create one final equation: *Skeletal muscle mass (kg) = (height²/(R * 0.401)) + (sex * 3.825) + (age * −0.071) + 5.102,* where height is in centimetres, *R* is BIA resistance in ohms, men = 1, women = 0, age is in years. This (Caucasian-derived) equation was then applied to Hispanics, African-Americans and Asians which resulted in a reasonable prediction of skeletal muscle in Hispanics and African-Americans (explained variance 74%, standard error of estimation 2.7 kg (9%)), but showed an underestimation of skeletal muscle mass in Asians. The average difference between MRI measured and BIA predicted skeletal muscle mass was 2.45 kg (SD 1.61, p < 0.001). These results indicate that the Caucasian-derived equation is not applicable to Asian populations and that individual prediction errors can be substantial.

In a second cross-sectional study [32], the prevalence of sarcopenia was investigated using data from the Third National Health and Nutrition Examination Survey (NHANES III). The predicted amount of muscle mass was expressed as the percentage of total body weight (termed skeletal muscle index) to adjust for stature and the mass of non-skeletal muscle tissues (fat, organ, bone). A potential disadvantage of the used index is that the ratio of whole body skeletal muscle mass divided by total body weight is largely dependent on the amount of body fat since the between-person variation in total body fat is much larger compared to the between-person variation in skeletal muscle. The mean skeletal muscle index in 3116 young men aged 18 to 39 years was 42.5% (SD 5.5%). The mean skeletal muscle index in 3298 young women aged 18 to 39 years was 33.1% (SD 5.5%). An index within one to two standard deviations from the sex-specific mean value was considered class I sarcopenia. An index less than two standard deviations from the young reference group was considered to indicate class II sarcopenia. This led to the following cut-off points: a normal skeletal muscle index in men was defined as an index greater than 37%, class I sarcopenia as an index between 31% and 37% and class II sarcopenia as an index of less than 31%. In women the cut-off points for normal skeletal muscle index, class I sarcopenia and class II sarcopenia were 28% or greater, between 22% and 28% and less than 22%, respectively. Using this approach, 45% and 59% of the older (≥60 years) men and women were classified as having class I (moderate) sarcopenia, and 7% and 10%, respectively, of the older men and women were classified as having class II (severe) sarcopenia.

In the same cross-sectional study [32], class II sarcopenia based on the skeletal muscle index was associated with functional impairment and disability in men and women. However, after adjustment for age, race, body mass index, health behaviors, and comorbidity, some of the associations disappeared. Of the 12 items, class II sarcopenia in men was only related to the tandem stand performance and self-reported limitations stooping/crouching/kneeling. In women, class II sarcopenia was associated with five items.

In another study by the same author, cut-off points were determined for identifying persons with increased risk of physical disability (difficulty performing activities of daily living) using data from NHANES III [33]. Receiver operating characteristics analysis was used to develop skeletal muscle cut-off points associated with physical disability. A skeletal muscle index of ≤6.75 kg/m^2 was selected as the moderately increased risk cut-off point (class I sarcopenia), and a skeletal muscle index of ≤5.75 kg/m^2 was selected as the high-risk cut-off point (class II sarcopenia) for physical disability in women. For men, a skeletal muscle index of ≤10.75 kg/m^2 was selected as the moderately increased risk cut-off point, and a skeletal muscle index of ≤8.50 kg/m^2 was selected as the high-risk cut-off point for physical disability. It should be noted that the skeletal muscle cut-off points determined in this study are similar to the arbitrary cut-off points based on two standard deviations below the mean of young adults determined in previous studies [10,34]. See paragraph on DXA cut-off points for more details. Also, the cut-off points determined in this study were for physical disability and might have been different if another outcome measure such as mobility limitations had been used. Furthermore, the cut-off points derived from the ROC analyses are population dependent and may be different in less healthy or institutionalized older persons.

Kyle et al. [35] developed a BIA prediction equation for appendicular skeletal muscle mass in a study sample of 444 healthy persons aged 22–94 years and 326 heart, lung or liver transplant patients aged 18–70 years which was validated against DXA. The correlation between appendicular skeletal muscle mass obtained by the BIA prediction equation and the DXA measurement was 0.95 in healthy persons and 0.91 in patients. The standard error of estimation was 1.1 kg (5%) in healthy persons and 1.5 kg (7.6%) in patients. The best fitted model to estimate skeletal muscle mass was: Appendicular skeletal muscle mass = −4.211 + (0.267 * height^2/(−0.012 * age) + (0.058 * reactance).

Recently, in a small cross-sectional study among older people in Taiwan, the BIA equation developed by Janssen to estimate skeletal muscle mass was used to investigate sarcopenia prevalence rates [36]. Despite the findings of Janssen that the BIA derived equation underestimates skeletal muscle mass in Asians, this study found only small differences between MRI measured and BIA estimated skeletal muscle in a small group of 41 volunteers (aged 22–90 years). The differences ranged from +2.84 kg to −2.81 kg, p = 0.15. Sarcopenia was defined as the SMI of two standard deviations or more below the normal sex-specific mean for young persons (n = 200, mean age 27 years). In this study an SMI of 8.87 kg/m^2 in men and 6.42 kg/m^2 in women or lower was considered as sarcopenia. The study shows a prevalence of sarcopenia of 23.6% in men and 18.6% in women. The sarcopenia prevalence rates found in this study are difficult to compare with other studies due to several issues. First, the current study only included community-dwelling volunteers without activities of daily living difficulties. Second, the cut-off points selected in this study are lower compared to the cut-off points in other studies [32,33], which obviously leads to lower prevalence rates of sarcopenia.

The equations by Janssen and Kyle were both validated against DXA in 98 non-institutionalized 75-year-old people [37]. The equation developed by Janssen overestimated total body skeletal muscle mass compared to DXA (mean difference of 1.02 (SD 1.39) in women, 4.05 (SD 2.22) in men, $p < 0.03$ in both groups). Also, the equation by Kyle over-estimated appendicular skeletal muscle mass (mean difference 0.64 (SD 1.41) in women, 1.23 (SD 1.63) in men, $p = 0.01$ and $p < 0.03$, respectively). It was suggested that these differences may be due to the fact that the equations by Janssen and Kyle were developed to include a wide range of ages, perhaps at the cost of less accuracy among older persons. Therefore, Tengvall developed a new age-specific equation to predict total body skeletal muscle mass by bioelectrical impedance spectrometry (BIS), which measures intracellular water, extracellular water, total body water and fat free mass. This equation could predict total body skeletal muscle mass (correlation with DXA 0.91), although with great individual variation and therefore needs to be validated in other populations. Cut-off points for sarcopenia were not selected in this study.

In 2009, the relationship between sarcopenia and cardiovascular disease risk was investigated [38] using skeletal muscle mass calculated with the equation developed by Janssen. Muscle mass was adjusted for height using a regression-based residual technique. Sarcopenia was defined as the lowest sex-specific tertile of muscle mass (mean muscle mass 18.9 kg (SD 4.5)) and was not significantly associated with increased risk of cardiovascular disease.

In conclusion, there are several BIA prediction equations and sarcopenia cut-off points in the current literature (see Table 15.2 for overview). Researchers should consider all options carefully with respect to the population under study.

DXA – METHOD DESCRIPTION

The dual-energy x-ray absorptiometry (DXA) method was originally developed to measure bone mineral density of the proximal femur, lumbar spine or forearm to allow a diagnosis of osteoporosis. Because of this application, the method is widespread and well-known in the clinical setting. The tissue attenuation of photons transmitted by the two x-ray beams with different energy levels also provides information on the composition of soft tissue. Whole body DXA therefore enables the precise derivation of the none-bone tissue into fat mass and fat-free mass. This can be determined for the total body as well as of specific regions of interest (such as the limbs) (Figure 15.2). The duration of the measurement depends on the type of DXA scanner, but can be less than five minutes for a whole body scan which enhances its feasibility in the clinical setting (39,40]. A detailed description of the DXA method can be found in Chapter 14 (Muscle imaging).

Heymsfield et al. were among the first to show that the bone-free, fat-free mass of the arms and legs provides an accurate assessment of appendicular skeletal muscle mass (ASMM) [41]. Using data from 44 healthy persons with a mean age of 52 (SD 20) years, they showed that ASMM was highly correlated with total body potassium as measured by whole body counting ($r = 0.94$) and total body nitrogen as estimated from prompt gamma-neutron-activation analysis ($r = 0.78$). Several years later, a high correlation between ASMM from

Table 15.2 Characteristics of studies that developed sarcopenia cut-off points based on BIA measurements

Reference	Study sample	N	Age range	Sex	BMI Mean (SD)	Ethnicity	Country	Muscle mass index		Cut-off points
Janssen, 2002	NHANES III	6414	18–39	M, F	—	Non-Hispanic whites, non-Hispanic blacks and Mexican Americans	USA	(Muscle mass/body mass)*100 Class I sarcopenia: within 1 to 2 SD Class II sarcopenia: > = 2 SD	M: F:	Class I: 31–37% Class II: ≤30% Class I: 22–28% Class II: ≤21%
Janssen, 2004	NHANES III	4509	≥60	M, F	M: 26.6 (4.3) F: 27.0 (5.5)	Non-Hispanic whites, non-Hispanic blacks and Mexican Americans	USA	Muscle mass/height^2 Cutpoints calculated by ROC analyses	M: F:	Class I: 8.51–10.75 kg/m^2 Class II: ≤8.51 kg/m^2 Class I: 5.76–6.75 kg/m^2 Class II: ≤5.75 kg/m^2
Chien, 2008	Healthy adults	200	18–40	M, F	M: 23.2 (3.5) F: 20.6 (2.5)	Asian	Taiwan	Muscle mass/height^2	M: F:	<8.87 kg/m^2 <6.42 kg/m^2

M: male; F: female; BMI: Body Mass Index; SD: standard deviation; ROC: receiver operating characteristics

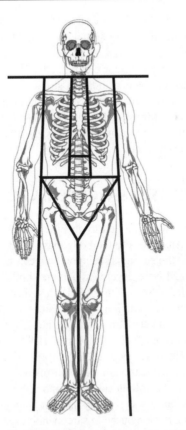

Figure 15.2 Schematic representation of the regions of interest commonly used in dual-energy x-ray absorptiometry. The tissue composition of the arms and legs is used to assess appendicular skeletal muscle mass.

DXA and total body skeletal muscle from computed tomography was shown in 17 healthy persons and eight AIDS patients [42].

DXA measurements of the amount of muscle mass of the leg only have also been validated against MRI and CT. Shih et al. [43] showed that the bone-free, fat-free soft tissue of the leg as determined by DXA in 207 adults was highly correlated with skeletal muscle mass as determined by multiple MRI scans of 1.0 cm thickness with a 4.0 cm space between scans (explained variance 89%). Age and body mass index also explained a small, but statistically significant, part of the variance and increased the total explained variance to 90.4%. The validity of leg muscle mass by DXA was validated in 60 men and women aged 70–79 years using multislice computer tomography of the legs [44]. The explained variance was 96% with a standard error of estimation of 0.7 kg. However, a study comparing a 1.3 cm mid-thigh slice by DXA with a 1.0 mm CT slice in 30 older women recovering from a hip fracture, showed a much lower explained variance (73%) [45]. In addition, the 8- to 12-month change in mid-thigh muscle mass by DXA was poorly correlated with the change assessed by CT, with an intraclass correlation coefficient of 0.51. In 50 sedentary older men and women the increase in total thigh skeletal muscle mass caused by single leg exercise training was measured by multislice CT as well as DXA [46]. Muscle mass at baseline and muscle mass after exercise training were highly correlated between the two methods (r = 0.88 and r = 0.90). The increase in thigh muscle mass due to exercise training was 3.9% by CT and 2.6% by DXA, with a poor correlation between the two methods (r = 0.52).

Based on these examples and other validation studies, DXA is currently considered a valid and accurate methodology to measure ASMM in humans. The method is being used in clinical as well as research settings. Although CT and MRI are more precise alternatives to detect small changes in muscle mass over time, DXA is frequently being used to test the effect of a specific intervention on muscle.

DXA – CUT-OFF POINTS IN SARCOPENIA RESEARCH

Baumgartner and colleagues were the first to develop a definition of sarcopenia based on DXA measurements (10). Analogous to the body mass index, the ASMM was divided by height squared to adjust for the strong association between body height and ASMM. The cut-off points for low ASMM were developed using a similar approach as for the cut-off points for osteoporosis. Older persons with a ASMM less than two standard deviations from the mean of a young reference population were considered sarcopenic. DXA data from a young (aged 18–40 years) volunteer sample of 229 non-Hispanic white men and women participating in the Rosetta Stone Study in New York [47] were used to determine the sarcopenia cut-off points. The developed ASMM cut-off points were 7.26 kg/m^2 for men and 5.45 kg/m^2 for women (10). Although these cut-off points are limited by the fact that the young reference group was a volunteer sample and might not have been representative for young US men and women (it was actually the first young sample with available DXA measurements) they are widely being used in sarcopenia research.

The Baumgartner cut-off points for sarcopenia were first applied to the New Mexico Elder Health Survey in which ASMM was predicted using an equation including sex, several anthropometric measures and grip strength (10). After adjustment for age, income, ethnicity, obesity, comorbidity, current smoking, physical activity and alcohol intake, sarcopenic men and women were more likely to have ≥3 physical disabilities on an Instrumental Activities of Daily Living scale. In men, but not in women, sarcopenia was also associated with >1 balance abnormality, the use of a cane or walker, and falling in the past year.

Using the same approach, based on two standard deviations below the mean of a young reference sample, sarcopenia cut-off points have also been developed in 111 young, health Chinese persons aged 20 to 39 years [48]. The mean reported ASMM was 7.4 (SD 0.84) for men and 6.4 (SD 0.79) for women, which would translate to ASMM cut-off points of <5.72 kg/m^2 for men and <4.82 kg/m^2 for women to indicate sarcopenia. These values are substantially lower than previously defined in young Caucasian persons (10) which suggests that sarcopenia cut-off points might be race-specific.

In 2003, a second approach was used to derive sarcopenia cut-off points [49]. This approach was initiated based on the finding in the Health, Aging and Body Composition Study that the sarcopenia prevalence using the original Baumgartner sarcopenia cut-off points was very high in normal weight older persons (>50%) but not present in obese older persons. In theory, obese older persons can also be sarcopenic and the term sarcopenic-obesity was developed to describe this condition [50]. The new method incorporated both body height and total body fat. The lowest 20th percentile of the residuals of the regression of total body height and body fat on ASMM derived in the older men and women separately was used to define sarcopenia. The percentile cut point was chosen arbitrarily. The residuals of the regression were thus used to identify those whose ASMM was much lower than the predicted value and had a negative residual. Separate models were fit for men: *ASMM (kg) = −22.48 + (24.14*height (m)) + (0.21*total fat mass (kg))* and for women: *ASMM (kg) = −13.19 + (14.75*height (m)) + (0.23*total fat mass (kg))*. This new definition was compared with the lowest 20th percentile of the ratio of ASMM divided by height squared (7.23 kg/m^2 in men, 5.67 kg/m^2 in women). These cut-off points turned out to be very similar to the original Baumgartner cut-off points (10). In men, sarcopenia according to both definitions increased the risk of having a low function. The risk of a low function score almost doubled in women with sarcopenia based on the residuals. In contrast, women with sarcopenia based on the ratio had a *lower* risk for having a low function. This is explained by the fact that the non-sarcopenic group includes obese women who have a low function score because of their excess body fat.

The association between sarcopenia using both these definitions and five-year change in physical function was also examined in the Health Aging and Body Composition Study (51). Again, sarcopenia based on the residual method was better for predicting incident lower-extremity mobility limitations compared to the ratio ASMM/height^2 method. In fact, men and women with sarcopenia based on the ratio method had a *lower* risk of developing incident mobility limitations which was attenuated after adjustment for total body fat. Based on these studies we can conclude that the amount of ASMM can only be correctly interpreted when considering not only body height but total body fat mass as well.

A third approach has been described to define a potential cut-off value for sarcopenia [52]. Receiver operating characteristic (ROC) curves were used to determine the optimal cut-off point for ASMM/height^2 based on the relationship with physical limitations in 3153 community-living, Chinese men and women aged 65 years and older [52]. A U-shaped association was observed between ASMM/height^2 and physical limitations for both men and women. However, the area under the ROC curve (AUC) was low (0.528), showing a very limited predictability of sarcopenia for the presence of physical limitations. ASMM/height^2 values below the range of 7.25–7.75 kg/m^2 in men and below the range of 6.00–6.25 kg/m^2 in women were associated with an increased risk of physical limitations. However, no clear, single cut-off value gave best sensitivity and specificity.

DXA data obtained in the National Health and Nutrition Examination Survey, collected from 1999 through 2004 in a representative sample of the United States population, have been recently used to determine reference values for body composition [53]. Mean values for ASMM/height^2 obtained in, for example, young persons aged 20–25 years could potentially be used to determine a cut-off value for sarcopenia using the approach of two standard deviations below the mean. This would result in the following cut-off points: <6.19 kg/m^2 for Caucasian men, <6.12 kg/m^2 for African-American men, <6.46 kg/m^2 for Mexican-American men, <4.73 kg/m^2 for Caucasian women, <5.29 kg/m^2 for African-American women, and <4.70 kg/m^2 for Mexican-American women. However, as explained before in this chapter, these cut-off points do not consider the amount of total body fat and may underestimate sarcopenia in obese persons. Furthermore, since this young NHANES sample also includes obese persons, the cut-off points might be overestimated.

Based on this literature overview, it can be concluded that there is no consensus on DXA derived sarcopenia cut-off points (Table 15.3). Even though the original cut-off points by Baumgartner are widely being used, these values have several drawbacks as discussed

Table 15.3 Characteristics of studies that developed sarcopenia cut-off points based on DXA measurements

Reference	Study sample	N	Age range	Sex	BMI mean (SD)	Ethnicity	Country	Muscle mass index		Cut-off points
Baumgartner, 1998	Rosetta Study	229	18–40	M, F	24.6 (3.8) 24.1 (5.4)	Non-Hispanic Whites	USA	$ASMM/ht^2$	M: F:	$<7.26 \, kg/m^2$ $<5.45 \, kg/m^2$
Newman, 2003	Health ABC Study	2984	70–79	M, F	Whites: M: 27.0 (3.7) F: 26.0 (4.6) Blacks: M: 27.1 (4.3) F: 29.7 (5.7)	Whites Blacks	USA	Residual of ASMM regressed on on ht and total body fat $ASMM/ht^2$	M: F: M: F:	$\leq -2.29 \, kg$ $\leq -1.73 \, kg$ $<7.23 \, kg/m^2$ $<5.67 \, kg/m^2$
Lau, 2005	Chinese community	111	20–39	M, F	M: 22.5 (9.5) F: 23.5 (3.9)	Asian	Hong Kong	$ASMM/ht^2$	M: F:	$<5.72 \, kg/m^2$ $<4.82 \, kg/m^2$
Woo, 2009	Chinese community	3153	65+	M, F	M: 23.5 (3.1) F: 24.0 (3.4)	Asian	Hong Kong	$ASMM/ht^2$	M: F:	$<7.25–7.75 \, kg/m^2$ $<6.00–6.25 \, kg/m^2$
Based on Kelly, 2009	NHANES 1999–2004	558	20–25	M, F	–	Non-Hispanic whites, non-Hispanic blacks and Mexican Americans	USA	$ASMM/ht^2$	NH Whites M: F: NH Blacks M: F: Mex. Americans M: F:	$<6.19 \, kg/m^2$ $<4.73 \, kg/m^2$ $<6.12 \, kg/m^2$ $<5.29 \, kg/m^2$ $<6.46 \, kg/m^2$ $<4.70 \, kg/m^2$

M: male; F: female; BMI: Body Mass Index; SD: standard deviation; ASMM: appendicular skeletal muscle mass; ht: body height.

above and cannot be applied to other race groups. A careful interpretation of ASMM from DXA, incorporating at least sex, race, body height and total body fat, is necessary to determine whether muscle mass is too low for an individual patient. This has unfortunately complicated the quick and easy determination of sarcopenia by DXA in clinical practice. A simple algorithm to interpret ASMM and high-quality research showing that sarcopenia according to this algorithm is clinically relevant with regard to future health and functioning of the older patient, are two important prerequisites for the future.

CT AND MRI – METHOD DESCRIPTION

Nowadays, computed tomography (CT) and magnetic resonance imaging (MRI) are more and more used for measurement of body composition and are considered the reference methods for studying skeletal muscle. The use of CT and MRI as reference methods is based on the main assumption that measured cross-sectional muscle area (CSA) is equivalent to actual skeletal muscle CSA. Information about the specific methods and usage of CT and MRI are discussed in detail in Chapter 14 (Muscle imaging). In short, the principle of CT is based on the use of a scanning an x-ray beam that passes through the participant/patient. The x-ray exit transmission intensity is monitored by a series of detectors, which results in the visual production of cross-sectional slices of about 10 mm thick. The average attenuation coefficient along the length of the x-ray beam is then calculated and expressed in Hounsfield Units (HU).

The principle of MRI involves a cylindrical magnet with an internal diameter large enough to enclose a human body to allow for an external magnetic field. The presence of gradient coils creates a smaller identification field, known as a gradient field. The radio frequency coil generated by these magnetic fields provides the force necessary to rotate nuclear spin away from the direction of the external magnetic field. Radio frequency signals are emitted, which are combined to form an image. Variations in the radio frequency pulse sequence are used to specific tissues, such as adipose tissue or skeletal muscle. Although multi-slice whole body imaging is generally considered the reference for measuring total body adipose tissue or skeletal muscle volumes, most researchers over the past two decades measured a single cross-sectional image of the abdomen. In a study by Shen et al., the correlation between single-slice abdominal CSAs and total body compartment volumes were examined in 328 healthy adults [54]. The highest correlation between a single-slice skeletal muscle area and total body skeletal muscle area was about 5 cm above the L4-L5 level (r = 0.924). Regression models based on this cross-sectional image accurately predicted total body skeletal muscle area. Effects of sex, age, ethnicity, body scanning position, BMI and waist circumference on the strength of the association were small, suggesting that a single slice image may be used to represent total body skeletal muscle mass across a wide range of healthy subjects.

CT and MRI are the most accurate imaging methods to assess muscle cross sectional area, muscle volume and muscle quality (muscle density and intramuscular fat infiltration). The assessment of muscle density using MRI or CT provides a reliable and valid measure of the fatty degeneration of muscle tissue [55]. A lower muscle density indicates more intramuscular fat, which is associated with lower muscle functioning/strength [56].

Caution should be taken with regard to using CT as an assessment of muscle mass in some patient populations. There is a variation of +30 to +80 Hounsfield units in the attenuation of normal muscle. There can be wide variation in the size or volume of muscles on each side of the body. Because of the variation in muscle size associated with physical training and nutrition status, general reductions in muscle size may be difficult to determine in the early stages of disease without baseline measurements [57]. The effect of energy restriction and exercise on appendicular skeletal muscle volume was examined recently with MRI [58]. Obese women treated with diet only showed a significant decrease in skeletal muscle volume in arms and legs compared with women treated with diet and aerobic exercise. This finding shows the ability to detect small changes in skeletal muscle mass by MRI. Another study by Song et al. [59] showed a significant loss of skeletal muscle mass (mean -0.72 (SD 0.71) measured by MRI after two years of follow-up in 29 African-American women aged 65 years and older. MRI and CT are costly, time consuming and are technically difficult to perform. CT also involves exposure to radiation. Therefore, their use is mostly restricted to body composition research and their use in clinical practice to assess sarcopenia is limited.

CT AND MRI – CUT-OFF POINTS IN SARCOPENIA RESEARCH

Only a few studies have used CT or MRI to investigate consequences of sarcopenia [60–63], and most of these studies did not use cut-off points but used rather population-specific tertiles or quartiles. Lauretani et al. [60] investigated calf muscle area, measured by peripheral quantitative CT (pQCT), in relationship to poor mobility in the InChianti study. The CSAs obtained at 66% of the tibia length was used in the analyses, as this has been suggested to be the region with the largest outer calf diameter, with little variability across individuals [64]. Sarcopenia cut-off points were developed in the participants aged 20–29 years. Persons were considered sarcopenic when their values were less than two standard deviations of the mean of the young reference group (83.3 cm^2 (95% CI 78.9—87.8) in men, 62.6 cm^2 (58.5 – 66.7) in women). Calf muscle area was divided into quintiles to investigate the relationship with poor mobility, but only showed weak associations. The area under the curve was 0.64 and 0.57 in women for the relationship between calf muscle area and walking slower than 0.8 m/s and unable to walk without difficulty for 1 km, respectively. For men these values were 0.84 and 0.69. The optimal cut-off value for low calf muscle area, yielding the highest sensitivity and specificity, was 54.97 and 56.67 cm^2 in women and 63.05 and 68.82 cm^2 in men for both these outcomes. However, after adjustment for age, low calf muscle area according to these cut-off points was not associated with an increased risk for poor mobility in women. In men, a low calf muscle area was only associated with a walking speed slower than 0.8 m/s and not with self-reported difficulty.

Several studies based on the Health, Aging, and Body Composition Study, have related measures of body composition derived by CT to indices of functional ability, quality of life and mortality in the well-functioning older persons. Visser et al. [61] used sex and race specific quartiles of mid-thigh muscle CSA and intramuscular fat infiltration to investigate the association with incident mobility limitations in 3075 well-functioning people aged 70–79 years. Persons in the lowest quartile (<230 cm^2 in white men, <245 cm^2 in black men, <152 cm^2 in white women, <181 cm^2 in black women) were more likely to develop mobility limitations compared to persons with a CSA in the highest quartile. In a study by Newman et al. [62], mid-thigh CSA (analysed as a continuous measure) was weakly associated with mortality in the same study population. This is in concordance with a

Table 15.4 Overview of methods to assess muscle mass in older persons

Method	Frequently used muscle mass measures	Regional muscle	Whole body muscle	Low cost	Availability	Radiation exposure	Precision	Accuracy
Anthropometry	Upper-arm muscle circumference	+++	+	+++	+++	+++	+	+
	Upper-arm muscle cross-sectional area	+++	+	+++	+++	+++	+	+
	Predicted ASMM	+	++	+++	+++	+++	+	+
Bioelectrical impedance	Predicted FFM	+	++	+++	+++	+++	+	+++
	Predicted ASMM	+	++	+++	+++	+++	+	+++
Dual-energy X-ray absorptiometry	ASMM	+++	++	++	++	++	++	++
Computed tomography	Mid-thigh cross-sectional muscle area	+++	+	+	+	+	+++	+++
Magnetic resonance imaging	Mid-thigh cross-sectional muscle area	+++	+	+	+	+++	+++	+++
	Total body muscle volume	+	+++	+	+	+++	+++	++

ASMM = appendicular skeletal muscle mass, FFM = fat-free mass. +++ indicates a very positive feature of the method, while + indicates a less positive feature.

study performed by Cesari et al [63]. In this study skeletal muscle mass was measured by peripheral quantitative CT (pQCT) of the calf and was then related to mortality in data from 934 participants (mean age 74.5 years (SD 7.0)). Sarcopenia was defined according to the lowest sex-specific tertile of the residuals of a linear regression model that predicted muscle mass from height (in cm) and fat mass area (log value of cm^2). Sarcopenia was not associated with an increased risk of mortality.

In conclusion, although CT and MRI are considered the reference methods for assessment of skeletal muscle mass, not many studies have yet used these methods to determine sarcopenia and its long-term consequences. No clinical cut-off points of muscle cross-sectional area have been developed to assess sarcopenia. Studies relating muscle mass by CT or MRI to specific outcomes mainly used population specific cut-off points like quartiles or tertiles or defined sarcopenia as muscle mass below two standard deviations of the mean muscle mass in a reference population. While low muscle area has been related to poorer functioning and mortality in some studies, no clear cut-off point has been established below which the risks are substantially increased.

OVERVIEW OF METHODS

In Table 15.4 an overview is provided of the discussed body composition methods to assess muscle mass in older persons. The most frequently used measures of muscle mass assessed by these methods are listed as well as the ability of the methods to measure regional and/or whole-body muscle mass. Furthermore, a rating of the cost of the method, the general availability of the method and the patient radiation exposure are provided. Also, the precision (validity) and accuracy (reproducibility) of each method are rated.

REFERENCES

1. Heymsfield SB, McManus C, Smith J, et al. (1982) Anthropometric measurement of muscle mass: revised equations for calculating bone-free arm muscle area. Am J Clin Nutr 36, 680–690.
2. Kuriyan R, Kurpad AV. (2004) Prediction of total body muscle mass from simple anthropometric measurements in young Indian males. Indian J Med Res 119, 121–128.
3. Kwok T, Woo J, Chan HHL, et al. (1997) The reliability of upper limb anthropometry in older Chinese people. Int J Obes 21, 542–547.
4. Baumgartner RN, Stauber PM, McHigh D, et al. (1995) Cross-sectional age differences in body composition in persons 60+ years of age. J Gerontol 50, M307–16.
5. Rolland Y, Lauwers-Cances V, Cournot M, et al. (2003) Sarcopenia, calf circumference, and physical function of elderly women: a cross-sectional study. J Am Geriatr Soc 51, 1120–1124.
6. Fuller NJ, Hardingham CR, Graves M, et al. (1999) Predicting composition of leg sections with anthropometry and bioelectrical impedance analysis, using magnetic resonance imaging as reference. Clin Sci 96, 647–657.
7. Elia M, Fuller J, Hardingham CR, et al. (2000) Modeling leg sections by bioelectrical impedance analysis, dual-energy x-ray absorptiometry, and anthropometry: assessing segmental muscle volume using magnetic resonance imaging as a reference. Ann N Y Acad Sci 904, 298–305.
8. Martin AD, Spenst LF, Drinkwater DT, et al. (1990) Anthropometric estimation of muscle mass in men. Med Sci Sports Exerc 22, 729–733.

9. Doupe MB, Martin AD, Searle MS, et al. (1997) A new formula for population-based estimation of whole body muscle mass in males. Can J Appl Physiol 22, 598–608.

10. Baumgartner RN, Koehler KM, Gallagher D, et al. (1998) Epidemiology of sarcopenia among the elderly in New Mexico. Am J Epidemiol 147, 755–763.

11. Landi F, Russo A, Liperoti R, et al. (2010) Midarm muscle circumference, physical performance and mortality: results from the aging and longevity study in the Sirente geographic area (ilSIRENTE study). Clin Nutr 29, 441–447.

12. Enoki H, Kuzuya M, Masuda Y, et al. (2007) Anthropometric measurements of mid-upper arm as a mortality predictor for community-dwelling Japanese elderly: the Nagoya Longitudinal Study of Frail Elderly (NLS-FE). Clin Nutr 26, 597–604.

13. Crotty M, Miller M, Giles L, et al. (2002) Australian Longitudinal Study of Aging: prospective evaluation of anthropometric indices in terms of four year mortality in community-living older adults. J Nutr Health Aging 6, 20–23.

14. Miller M, Crotty M, Giles LC, et al. (2002) Corrected arm muscle area: an independent predictor of long-term mortality in community-dwelling older adults? J Am Geriatr Soc 50, 1272–1277.

15. Mühlethaler R, Stuck AE, Minder CE, et al. (1995) The prognostic significance of protein-energy malnutrition in geriatric patients. Age Ageing 24, 193–197.

16. Wijnhoven HAH, van Bokhorst-de van der Schueren MAE, Heymans MW, et al. (2010) Low mid-upper arm circumference, calf circumference, and body mass index and mortality in older persons. J Gerontol Med Sci 65A, 1107–1114.

17. Izawa S, Enoki H, Hirakawa Y, et al. (2010) The longitudinal change in anthropometric measurements and the association with physical function decline in Japanese community-dwelling frail elderly. Br J Nutr 103, 289–294.

18. Elia M. (1992) Organ and tissue contribution to metabolic rate. In: Kinney JM, Tucker HN (eds). Energy metabolism: tissue determinants and cellular corollaries. Raven, New York; 1992. pp 19–59.

19. Schols AMWJ, Mostert R, Soeters PB, et al. (1991) Body composition and exercise performance in patients with chronic obstructive pulmonary disease. Thorax 46, 695–699.

20. Haapala I, Hirvonen A, Niskanen L, et al. (2002) Anthropometry, bioelectrical impedance and dual-energy X-ray absorptiometry in the assessment of body composition in elderly Finnish women. Clin Physiol Funct Imaging 22, 383–391.

21. Visser M, Deurenberg P, van Staveren WA. (1995) Multi-frequency bioelectrical impedance for assessing total body water and extracellular water in elderly subjects. Eur J Clin Nutr 49, 256–266.

22. Deurenberg P, van der Kooy K, Leenen R, et al. (1989) Body impedance is largely dependent on the intra- and extra-cellular water distribution. Eur J Clin Nutr 43, 845–853.

23. Pietrobelli A, Morini P, Battistini N, et al. (1998) Appendicular skeletal muscle mass: prediction from multiple frequency segmental bioimpedance analysis. Eur J Clin Nutr 52, 507–511.

24. Roubenoff R, Baumgartner RN, Harris TB, et al. (1997) Application of bioelectrical impedance analysis to elderly populations. J Gerontol A Biol Sci Med Sci 52, M129–36.

25. Rech CR, Cordeiro BA, Petroski EL, et al. (2008) Validation of bioelectrical impedance for the prediction of fat-free mass in Brazilian elderly subjects. Arq Bras Endocrinol Metabol 52, 1163–1171.

26. Genton L, Karsegard VL, Kyle UG, et al. (2001) Comparison of four bioelectrical impedance analysis formulas in healthy elderly subjects. Gerontology 47, 315–323.

27. Kyle UG, Genton L, Karsegard L, et al. (1990) Single prediction equation for bioelectrical impedance analysis in adults aged 20–94 years. Nutrition 17, 248–253.

28. Deurenberg P, van der Kooij K, Evers P, et al. (1990) Assessment of body composition by bioelectrical impedance in a population aged >60 years. Am J Clin Nutr 51, 3–6.

29. Dey DK, Bosaeus I, Lissner L, et al. (2003) Body composition estimated by bioelectrical impedance in the Swedish elderly. Development of population-based prediction equation and reference values of fat-free mass and body fat for 70- and 75-y olds. Eur J Clin Nutr 57, 909–916.

30. Lustgarten MS, Fielding RA. (2011) Assessment of analytical methods used to measure changes in body composition in the elderly and recommendations for their use in phase II clinical trials. J Nutr Health Aging 15, 368–375.

31. Janssen I, Heymsfield SB, Baumgartner RN, et al. (2000) Estimation of skeletal muscle mass by bioelectrical impedance analysis. J Appl Physiol 89, 465–471.

32. Janssen I, Heymsfield SB, Ross R. (2002) Low relative skeletal muscle mass (sarcopenia) in older persons is associated with functional impairment and physical disability. J Am Geriatr Soc 50, 889–896.

33. Janssen I, Baumgartner RN, Ross R, (2004). Skeletal muscle cut-off points associated with elevated physical disability risk in older men and women. Am J Epidemiol 159, 413–421.

34. Tankó LB, Movsesyan L, Mouritzen U, et al. (2002) Appendicular lean tissue mass and the prevalence of sarcopenia among healthy women. Metabolism 51, 69–74.

35. Kyle UG, Genton L, Hans D, et al. (2003) Validation of a bioelectrical impedance analysis equation to predict appendicular skeletal muscle mass (ASMM). Clin Nutr 22, 537–543.

36. Chien MY, Huang TY, Wu YT. (2008) Prevalence of sarcopenia estimated using a bioelectrical impedance analysis prediction equation in community-dwelling elderly people in Taiwan. J Am Geriatr Soc 56, 1710–1715.

37. Tengvall M, Ellegård L, Malmros V, et al. (2009) Body composition in the elderly: reference values and bioelectrical impedance spectroscopy to predict total body skeletal muscle mass. Clin Nutr 28, 52–58.

38. Stephen WC, Janssen I. (2009) Sarcopenic-obesity and cardiovascular disease risk in the elderly. J Nutr Health Aging 13, 460–466.

39. Laskey MA, Phil D. (1996) Dual-energy x-ray absorptiometry and body composition. Nutrition 12, 45–51.

40. Albanese CV, Diessel E, Genant HK. (2003) Clinical applications of body composition measurements using DXA. J Clin Densitom 6, 75–85.

41. Heymsfield SB, Smith R, Aulet M, et al. (1990) Appendicular skeletal muscle mass: measurement by dual-photon absorptiometry. Am J Clin Nutr 52, 214–218.

42. Wang ZM, Visser M, Ma R, et al. (1996) Skeletal muscle mass: evaluation of neutron activation and dual-energy X-ray absorptiometry methods. J Appl Physiol 80, 824–831.

43. Shih R, Wang Z, Heo M, et al. (2000) Lower limb skeletal muscle mass: development of dual-energy X-ray absorptiometry prediction model. J Appl Physiol 89, 1380–1386.

44. Visser M, Fuerst T, Lang T, et al. (1999) Validity of fan-beam dual-energy x-ray absorptiometry for measuring fat-free mass and leg muscle mass. J Appl Physiol 87, 1513–1520.

45. Hansen RD, Williamson DA, Finnegan TP, et al. (2007) Estimation of thigh muscle cross-sectional area by dual-energy X-ray absorptiometry in frail elderly patients. Am J Clin Nutr 86, 952–958.

46. Delmonico MJ, Kostek MC, Johns J, et al. (2008) Can dual energy X-ray absorptiometry provide a valid assessment of changes in thigh muscle mass with strength training in older adults? Eur J Clin Nutr 62, 1372–1378.

47. Gallagher D, Visser M, De Meersman RE, et al. (1997) Appendicular skeletal muscle mass: effects of age, gender, and ethnicity. J Appl Physiol 83, 229–239.

48. Lau EM, Lynn HS, Woo JW, et al. (2005) Prevalence of and risk factors for sarcopenia in elderly Chinese men and women. J Gerontol A Biol Sci Med Sci 60, 213–216.

49. Newman AB, Kupelian V, Visser M, et al. (2003) Sarcopenia: alternative definitions and associations with lower extremity function. J Am Geriatr Soc 51, 1602–1609.

50. Zamboni M, Mazzali G, Fantin F, et al. (2008) Sarcopenic obesity: a new category of obesity in the elderly. Nutr Metab Cardio Diseases 18, 388–395.

51. Delmonico MJ, Harris TB, Lee JS, et al. (2007) Alternative definitions of sarcopenia, lower extremity performance, and functional impairment with aging in older men and women. J Am Geriatr Soc 55, 769–774.

52. Woo J, Leung J, Sham A, et al. (2009) Defining sarcopenia in terms of risk of physical limitations: a 5-year follow-up study of 3,153 Chinese men and women. J Am Geriatr Soc 57, 2224–2231.

53. Kelly TL, Wilson KE, Heymsfield SB. (2009) Dual energy x-ray absorptiometry body composition reference values from NHANES. PloS ONE 4, e7038.

54. Shen W, Punyanitya M, Wang Z, et al. (2004) Total body skeletal muscle and adipose tissue volumes: estimation from a single abdominal cross-sectional image. Appl Physiol 97, 2333–2338.

55. Goodpaster BH, Kelley DE, Thaete FL, et al. (2000) Skeletal muscle attenuation determined by computed tomography is associated with skeletal muscle lipid content. J Appl Physiol 89, 104–110.

56. Goodpaster BH, Carlson CL, Visser M, et al. (2001) Attenuation of skeletal muscle and strength in the elderly: The Health ABC Study. J Appl Physiol 90, 2157–2165.

57. Lukaski H. (1997) Sarcopenia: assessment of muscle mass. J Nutr 127(5 Suppl), 994S–997S.

58. Ross R, Pedwell H, Rissanen J. (1995) Response of total and regional lean tissue and skeletal muscle to a program of energy restriction and resistance exercise. Int J Obes Relat Metab Disord 19, 781–787.

59. Song MY, Ruts E, Kim J, et al. (2004) Sarcopenia and increased adipose tissue infiltration of muscle in elderly African American women. Am J Clin Nutr 79, 874–880.

60. Lauretani F, Russo CR, Bandinelli S, et al. (2003) Age-associated changes in skeletal muscles and their effect on mobility: an operational diagnosis of sarcopenia. J Appl Physiol 95, 1851–1860.

61. Visser M, Goodpaster BH, Kritchevsky SB, et al. (2005) Muscle mass, muscle strength, and muscle fat infiltration as predictors of incident mobility limitations in well-functioning older persons. J Gerontol Med Sci 60, 324–333.

62. Newman AB, Kupelian V, Visser M, et al. (2006) Strength, but not muscle mass, is associated with mortality in the health, aging and body composition study cohort. J Gerontol Med Sci 61, 72–77.

63. Cesari M, Pahor M, Lauretani F, et al. (2009) Skeletal muscle and mortality results from the InCHIANTI Study. J Gerontol Med Sci 64, 377–384.

64. Rittweger J, Beller G, Ehrig J, et al. (2000) Bone-muscle strength indices for the human lower leg. Bone 27, 319–326.

CHAPTER 16

Measurement of Muscle Strength and Power

Michael Drey

Institute for Biomedicine of Aging, Friedrich-Alexander University, Erlangen-Nürnberg, Germany

Jürgen M. Bauer

Institute for Biomedicine of Aging, Friedrich-Alexander University, Erlangen-Nürnberg, Germany; and Geriatrics Center, Oldenburg, Germany

INTRODUCTION

As has been shown in Chapter 5 loss of muscle mass is not inevitably associated with loss of muscle strength. In fact, a correlation of the two parameter amounts can only be found between 0.3 and 0.6 [1]. Consequently the European Consensus definition of sarcopenia now also includes physical performance instead of relying solely on muscle mass as in older definitions. (Chapter 2: Definition of sarcopenia). Besides muscle strength muscle power also shows an age-related decline. Furthermore, it could be shown that muscle power declines faster than muscle strength [2]. These observations are of practical relevance, as lower power of the lower extremities has been shown to be associated with a two to three times higher risk for the development of functional deficits. This association is much stronger than between muscular strength and future functional deficits [3]. In addition increases in muscle power have a higher impact on improvements of functionality when compared to increases of muscle strength [4]. These findings have a strong influence on exercise concepts which are developed for the therapy of sarcopenia (see Chapter 18: Exercise interventions to improve sarcopenia).

The above introduction underlines the relevance of measuring muscle strength and muscle power. In this chapter the different options of measurement that are applicable in science and in clinical routine will be presented. First, the terminology of physical parameters that are relevant in this context will be outlined. These parameters differentiate from those measured for the evaluation of physical performance. The latter will be discussed in Chapter 17. In the second part the different methods of measurement that are relevant for research and clinical practice will be presented.

Sarcopenia, First Edition. Edited by Alfonso J. Cruz-Jentoft and John E. Morley.
© 2012 John Wiley & Sons, Ltd. Published 2012 by John Wiley & Sons, Ltd.

TERMINOLOGY

Muscular activity

The interaction between muscle-generated strength and external forces can lead to dynamic or isometric activity. Isometric activity is characterized by a pure increase of tension while the distance between muscle origin and muscle attachment remains constant. Strength is generated, but no outside work is performed, as no muscle shortening occurs. In contrast all muscle activity that is associated with changes of muscle length – not taking into account the direction – is described as dynamic.

Dynamic activity is always associated with changes of joint angles, whether increases or decreases. They are described as concentric if they cause muscle shortening, and as eccentric if despite muscle activity muscle lengthening is observed which is caused by external factors, e.g. weights. When defining a specific dynamic muscle activity the type of change of length – muscle shortening or muscle lengthening –, the speed of the respective change and the movement of involved body parts against each other has to be mentioned. In principal the muscle's operating strength is never constant; when changing joint angles the conditions under which the muscle is working do not stay constant and its ability to generate strength is changing. Therefore, isotonic muscle activity with constant tension is not found in everyday movements. Likewise, one does not normally come across isokinetic muscle activity with constant speed of contraction. Even if a certain movement would be realized with constant velocity – which would mean isokinetically – maybe with the help of a specifically constructed power machine or an ergometer this would not imply that the individual muscle would contract with constant velocity. Furthermore, in practice conditions rarely occur, under which pure concentric, eccentric or isometric activities are realized. In fact combinations of all these actions are observed in the context of everyday movements.

Quantification of muscular action

In the context of muscular actions several physical parameters can be measured. Strength describes the capacity to alter the passive and / or motion state of an object (standard unit = Newton N). Moment of force or torque describes the rotary impact of a force exerted on an object. It is calculated by multiplying the operating force and the vertical distance of the force vector to the axis of rotation (standard unit = Newton × meter Nm). Work is defined as the product of strength and distance without taking into account the time factor (standard unit = Joule J). Power describes the velocity, by which a certain work is performed (standard unit = Watt W).

Strength and power

Muscular strength is globally defined as the physical force that a muscle can exert on specific parts of the body. Here, the muscle may develop different sized forces, depending on the realized form of action (isometric, concentric, eccentric, etc.).

Therefore, it is necessary to specify the form of action under which the force was measured. Besides the form of action, information on the initial muscle length or joint angle must also be available.

Another form to determine muscular strength was proposed by De Lorme [5]. He assumed that even with known terms and conditions of muscle length and/or joint angle, precise determination of muscle strength and torque can still only be carried out with difficulty. From a practical point of view his method offers clear advantages to the physically-based approach for the determination of musclar strength. The basic idea is to define strength by the maximum load that can be lifted once (1RM = One repetition maximum).

Power, however, can be determined for a single movement, a series of movements, or, as in the case of endurance, for a large number of repetitive movements. This can occur continuously at any point in time of the movement sequence, or transmitted over certain movement sections. Power (W) is the outcome of work (J) per time, or the product of operating strength (N) and the distance covered (m) divided by time (s). Calculating power is easily possible on strength-training equipment, as it is common in research, since the resistance needed to overcome the muscular action is known. For measurements in clinical routine this is usually not an option.

METHODS OF MEASUREMENT

In the following section several methods for measurement of muscle strength and muscle power will be described. These methods represent only a selection and are by no means complete. We will describe both kinds of methods – those that are used almost exclusively for research and also those that can be applied in clinical practice as well.

Methods used for research purposes

Computerized pneumatic strength training equipment

Limb strength and power can be measured using computerized pneumatic strength training equipment. Specific training machines are available for different movements of upper and lower extremities, e.g. arm curl, triceps extension, triceps flexion, leg extension, leg press, leg curl, hip abductor and hip adductor.

For strength measurement the use of the so-called one repetition maximum (1RM) has become a standard. The 1RM is defined as the maximum load that can be moved one time only throughout the full range of motion while maintaining proper form.

The double leg press may serve as an example to explain how these measurements are actually taken (Figure 16.1). In the starting position, the seat of the machine is usually positioned to place the knee joint between 90° and 100° of flexion. The hips are kept in a similar degree of flexion. Test persons are instructed to extend both legs fully but without locking the knee joint. They perform the concentric phase, maintain full extension, and perform the eccentric phase of each repetition over 2, 1, and 2 seconds, respectively. The resistance is then progressively increased until the participant is no longer able to move the lever arm one time through the full range of motion.

For measurement of power and velocity the test persons are instructed to perform the lift at each established percentage of 1RM as fast as possible through the full range of motion. Power may be assessed at different percentages of 1RM (40%, 50%, 60%, 70%, 80%, and 90%). Specifically developed software assists in the calculation of power and velocity. In

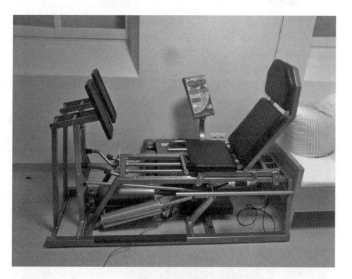

Figure 16.1   Double leg press.

many studies 40% of 1RM and 70% of 1RM have been chosen as outcome variables as they represent power production at relatively high force and low velocity – 70% 1RM – and at low force and high velocity – 40% 1RM. Similar test protocols as above have been applied in several well-designed studies on power and velocity in older individuals. Among others Fielding and co-workers have published several highly relevant papers in this field [6–8].

Nottingham power rig

The leg extensor power rig provides a safe and convenient method for assessing explosive power output from the lower limb [9] (Figure 16.2). The measurement of leg extensor power is functionally relevant, as it has been shown to be related to mobility [10] and instrumental activities of daily living [11] and has been identified as a risk factor for falls [12]. This measurement is also thought to be related to functional activities such as stair climbing [9,13]. It allows an acceptable and useful measurement of muscle power in the elderly, which is not confounded by balance. It is sensitive to the loss of muscle with age and to improvements with training. The equipment was designed in the School of Biomedical Sciences at the University of Nottingham Medical School in 1990. Measurement is made seated using one leg at a time. There is minimal involvement of back muscles. The extension movement takes 0.25-0.40 s in a push through 0.165 m against a flat pedal. At the end of the push the leg is fully extended. As the movement is made seated the forces are contained between the buttocks and the foot. The seat position is adjusted for leg length and the push is transmitted by a lever and chain to spin a flywheel. The gearing is such that resistance to the movement remains nearly constant throughout the extension. The final angular velocity of the flywheel is measured by an optoswitch and is used to calculate the average leg extensor power (LEP) in the push.

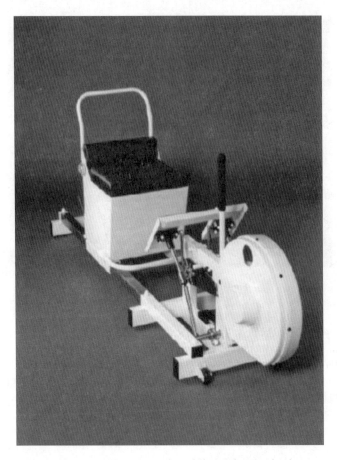

Figure 16.2 Nottingham Power Rig. Reproduced from the Medical Engineering Unit of the University of Nottingham Medical School, http://www.nottingham.ac.uk/biomedsci/documents/meu/legrig.pdf.

STS-transfer

When compared to the aforementioned methods, power measurement of the sit-to-stand transfer on a force platform represents a movement that is also relevant for everyday practice. Simultaneously additional capabilities with regard to balance have to be met by test persons. Furthermore, the transfer has to be executed without any support by the arms. The procedure to measure muscular power of the lower limb by the sit-to-stand transfer test was described by Lindemann et al. for the first time in 2003 [14]. According to their protocol subjects were seated on the front part of a chair with defined height. The arms were crossed over the chest and the eyes were fixed straight ahead while both feet rested on a force plate. The force plate measures the vertical ground reaction force. Test persons were then asked to rise as fast as possible into a standing position and to stand as quiet as possible until the end of data recording. The test should be performed three times with a one minute rest between the trials. For all trials the subjects were encouraged by the investigator to ensure the explosive movement. Sit-to-stand transfer power is defined as $P = F \cdot s/t$ and is calculated by using the changes of vertical ground reaction force during the rising phase (time in seconds between peak force and end of the rising phase: t), vertical ground reaction force during quiet standing (F = m·g, m: weight of subject in kg, g: 9,81m/s^2) and the difference between body height standing and body height sitting in meters (s). The trial that showed the highest power should be used as maximum power. Other studies could show that power measurement based on the sit-to-stand transfer correlated well with power measured by the Nottingham power rig [14].

Vertical jump

Muscle power can be derived from ground reaction force resulting from a vertical jump. For measurement a commercially available mechanographic system may be used. A rather simple jumping paradigm can be applied in older individuals ranging between senior athletes and frail individuals. The following protocol which has originally been described by Rittweger et al. may be followed [15]. Jumping has to be performed as a counter-movement jump (i.e. brief squat before the jump) with freely moving arms. Subjects are usually allowed to make themselves acquainted with several submaximal jumps. The instruction should be to jump with the head and chest as high as possible, thus producing the maximum elevation of the center of mass. As a variable of interest, the peak power out of three two-legged counter-movement jumps should be identified. The authors noticed in their studies that the peak force is 10% greater if the jumping takes place on one leg only. Therefore, peak force may be assessed as the best of three one-legged jumps on the dominant leg. This test can be performed on a ground reaction force platform with a personal computer and an integrated analog-digital board and software. Such a system computes the subject's vertical velocity by integrating the ground reaction force. Body mass and starting point are assessed during quiet stance immediately before the jump. Instantaneous power is calculated as the product of force and velocity. For further information the reader may refer to the original publications [15,16].

Methods for clinical routine

The methods that have been described in the previous section require equipment that will be regarded as too costly and sophisticated for application in clinical practice. Here the ideal approach should be simple and quick. In addition costs should be low and the method should also be applicable in frail older adults. The following methods do at least partly meet these expectations.

Hand grip strength

The measurement of hand grip strength is a common procedure in the course of geriatric assessments and used in both research and clinical practice. Primarily two measuring methods are used. On the one hand dynamometers (e.g. Jamar dynamometer, Figure 16.3) are used to measure the isometric hand grip strength. Often the measured values are given in kg, although the physical quantity measured is a force. The measurement should be done in a sitting position with the shoulder adducted and neutrally rotated, elbow flexed at 90°, forearm in neutral position, and wrist between 0° and 30° dorsiflexion and between 0° and 15° ulnar deviation to avoid overlapping with other motoric tasks, as is the case

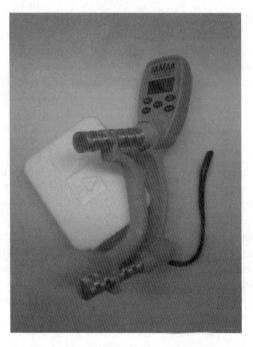

Figure 16.3 The Jamar dynamometer.

when standing. When measuring, make sure a constant muscle length or joint angle by adjustment of the thrust bearing is set depending on the size of the hand. Individuals' ability to use their hand functionally needs to be considered when interpreting hand grip strength (e.g. osteoarthritis, rheumatoid arthritis). Measurement of the maximum strength requires repeated measurements, usually three on each side. The subject should be verbally motivated by a standard command to carry out the contraction with maximum force. The maximum value of these measurements corresponds to the maximum hand grip strength of this person. Table 16.1 shows standard values of the isometric hand grip strength on the dynamometer.

On the other hand, the hand grip strength can be measured with a vigorimeter (e.g. Martin Vigorimeter, Figure 16.4). Here the subjects are given a type of rubber ball in their hand to

Table 16.1 Standard values of the isometric hand grip strength on the dynamometer according to [17]

| | | | Hand grip strength | | | |
| | | | Male | | Female | |
Age	Number	Hand	Mean value [kg]	SD [kg]	Mean value [kg]	SD [kg]
65-69	55	R	41.3	9.3	22.5	4.4
		L	34.8	9.0	18.6	3.7
70-74	55	R	34.2	9.8	22.5	5.3
		L	29.4	8.2	18.8	4.6
75+	51	R	29.8	9.5	19.3	5.0
		L	24.9	7.7	17.1	4.0

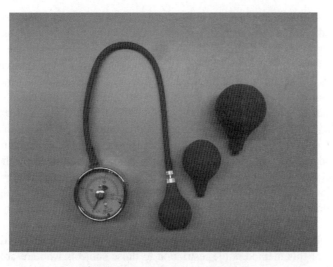

Figure 16.4 Martin vigorimeter.

Table 16.2 Standard values of the Martin vigorimeter. Modified from [19]

Age (yr)	Males Median values (kPa) per age span	Females Median values (kPa) per age span
60 – 64	106	76
65 – 69	97	71
70 – 74	91	67
75 – 79	82	63
80 – 84	75	59
≥85	64	64

contract. This rubber ball is connected to a manometer. The maximum increased pressure reached in this ball is equivalent to the maximum hand grip strength and is expressed in kPa. The instruction on carrying out measurements of isometric hand grip strength outlined above also applies to the vigorimeter. Different ball sizes are used to adapt to different hand sizes, thus enabling uniform pretension of the muscles. This form of action is a dynamic contraction process. Therefore, the two measurements are not directly convertible with each other. Comparative studies show a good correlation between the two methods, although the isometric hand grip measurement depends strongly on the hand anthropometry, as it is the case with the vigorimeter [18]. Table 16.2 shows standard values for the Vigorimeter Martin.

The relevance of the measurement of hand strength lies in its high predictive value of mortality, morbidity and cognitive decline [20].

Chair rise

Often the ability to stand up from a chair is used to gauge the power of the lower extremities. From a practical point of view this is very appealing for use in clinical practice, but also for examinations / assessments outside of the clinic. Generally, it must be stressed that from a biomechanical point of view such an assessment determines far more than just the power of the lower extremities. Similar to the STS-transfer on the force plate and the vertical jump, further coordinative and cognitive exertions are needed to perform this activity.

A standard seat height is recommended. In order to confine the power measurement to the lower extremities, it is important that the subject's arms are not used in supporting the upward movement. Therefore, the exercise should be carried out with folded arms. For this purpose a chair without armrests is recommended. A standard command, that accentuates the explosive movement of standing up is very important. The time span between the command and upright standing of the subject should be determined by the investigator using a stopwatch. In practice the time of five consecutive sit-stand phases is measured. The calculation of power in Watt with the involvement of body weight and height difference is often not done in clinical application. Rather, the immediately measured time value is used to estimate the power. This conclusion also seems feasible as the muscle power measured by the Nottingham power rig correlated well with the chair rise time [21]. The disadvantage of this method is the restriction to those subjects who are able to stand up without using their arms. Nevertheless, the fact alone that those subjects, who cannot get up without assistance, already have an increased risk for a prolonged hospital stay than those who can carry out the exercise [22] is interesting.

Stair climbing

The stair climb power (SCP) test can be considered as an inexpensive test which is easy to perform. This test can be completed in less than one minute and requires only access

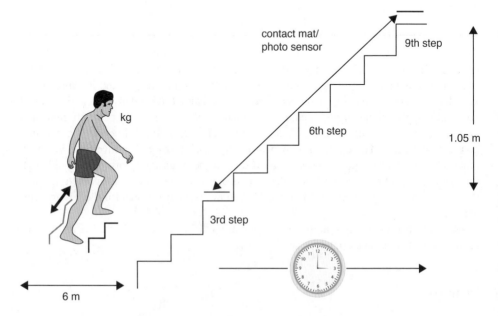

Figure 16.5   Principles of the stair climb test.

to a flight of stairs, a scale and a stopwatch. Stair climb power is calculated based on the following formula: power equals force times velocity. Stair climb time and vertical height of stairs are used to calculate velocity (distance/time), while body mass and acceleration due to gravity are used to calculate force (see Figure 16.5). The stairs should be well-lighted and a number around ten would be appropriate. Test persons are instructed to safely ascend the stairs as fast as they can. For safety purposes they are allowed to use a handrail if they find it necessary. Very clear orders are indicated. Timing starts when the test person begins moving and it is stopped when both feet of the test person reach the top step. Excellent test-retest reliability could be shown for this approach. Stair climb power is usually expressed as SCP/kg. Stair climb power is well correlated with the score of the short physical performance battery (SPPB) [23]. When the components of the SPPB were analysed separately a much higher correlation could be shown with the results of the chair rise test than for gait speed [24].

Summary

It should have been become clear from the above that we have to have a clear understanding of what muscle strength and power are from a physiological standpoint and how difficult it can be to measure both parameters correctly without interference of other parameters like balance etc. Muscle strength and power are associated with more complex tasks like gait speed and 6 minute walking distance as has been underlined by recent publications [25–27]. However, although we associate muscle strength and muscle power directly with muscle function, one has to be aware that these more complex tasks also involve other aspects like cerebral and spinal processing, characteristics of the neuromuscular junction and psychological traits. Therefore measurements of muscle strength and power are not directly comparable with measurements of physical performance. On the other hand measurements of physical performance may be regarded as superior predictors for morbidity, institutionalization and mortality [28, 29] and may therefore be more suitable as primary outcomes in clinical trials.

REFERENCES

1. Goodpaster BH, Park SW, Harris TB et al. (2006) The loss of skeletal muscle strength, mass, and quality in older adults: the health, aging and body composition study. J Gerontol A Biol Sci Med Sci. 61, 1059–1064.
2. Metter EJ, Conwit R, Tobin J et al. (1997) Age-associated loss of power and strength in the upper extremities in women and men. J Gerontol A Biol Sci Med Sci. 52, B267–76.
3. Bean JF, Leveille SG, Kiely DK et al. (2003) A comparison of leg power and leg strength within the InCHIANTI study: which influences mobility more? J Gerontol A Biol Sci Med Sci. 58, 728–733.
4. Bean JF, Kiely DK, LaRose S et al. (2010) Are changes in leg power responsible for clinically meaningful improvements in mobility in older adults? J Am Geriatr Soc. 58, 2363–2368.
5. Delorme TL. (1945) Restoration of muscle power by heavy resistance exercises. J. Bone Jt. Surg. 27, 645–667.

6. Thomas M, Fiatarone MA, Fielding RA. (1996) Leg extensor power in young women: functional correlates and relationship to body composition and strength. Med Sci Sports Exerc. 28, 1321–1326.

7. Fielding R, LeBrasseur N, Cuoco A et al. (2002) High-velocity resistance training increases skeletal muscle peak power in older women. J Am Geriatr Soc. 50, 655–662.

8. Cuoco A, Callahan DM, Sayers S et al. (2004) Impact of muscle power and force on gait speed in disabled older men and women. J Gerontol A Biol Sci Med Sci. 59, 1200–1206.

9. Bassey EJ, Short AH. (1990) A new method for measuring power output in a single leg extension: Feasibility, reliability and validity. Eur J Appl Physiol Occup Physiol 60, 385–390.

10. Bean JF, Kiely DK, LaRose S et al. (2007) Is stair climb power a clinically relevant measure of leg power impairments in at-risk older adults? Arch Phys Med Rehabil. 88, 604–609.

11. Kuo HK, Leveille SG, Yen CJ, et al. (2006) Exploring how peak leg power and usual gait speed are linked to late-life disability: Data from the National Health and Nutrition Examination Survey (NHANES), 1999–2002. Am J Phys Med Rehabil 85, 650–658.

12. Skelton DA, Kennedy J, Rutherford OM. (2002) Explosive power and asymmetry in leg muscle function in frequent fallers and non-fallers aged over 65. Age Ageing 31, 119–125.

13. Bassey EJ, Tay G, West F. (1990) A comparison between power output in a single leg extension and in weightbearing activities of brief duration such as stair running in man. J Physiol (London) 427: 12P

14. Lindemann U, Claus H, Stuber M et al. (2003) Measuring power during the sit-to-stand transfer. Eur J Appl Physiol 89, 466–470.

15. Rittweger J, Schiessl H, Felsenberg D et al. (2004) Reproducibility of the jumping mechanography as a test of mechanical power output in physically competent adult and elderly subjects. J Am Geriatr Soc. 52, 128–131.

16. Runge M, Rittweger J, Russo CR et al. (2004) Is muscle power output a key factor in the age-related decline in physical performance? A comparison of muscle cross section, chair-rising test and jumping power. Clin Physiol Funct Imaging. 24, 335–340.

17. Mathiowetz V, Kashman N, Volland G et al. (1985) Grip and pinch strength: normative data for adults. Arch Phys Med Rehabil. 66, 69–74.

18. Desrosiers J, Hébert R, Bravo G et al. (1995) Comparison of the Jamar dynamometer and the Martin vigorimeter for grip strength measurements in a healthy elderly population. Scand J Rehabil Med. 27, 137–143.

19. Merkies IS, Schmitz PI, Samijn JP et al. (2000) Assessing grip strength in healthy individuals and patients with immune-mediated polyneuropathies. Muscle Nerve. 23, 1393–1401.

20. Ling CH, Taekema D, de Craen AJ et al. (2010) Handgrip strength and mortality in the oldest old population: the Leiden 85-plus study. CMAJ. 182, 429–435.

21. Hardy R, Cooper R, Shah I et al. (2010) Is chair rise performance a useful measure of leg power? Aging Clin Exp Res. 22, 412–418.

22. Fisher SR, Ottenbacher KJ, Goodwin JS et al. (2009) Chair rise ability and length of stay in hospitalized older adults. J Am Geriatr Soc. 57, 1938–1940.

23. Guralnik JM, Simonsick EM, Ferrucci L et al. (1994) A short physical performance battery assessing lower extremity function: association with self-reported disability and prediction of mortality and nursing home admission. J Gerontol. 49, M85–94.

24. Bean JF, Kiely DK, LaRose S et al. (2007) Is stair climb power a clinically relevant measure of leg power impairments in at-risk older adults? Arch Phys Med Rehabil. 88, 604–609.

25. Mänty M, Mendes de Leon CF, Rantanen T et al. (2011) Mobility-Related Fatigue, Walking Speed, and Muscle Strength in Older People. J Gerontol A Biol Sci Med Sci. Oct 19. [Epub ahead of print]

26. LaRoche DP, Millett ED, Kralian RJ. (2011) Low strength is related to diminished ground reaction forces and walking performance in older women. Gait Posture. 233, 668–672.

27. Cooper R, Kuh D, Cooper C *et al*, FALCon and HALCyon Study Teams. (2011) Objective measures of physical capability and subsequent health: a systematic review. Age Ageing. 40: 14–23.

28. Kwon S, Perera S, Pahor M et al. (2009) What is a meaningful change in physical performance? Findings from a clinical trial in older adults (the LIFE-P study). J Nutr Health Aging. 13(6):538–544.

29. Perera S, Studenski S, Chandler JM et al. (2005) Magnitude and patterns of decline in health and function in 1 year affect subsequent 5-year survival. J Gerontol A Biol Sci Med Sci. 60(7):894–900.

CHAPTER 17

Measurements of Physical Performance

Rolland Yves, Gabor Abellan van Kan and Matteo Cesari

INSERM Unit 1027, Toulouse, France; Université de Toulouse, Toulouse, France; Gérontopôle, Centre Hospitalier Universitaire de Toulouse, Toulouse, France

INTRODUCTION

In hospitalized and community-dwelling older people, the comprehensive geriatric assessment (CGA) is one of the most effective clinical approaches to prevent functional decline and disability. The first researches on this topic were performed more than 20 years ago [1] and several meta-analyses have confirmed numerous benefits from routinely adopting the CGA in the evaluation of older persons [2].

Physical performance can be defined as the degree to which the organism is capable of accomplishing specific and independent physical tasks. It is a function of body shape, gender and age, but also affected by endogenous and exogenous stimuli. Physical performances should be differentiated from physical impairment, which can be considered as an early and preclinical state of disability. Physical performance measures are, among the multiple determinants of functional decline, key factors predicting disability; they also represent secondary endpoints (or surrogates markers) for interventions aimed at preventing the onset of major health-related events, including hospitalization, institutionalization, disability and death. In the classical model of disability proposed by Jette and Nagi [3] functional limitations such as the impossibility of performing basic physical tasks (walking, rising from a chair, climbing stairs. . .) represent relevant early phases of the disabling process. Initial functional impairments may be assessed using physical performance tests in which patients are asked to perform a specific physical task. Physical performance measures are performed in a standardized manner and objectively evaluate the capacity of the individual to accomplish specific physical tasks characterized by different degrees of difficulty. Thus, the adopted test can be chosen according to the functional status of the individual and the objectives of the assessment. This approach limits environmental influences and provides objective estimates which may be more reliable than self- or proxy reports of functional limitations [4].

The interest in the physical performance measures is linked to the reversible nature of the disability process, especially if interventions are promptly put in place at the very early phases of it [5]. In fact, early detection of physical impairment may prevent a progression to more severe stages of the disabling process [6]. For example, it has been demonstrated that physical exercise interventions in frail older people can prevent disability and prolong functional independence [6]. On the other hand, once disability appears, it is rarely reversible despite difficult and costly interventions.

During the past two decades, physical performances measures have been included in most longitudinal studies to measure functional limitations [7]. The physical performance measures are clinically meaningful outcomes in pharmacological and non pharmacological researches. Unfortunately, physical performance measures are rarely considered in a routine fashion. However, preventing the functional decline of the older people represents a primary goal of geriatric care, and is a well-recognized priority for public health. Assessment of the functional status of older people is now recommended in clinical practice as a 'sixth vital sign' [8].

WHAT INFORMATION IS PROVIDED TO A CLINICIAN WHEN ADOPTING PHYSICAL PERFORMANCE MEASURES?

Physical performance measures are relevant both in clinical and research settings because they are strong predictors of clinically meaningful adverse health events in older people. During the past 20 years, large numbers of data have demonstrated that low scores on standardized physical performance measures (such as the short physical performance battery, SPPB [4,9–14]) are able to independently predict adverse outcomes (including physical disability, hospitalization, institutionalization. and death), even in non-disabled older persons [4,11,14–18]. The short-walk tests (e.g. 4 meter walk test) are also appropriate for frail elderly people to predict adverse events. Walking speed predicts future onset of ADL and lower body disability [9,12,19], cognitive decline and dementia [20–22], institutionalization and hospitalization [17,23] and mortality [14,17,24]. In nine pooled cohort studies of older people, gait speed was associated with survival with significant increments per 0.1 m/s [25]. All of this information is relevant to improve clinical decisions in geriatrics, but also in other medical disciplines increasingly involved in the health care of older persons (e.g., oncology or surgery). The validity of physical performance tests for major health-related events has been shown to be remarkably consistent throughout multiple cohorts and in extremely different populations [26].

Several reasons can explain the predicting value of poor physical performance measures for adverse outcomes. Prevalence of comorbidity increases with advancing age and results in poor physical performances. In patients with congestive heart failure [27,28] or lung disease [29] the distance covered at the 6-minute walk test is a reliable marker of mortality. However, even in well functioning older adults, slow walking speed is strongly associated with an increased risk of cardiovascular mortality [30]. This suggests that poor physical performance measures could also represent a marker of underlying subclinical disease. It has been repeatedly reported that poor results of physical performance measures remain strong predictors of hospitalization [10] or death [11] in non-disabled older persons even after adjustment for baseline comorbidity or blood test parameters. Moreover, poor physical performances may also reflect a hidden underlying component of vulnerability (e.g., genetic factors [31]) or psychological components (e.g., motivation, mood, personality traits) reflecting the capacity to cope with psychological, clinical, or social stressors. It has been estimated that about half of the individual differences in walking speed might account for both genetic and nongenetic familial effects [32].

In addition to delivering a reliable and efficient measure to classify performance, the physical performance tests are also responsive to changes over time, and might be helpful in monitoring the efficacy of interventions. These tests are sensible to small changes [33]. The efficacy of rehabilitation or physical exercise programs or a new treatment for sarcopenia can objectively be assessed with these measures [34]. A treatment for sarcopenia would be much more convincing if it improves physical performance measures rather than muscle mass only.

SARCOPENIA AND PHYSICAL PERFORMANCE

Sarcopenia is considered responsible in a large part for the age associated decline in functional capacity. The age-related loss of muscle mass and quality occurring with aging is characterized by decreased strength and performance. Several methods have been developed to assess skeletal muscle mass, strength, and quality [35]. Physical performance measures are commonly considered in the operative definitions of sarcopenia mainly because they are directly related to skeletal muscle quality [35]. For clinicians, the integration of the physical performance tests into the routine clinical practice is facilitated by their non-invasiveness [35].

Since the first description of sarcopenia as an age-related decline in muscle mass among the elderly [36], its definition has continued to evolve. Several groups of experts have recently proposed operational definitions of sarcopenia. Each group recognized physical performance measures as a key component for the operational definition of this age-related phenomenon.

The ESPEN SIG (*European Society of Clinical Nutrition and Metabolism Special Interest Groups*) sought to define sarcopenia on the basis of a low muscle mass and low physical performance score (lower quartile score of walking speed [0.8 m/s] from the short physical performance battery). This cut-off has been reported as predictive of mobility disability and adverse events [37]. The *European Working Group on Sarcopenia in Older People* (EWGSOP) [38], recommended different muscle strength and physical performance tests, suggesting different thresholds for the considered adverse outcomes. A 1 m/s walking speed (4 seconds to walk 4 meters) has also been recommended to define sarcopenia by the *International working group on sarcopenia* [39]. This faster gait speed results in a less specific but more sensitive screening tool. The *Cachexia and Wasting Disorders Trialist Workshop* added to slow walking speed (equal to or less than 1 m/s), also the assessment of the 6-minute walk to identify older people simultaneously experiencing sarcopenia and limited mobility [40]. The relevance of these different screening approaches will have to be demonstrated in future cohort researches studies performed in different populations.

All these approaches are substantially consistent. They combine both muscle mass and function evaluations in defining sarcopenia. Although future cohort research studies will have to validate and hopefully unify these different approaches into one single diagnostic instrument/algorithm, they all suggest that physical performance measures (in particular the walking speed test) is the first screening tool to identify sarcopenia in older persons. Interestingly, the walking speed test is extremely appealing in clinical and research settings because it is a simple, quick, well tolerated, inexpensive, and highly reliable test [37], in addition to being predictive of disability, institutionalization, falls, and mortality.

The links between physical performance (such as walking speed) and muscle mass and strength are complex [41]. An increase in muscle mass usually results in an increase in muscle strength, but an increase in muscle mass does not automatically result in improved physical performance (for example, gait speed). The decline in muscle mass affects physical performance only when such loss falls under a critical threshold. This cut-off point is specific for each single physical function test. This relationship between muscle mass and physical performance measures has important implications on the definition of sarcopenia and on the selection of volunteers for clinical trials. In fact, current evidence clearly demonstrates that muscle function is a better predictor of clinical outcomes than muscle mass. The inclusion of physical performance measures in the definition of sarcopenia is due to the importance of capturing a dynamic measure of the muscle rather than just a single static parameter (provided by Dual X-ray Absorptiometry [DXA] or magnetic resonance imaging [MRI]).

THE PHYSICAL PERFORMANCE MEASURES

The Short Physical Performance Battery (SPPB)

The Short Physical Performance Battery (SPPB) is probably the most validated and used physical performance test. It was originally developed at the National Institute on Aging for use in the Established Population for the Epidemiologic Studies of the Elderly (EPESE) [4]. The SPPB is a composite measure of the physical performance of lower extremities. It is a standardized measure that can be adopted both in research and clinical practice.

The SPPB is based on three timed tests: the walking speed (performed on a short distance course), the repeated chair stands, and the balance tests. The instructions to administer this test, developed by the National Institute on Aging, can be downloaded for free on the web (http://www.grc.nia.nih.gov/branches/ledb/sppb/).

For the walking speed test, the subject is asked to walk at his/her usual pace over a 4-meter course [42] (originally 8 feet or 2.4 meter [4]). He/she is instructed to stand with both feet touching the starting line and to start walking after a verbal command. The subject is allowed to use walking aids (cane, walker, or other walking aid) if necessary, but no assistance by another person can be provided. Timing began when the starting command is given, and time in seconds needed to complete the entire distance is recorded. The faster of two walks is usually considered in computing the SPPB score.

The repeated chair stands test is performed using a straight-backed chair, placed with its back against a wall. The subject is first asked to stand from a sitting position without using their arms. If he/she is able to perform the task, he/she is then asked to stand up and sit down five times, as quickly as possible with arms folded across their chests. The time to complete five stands is recorded.

For the balance test, the subject is asked to hold three increasingly challenging standing positions for 10 seconds each: 1) a side-by-side position; 2) semi-tandem position (the heel of one foot beside the big toe of the other foot); 3) tandem position (the heel of one foot in front of and touching the toes of the other foot). Balance test score (in seconds) is given by the total time for which positions are held (range 0 to 30 seconds).

These three physical performance subtasks are used to calculate a summary score by using a pre-determined cut-off point identifying different degrees of physical capacity. The score is ranging from 0 to 4 for each of the three physical performance subtasks, whereas 4 indicates the best performers and 0 the worst performers. Therefore, a summary score ranging from 0 (worst performers) to 12 (best performers) is calculated by adding the categorical results derived from the three timed physical performance subtasks. This scale has proved its reliability [43] and validity for predicting institutionalization, hospital admission and physical disability [4,9,11–13]. These tests have been performed in large studies, with no significant adverse events reported. For clinical research, an arithmetic summary performance score can also be calculated to obtain a continuous measure. This scoring is more sensitive to change, as compared to the quantile score.

The cut-off point identifying older persons with physical impairment is usually set to 8 or lower [9]. The *lifestyle interventions and independence for elders* (LIFE) study selected community-dwelling participant at higher risk of experiencing future disability by adopting a SPPB score of 9 or lower as primary inclusion criteria [6]. Using a SPPB score ranging between 4 and 9 in community-dwelling older people as a strategy of recruitment has been successful to identify large samples of older persons with initial mobility impairment, but not yet disabled. Other epidemiological studies have proposed to define good performers, participants with a SPPB score between 10 and 12, fair performers between 7 and 9 and poor performers between 0 and 6 [26]. Older people with SPPB scores of 10 or lower experience a three-fold higher risk (OR $= 3.38$, 95% confidence interval [CI]: $1.32 - 8.65$) of losing their ability to walk a 400 meter distance over three years compared to those with a SPPB of 12 [44].

It is important to properly design clinical trials and demonstrate the efficacy of pharmacological or non-pharmacological interventions. The estimated lower threshold of clinical meaningful modification for the SPPB is between 0.3 and 0.8 points. A substantial change of the SPPB is estimated at 0.4 to 1.5 points [45]. Gill and colleagues have proposed the criteria of responsiveness to be 0.5 (small meaningful change) and 1 point (substantial meaningful change) [42]. A meaningful improvement of the SPPB would be a strong argument when examining the indication for any new drug that targets low muscle mass or muscle functional decline [46].

In high functioning older adults, the SPPB (or the short distance walk tests) may have a ceiling effect (all individuals may have a high gait speed and a SPPB score at 12). More challenging tests of physical performance must be performed in this population to cover the whole functional spectrum, especially at the high end. These measures may better discriminate amongst higher functioning study participants. In this case, 6-minute walk test, 400 meter tests can be proposed. In the Three-City (3C) study, community-dwelling participants were asked to walk down the corridor as fast as possible without running [30]. In the Health, Aging and Body Composition (Health ABC) Study, time to walk 400 m was measured, and a more challenging SPPB was performed by extending the times from 10 to

30 seconds for the three standard balance tests [47]. This approach is relevant to characterize the wide range of function at baseline among fit older participants of cohort studies.

Timed-get-up-and-go test

The Timed-get-up-and-go (TGUG) test is a physical performance measure that has been mainly used to assess dynamic balance [48]. It is a single test measuring the time a person takes to complete a complex series of different motor tasks (i.e., standing up from a standard armchair, walking three meters, turning, walking back to the chair, and sitting down again). The stopwatch is started on the word 'go' and stopped at the moment the subject sits down. The time to perform the task is compared to normative values for age, gender, and research-based guidelines that measure increased risk of falls and functional decline. The TGUG test has been repeatedly used in persons with frailty, Parkinson's disease, cognitive impairment, recent joint surgery, and osteoarthritis.

The test is easy to learn and perform in clinical settings. The PDF form can be downloaded from the following website: http://foxrehab.org/uploads/pdf/2008_ AssitedLiving-Consult_TUGTest.pdf. The TGUG test can be performed by physicians, nurses, occupational or physical therapists. The patient wears his regular footwear, uses his usual assistive device, if needed (it has to be reported on the form), and walks at a usual pace. No physical assistance is given. A practice trial is given first and the averaged times of two following trials are recorded.

A TGUG score of 14 seconds is sensitive (87%) and specific (87%) for identifying elderly individuals who are at risk for falls [49]. The test-retest reliability (intraclass correlation 0.97–0.99 and Spearmans = 0.93) [48,50,51] and the inter-rater reliability (ICC = 0.99) [48] are good. The performance of the patient can also be summarized into a five-point scaled score [52].

Stair climb power test

The stair climbing exercise tests were developed more than 40 years ago as an anaerobic power test aimed at assessing athletic performance. They have also been widely used to evaluate respiratory function in people with chronic respiratory diseases. More recently, the stair climb power test (SCPT) has been proposed as a clinically relevant measure of leg power impairment [53]. The SCPT may also be helpful, inexpensive, and simple in establishing the diagnosis of sarcopenia [38,54] in community dwelling older people or nursing home residents [53,55,56]. SCPT results are consistent with the SPPB and a more complex measurement of leg power obtained on a leg press resistance machine [53]. This test requires only a flight of stairs and a scale to measure the height of a stair. Test-retest reliability for the SCPT measure has been reported as excellent (r = 0.99) [53]. The procedure is simple and can be completed in less than one minute. The subject is asked to climb a 10-stair flight of stairs as fast as he/she can. For safety reasons, the examiner stands close to him/her. The subject is instructed to use the handrail if needed. After command 'Ready, set, go' the examiner starts timing when the subject starts to move and stops timing when both feet have reached the 10th step. The average time of two trials is recorded.

The SCPT measure (in watt, W) is calculated by multiplying the vertical height of the 10 steps (meter, m) by the body weight of the patient (kilogram, kg) by the acceleration due to gravity ($g = 9.80$ m.s^{-2}) divided by the stair climb time (seconds).

$$\text{SCPT} = \text{strength (F)} \times \text{speed (V)} = [\text{body weight (M)} \times \text{acceleration}$$
$$(g) \times \text{distance (d)}] / \text{time (t)}$$

This clinically meaningful test may be useful both in clinical and research settings.

Gait speed tests

The 6-minute walk test has been widely used in geriatric research settings because it is a reliable physical performance measure [57–61]. During this test, participants are encouraged to walk at a regular pace for as much as possible over a 6-minute period [62]. The 6-minute walk test captures a hierarchy of functioning in healthy elderly subjects. A 20 meter change at the 6-minute test results is considered to be of minimum clinical meaning, while a 50 meter modification is considered as a substantial variation [42].

The benefit of the resistance testing is limited in elderly people who may have multiple reasons for performing poorly beyond simple exhaustion. Moreover, by soliciting the organism with a major effort may increase the risk of adverse events from its assessment among the frailest persons. On the other hand, the 6-minute walk test as well as the 400-meter long-distance corridor walk [63] may become extremely useful in discriminating different categories of risk among older individuals in healthy conditions (by demanding more challenging tasks compared to the short-course walking tests).

In the Health, Aging, and Body Composition (Health ABC) study, 13% of the community-dwelling elderly participants did not complete the 400 m-long distance corridor walk. This test consisted of walking 400 m in a hallway on a 20 m per segment course for 10 laps ([40] m per lap) after a 2-minute warm-up with standard encouragement given at each lap. Patient has to walk as quickly as possible, without running, at a pace they can maintain. The maximum time allowed for the test is 15 minutes. Time to complete the 400 m walk is recorded [64].

Gait speed is one of the three components of the SPPB, but it can also be used as a single parameter for clinical practice and research settings [46]. This simple assessment tool can easily identify large high-risk groups in the community that can benefit from primary preventive measures (Figure 17.1). Gait speed has a good sensitivity to change and can be used to evaluate effect of pharmacological or non pharmacological intervention. The estimated minimally significant magnitude of meaningful change of gait speed is 0.05 m/s while a substantial change of gait speed is 0.10 m/s [42].

Moreover they can be administered in restrictive areas, such as homes and they take less time than long distance walk tests. The 4 m walk test is currently the most commonly used short-walk test validated in elderly adults. It has also shown high reliability [57,65] and the test-retest reliability is also high (intraclass $r = 0.9$) [66]. Short walking test such as the 4 m test can also be used as a single parameter for clinical practice and research. This short walk test can be used as a surrogate for the long distance walk tests to measure the overall functional status in elderly adults [66]. On the other hand, gait speed assessed in a short

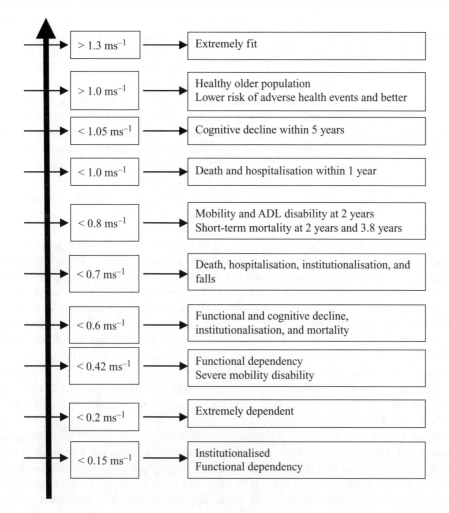

Figure 17.1 Cut-off points of gait speed at usual pace and risk of adverse outcomes
Adapted from Abellan van Kan G. and *al. with permission from JNHA* [37].

walk test is not a surrogate for the whole SPPB. The standing balance and the time to rise from a chair five times, the two other components of the SPPB, have been reported to add valuable information to the gait speed [67] and to be a similarly strong predictor of adverse health events [68].

Self-reported functional limitations assessment

Several self- or proxy physical function tools have been developed. Few of them focus on functional limitations. These tools are practical, safe, not time-consuming, and have a lower cost than the usual physical performance measures. Self-report of difficulty in performing functional activities identifies older persons with physical disability not ascertained by self-report of the need for help [69]. The validity of self-report of difficulty in performing functional activities has to be demonstrated compared to objective physical performance measures. However, these questionnaires may also capture different aspects of the health status than those evaluated by the physical performance measures.

The Late-life Function and Disability Instrument (LLFDI) is currently the most validated self-reported functional limitation assessment measure [70]. The LLFDI lists items evaluating 32 physical activities and the capacity to accomplish 16 major life tasks. The basic and advanced lower extremity functional limitation and upper extremity functional limitation are self-reported in questionnaires. The reliability and validity of this comprehensive measure has been demonstrated compared to the SPPB and the 400 meter test [70]. It has been translated into several languages, a short form has been developed, and it has been reported to be more sensitive to change than the Bartel index [71]. However, its responsiveness to clinically meaningful changes still warrants further research.

Other promising measurement technologies have been developed during the past ten years to measure functional limitations while avoiding floor or ceiling effect. These approaches rely on a large set of questions related to functional tasks which are hierarchically ordered by a computer-adaptive testing (CAT) system [72,73]. This tool creates directly an algorithm adapted to the patient functional level that avoids unnecessary questions (so called *item response theory* [IRT]). Then, this adaptive testing results in a shorter time of drawing-up without losing the precision of the assessment. This approach has been initially supported by the Patient-Reported Outcomes Measurement Information System (PROMIS) initiative, funded by the National Institutes of Health to both, improve the precision of physical function assessment and reducing respondent burden [74]. Compared to the LLFDI, using IRT and CAT results in a small loss in accuracy and sensitivity to change but a substantial reduction in time of administration [75].

Apart from the reduction of the amount of time required to complete a functional assessment, this approach is relevant in longitudinal studies on aging because it can be performed across multiple settings (from community-dwelling to nursing home resident) and because it tends to cover the whole spectrum of functioning. However, a simple instrument that can accurately measure physical performances from bedridden patients to higher levels of independent mobility in hospital or community settings is still lacking [76,77]. The De Morton Mobility Index (DEMMI) has recently been proposed as a mobility instrument developed in the acute hospital setting to overcome this limitation [78]. This score has been reported to be valid and reliable [78]. The scores ranged from 0 (poor mobility) to 100 (good mobility) relying on clinician observation of performance on 15 hierarchical mobility tasks.

To avoid the lack of specificity in item content of the self-report measures that creates error in measurements, new approaches have been proposed. A short form video-animated tool for assessing mobility, the Mobility Assessment Tool—MAT-sf, has been recently developed and validated [79]. The MAT-sf consists of 10 animated video clips that assess respondents' level of proficiency in performing mobility tasks. Several video clips present standardized representation of task performance along dimensions of speed, the slope of inclines, and other environmental challenges. This promising MAT-sf test takes <5 minutes to complete. A demo of the measure can be downloaded from the following website: http://mat-sf.wfuhs.arane.us/.

CONCLUSION

The administration of physical performance measures is crucial for the proper and complete assessment of older people. It allows the heterogeneity of older persons' health status to be captured clearly and objectively estimates the risk of negative health-related events. These measures differently identify high-risk groups from self-reported difficulties, and support the selection and evaluation of older people in both clinical and research settings. The additional information provided by these measures may significantly affect clinical decisions.

Physical performance measures can also serve as important outcomes when evaluating the efficacy of implemented intervention because they are considered as markers of well-being.

Physical performance can be improved at any age even in frail elderly populations. Interventional studies have demonstrated that physical activity programs result in better walking ability, balance and strength. Physical performance measures can be used as surrogate biomarkers of functional decline.

Evaluation of physical performance measures in older people is still not performed in daily practice as are other clinical or biochemical parameters. Among the different tools developed during the past ten years, the walking speed test is easy to perform in a short time and small space without any equipment. It appears to be a simple, reliable screening tool to predict bad outcomes in large populations. This test alone could routinely identify high-risk groups in geriatric clinical settings.

REFERENCES

1. Rubenstein LZ, Josephson KR, Wieland GD, English PA, Sayre JA, Kane RL. Effectiveness of a geriatric evaluation unit. A randomized clinical trial. N Engl J Med. 1984 Dec 27;311(26):1664–1670.

2. Stuck AE, Siu AL, Wieland GD, Adams J, Rubenstein LZ. Comprehensive geriatric assessment: a meta-analysis of controlled trials. Lancet. 1993 Oct 23;342(8878):1032–6.

3. Jette AM. Disablement outcomes in geriatric rehabilitation. Med Care. 1997 Jun;35(6 Suppl):JS28–37; discussion JS8–44.

4. Guralnik JM, Simonsick EM, Ferrucci L, Glynn RJ, Berkman LF, Blazer DG, et al. A short physical performance battery assessing lower extremity function: association with self-reported disability and prediction of mortality and nursing home admission. J Gerontol. 1994 Mar;49(2):M85–94.

5. Gill TM, Gahbauer EA, Allore HG, Han L. Transitions between frailty states among community-living older persons. Arch Intern Med. 2006 Feb 27;166(4):418–423.

6. Pahor M, Blair SN, Espeland M, Fielding R, Gill TM, Guralnik JM, et al. Effects of a physical activity intervention on measures of physical performance: Results of the lifestyle interventions and independence for Elders Pilot (LIFE-P) study. J Gerontol A Biol Sci Med Sci. 2006 Nov;61(11):1157–1165.

7. Gill TM. Assessment of function and disability in longitudinal studies. J Am Geriatr Soc. Oct;58 Suppl 2: S308–12.

8. Bierman AS. Functional status: the six vital sign. J Gen Intern Med. 2001 Nov;16(11):785–786.

9. Guralnik JM, Ferrucci L, Pieper CF, Leveille SG, Markides KS, Ostir GV, et al. Lower extremity function and subsequent disability: consistency across studies, predictive models, and value of

gait speed alone compared with the short physical performance battery. J Gerontol A Biol Sci Med Sci. 2000 Apr;55(4):M221–31.

10. Ferrucci L, Penninx BW, Leveille SG, Corti MC, Pahor M, Wallace R, et al. Characteristics of nondisabled older persons who perform poorly in objective tests of lower extremity function. J Am Geriatr Soc. 2000 Sep;48(9):1102–1110.

11. Penninx BW, Ferrucci L, Leveille SG, Rantanen T, Pahor M, Guralnik JM. Lower extremity performance in nondisabled older persons as a predictor of subsequent hospitalization. J Gerontol A Biol Sci Med Sci. 2000 Nov;55(11):M691–7.

12. Guralnik JM, Ferrucci L, Simonsick EM, Salive ME, Wallace RB. Lower-extremity function in persons over the age of 70 years as a predictor of subsequent disability. N Engl J Med. 1995 Mar 2;332(9):556–561.

13. Guralnik JM, Seeman TE, Tinetti ME, Nevitt MC, Berkman LF. Validation and use of performance measures of functioning in a non-disabled older population: MacArthur studies of successful aging. Aging (Milano). 1994 Dec;6(6):410–419.

14. Cooper R, Kuh D, Hardy R. Objectively measured physical capability levels and mortality: systematic review and meta-analysis. Bmj. 2011;341:c4467.

15. Rantanen T. Muscle strength, disability and mortality. Scand J Med Sci Sports. 2003 Feb;13(1):3–8.

16. Williams ME, Gaylord SA, Gerritty MS. The Timed Manual Performance test as a predictor of hospitalization and death in a community-based elderly population. J Am Geriatr Soc. 1994 Jan;42(1):21–27.

17. Woo J, Ho SC, Yu AL. Walking speed and stride length predicts 36 months dependency, mortality, and institutionalization in Chinese aged 70 and older. J Am Geriatr Soc. 1999 Oct;47(10):1257–1260.

18. Fujita Y, Nakamura Y, Hiraoka J, Kobayashi K, Sakata K, Nagai M, et al. Physical-strength tests and mortality among visitors to health-promotion centers in Japan. J Clin Epidemiol. 1995 Nov;48(11):1349–1359.

19. Ostir GV, Markides KS, Black SA, Goodwin JS. Lower body functioning as a predictor of subsequent disability among older Mexican Americans. J Gerontol A Biol Sci Med Sci. 1998 Nov;53(6):M491–5.

20. Alfaro-Acha A, Al Snih S, Raji MA, Markides KS, Ottenbacher KJ. Does 8-foot walk time predict cognitive decline in older Mexican Americans? J Am Geriatr Soc. 2007 Feb;55(2):245–251.

21. Waite LM, Grayson DA, Piguet O, Creasey H, Bennett HP, Broe GA. Gait slowing as a predictor of incident dementia: 6-year longitudinal data from the Sydney Older Persons Study. J Neurol Sci. 2005 Mar 15;229–230:89–93.

22. Wang L, Larson EB, Bowen JD, van Belle G. Performance-based physical function and future dementia in older people. Arch Intern Med. 2006 May 22;166(10):1115–1120.

23. Cesari M, Kritchevsky SB, Penninx BW, Nicklas BJ, Simonsick EM, Newman AB, et al. Prognostic value of usual gait speed in well-functioning older people–results from the Health, Aging and Body Composition Study. J Am Geriatr Soc. 2005 Oct;53(10):1675–1680.

24. Laukkanen P, Heikkinen E, Kauppinen M. Muscle strength and mobility as predictors of survival in 75–84-year-old people. Age Ageing. 1995 Nov;24(6):468–473.

25. Studenski S, Perera S, Patel K, Rosano C, Faulkner K, Inzitari M, et al. Gait speed and survival in older adults. Jama. Jan 5;305(1):50–58.

26. Rolland Y, Lauwers-Cances V, Cesari M, Vellas B, Pahor M, Grandjean H. Physical performance measures as predictors of mortality in a cohort of community-dwelling older French women. Eur J Epidemiol. 2006;21(2):113–122.

27. Rostagno C, Olivo G, Comeglio M, Boddi V, Banchelli M, Galanti G, et al. Prognostic value of 6-minute walk corridor test in patients with mild to moderate heart failure: comparison with other methods of functional evaluation. Eur J Heart Fail. 2003 Jun;5(3):247–252.

28. Bettencourt P, Ferreira A, Dias P, Pimenta J, Frioes F, Martins L, et al. Predictors of prognosis in patients with stable mild to moderate heart failure. J Card Fail. 2000 Dec;6(4):306–313.

29. Bowen JB, Votto JJ, Thrall RS, Haggerty MC, Stockdale-Woolley R, Bandyopadhyay T, et al. Functional status and survival following pulmonary rehabilitation. Chest. 2000 Sep;118(3):697–703.

30. Dumurgier J, Elbaz A, Ducimetiere P, Tavernier B, Alperovitch A, Tzourio C. Slow walking speed and cardiovascular death in well functioning older adults: prospective cohort study. Bmj. 2009;339:b4460.

31. Carmelli D, Kelly-Hayes M, Wolf PA, Swan GE, Jack LM, Reed T, et al. The contribution of genetic influences to measures of lower-extremity function in older male twins. J Gerontol A Biol Sci Med Sci. 2000 Jan;55(1):B49–53.

32. Pajala S, Era P, Koskenvuo M, Kaprio J, Alen M, Tolvanen A, et al. Contribution of genetic and environmental factors to individual differences in maximal walking speed with and without second task in older women. J Gerontol A Biol Sci Med Sci. 2005 Oct;60(10):1299–1303.

33. Reuben DB, Laliberte L, Hiris J, Mor V. A hierarchical exercise scale to measure function at the Advanced Activities of Daily Living (AADL) level. J Am Geriatr Soc. 1990 Aug;38(8):855–861.

34. Schwartz RS. Sarcopenia and physical performance in old age: introduction. Muscle Nerve Suppl. 1997;5:S10–2.

35. Pahor M, Manini T, Cesari M. Sarcopenia: clinical evaluation, biological markers and other evaluation tools. J Nutr Health Aging. 2009 Oct;13(8):724–728.

36. Rosenberg IH. Sarcopenia: origins and clinical relevance. Clin Geriatr Med. 2011 Aug;27(3):337–339.

37. Abellan van Kan G, Rolland Y, Andrieu S, Bauer J, Beauchet O, Bonnefoy M, et al. Gait speed at usual pace as a predictor of adverse outcomes in community-dwelling older people: an International Academy on Nutrition and Aging (IANA) Task Force. J Nutr Health Aging. 2009 Dec;13(10):881–889.

38. Cruz-Jentoft AJ, Baeyens JP, Bauer JM, Boirie Y, Cederholm T, Landi F, et al. Sarcopenia: European consensus on definition and diagnosis: Report of the European Working Group on Sarcopenia in Older People. Age Ageing. 2011 Jul;39(4):412–423.

39. Fielding RA, Vellas B, Evans WJ, Bhasin S, Morley JE, Newman AB, et al. Sarcopenia: an undiagnosed condition in older adults. Current consensus definition: prevalence, etiology, and consequences. International working group on sarcopenia. J Am Med Dir Assoc. 2011 May;12(4):249–256.

40. Morley JE, Abbatecola AM, Argiles JM, Baracos V, Bauer J, Bhasin S, et al. Sarcopenia with limited mobility: an international consensus. J Am Med Dir Assoc. 2011 Jul;12(6):403–409.

41. Buchner DM, Larson EB, Wagner EH, Koepsell TD, de Lateur BJ. Evidence for a non-linear relationship between leg strength and gait speed. Age Ageing. 1996 Sep;25(5):386–391.

42. Gill TM. Assessment of function and disability in longitudinal studies. J Am Geriatr Soc. 2010 Oct;58 Suppl 2: S308–12.

43. Ostir GV, Volpato S, Fried LP, Chaves P, Guralnik JM. Reliability and sensitivity to change assessed for a summary measure of lower body function: results from the Women's Health and Aging Study. J Clin Epidemiol. 2002 Sep;55(9):916–921.

44. Vasunilashorn S, Coppin AK, Patel KV, Lauretani F, Ferrucci L, Bandinelli S, et al. Use of the Short Physical Performance Battery Score to predict loss of ability to walk 400 meters: analysis from the InCHIANTI study. J Gerontol A Biol Sci Med Sci. 2009 Feb;64(2):223–229.

45. Kwon S, Perera S, Pahor M, Katula JA, King AC, Groessl EJ, et al. What is a meaningful change in physical performance? Findings from a clinical trial in older adults (the LIFE-P study). J Nutr Health Aging. 2009 Jun;13(6):538–544.

46. Working group on functional outcome measures for clinical trials. Functional outcomes for clinical trials in frail older persons: time to be moving. J Gerontol A Biol Sci Med Sci. 2008 Feb;63(2):160–164.

47. Simonsick EM, Newman AB, Nevitt MC, Kritchevsky SB, Ferrucci L, Guralnik JM, et al. Measuring higher level physical function in well-functioning older adults: expanding familiar approaches in the Health ABC study. J Gerontol A Biol Sci Med Sci. 2001 Oct;56(10):M644–9.

48. Podsiadlo D, Richardson S. The timed "Up & Go": a test of basic functional mobility for frail elderly persons. J Am Geriatr Soc. 1991 Feb;39(2):142–148.

49. Shumway-Cook A, Brauer S, Woollacott M. Predicting the probability for falls in community-dwelling older adults using the Timed Up & Go Test. Phys Ther. 2000 Sep;80(9):896–903.

50. Schoppen T, Boonstra A, Groothoff JW, de Vries J, Goeken LN, Eisma WH. The Timed "up and go" test: reliability and validity in persons with unilateral lower limb amputation. Arch Phys Med Rehabil. 1999 Jul;80(7):825–828.

51. Steffen TM, Hacker TA, Mollinger L. Age- and gender-related test performance in community-dwelling elderly people: Six-Minute Walk Test, Berg Balance Scale, Timed Up & Go Test, and gait speeds. Phys Ther. 2002 Feb;82(2):128–137.

52. Mathias S, Nayak US, Isaacs B. Balance in elderly patients: the "get-up and go" test. Arch Phys Med Rehabil. 1986 Jun;67(6):387–389.

53. Bean JF, Kiely DK, LaRose S, Alian J, Frontera WR. Is stair climb power a clinically relevant measure of leg power impairments in at-risk older adults? Arch Phys Med Rehabil. 2007 May;88(5):604–609.

54. von Haehling S, Morley JE, Anker SD. An overview of sarcopenia: facts and numbers on prevalence and clinical impact. J Cachex Sarcopenia Muscle. 2010 Dec;1(2):129–133.

55. Bean J, Herman S, Kiely DK, Callahan D, Mizer K, Frontera WR, et al. Weighted stair climbing in mobility-limited older people: a pilot study. J Am Geriatr Soc. 2002 Apr;50(4):663–670.

56. Fiatarone MA, O'Neill EF, Ryan ND, Clements KM, Solares GR, Nelson ME, et al. Exercise training and nutritional supplementation for physical frailty in very elderly people. N Engl J Med. 1994 Jun 23;330(25):1769–1775.

57. Demers C, McKelvie RS, Negassa A, Yusuf S. Reliability, validity, and responsiveness of the six-minute walk test in patients with heart failure. Am Heart J. 2001 Oct;142(4):698–703.

58. Hamilton DM, Haennel RG. Validity and reliability of the 6-minute walk test in a cardiac rehabilitation population. J Cardiopulm Rehabil. 2000 May-Jun;20(3):156–164.

59. Rejeski WJ, Foley KO, Woodard CM, Zaccaro DJ, Berry MJ. Evaluating and understanding performance testing in COPD patients. J Cardiopulm Rehabil. 2000 Mar-Apr;20(2):79–88.

60. King S, Wessel J, Bhambhani Y, Maikala R, Sholter D, Maksymowych W. Validity and reliability of the 6 minute walk in persons with fibromyalgia. J Rheumatol. 1999 Oct;26(10):2233–2237.

61. Harada ND, Chiu V, Stewart AL. Mobility-related function in older adults: assessment with a 6-minute walk test. Arch Phys Med Rehabil. 1999 Jul;80(7):837–841.

62. Guyatt GH, Sullivan MJ, Thompson PJ, Fallen EL, Pugsley SO, Taylor DW, et al. The 6-minute walk: a new measure of exercise capacity in patients with chronic heart failure. Can Med Assoc J. 1985 Apr 15;132(8):919–923.

63. Simonsick EM, Montgomery PS, Newman AB, Bauer DC, Harris T. Measuring fitness in healthy older adults: the Health ABC Long Distance Corridor Walk. J Am Geriatr Soc. 2001 Nov;49(11):1544–1548.

64. Newman AB, Simonsick EM, Naydeck BL, Boudreau RM, Kritchevsky SB, Nevitt MC, et al. Association of long-distance corridor walk performance with mortality, cardiovascular disease, mobility limitation, and disability. Jama. 2006 May 3;295(17):2018–2026.

65. Ferrucci L, Guralnik JM, Salive ME, Fried LP, Bandeen-Roche K, Brock DB, et al. Effect of age and severity of disability on short-term variation in walking speed: the Women's Health and Aging Study. J Clin Epidemiol. 1996 Oct;49(10):1089–1096.

66. Rolland YM, Cesari M, Miller ME, Penninx BW, Atkinson HH, Pahor M. Reliability of the 400-m usual-pace walk test as an assessment of mobility limitation in older adults. J Am Geriatr Soc. 2004 Jun;52(6):972–976.

67. Cesari M, Kritchevsky SB, Newman AB, Simonsick EM, Harris TB, Penninx BW, et al. Added value of physical performance measures in predicting adverse health-related events: results from the Health, Aging And Body Composition Study. J Am Geriatr Soc. 2009 Feb;57(2):251–259.

68. Cesari M, Onder G, Zamboni V, Manini T, Shorr RI, Russo A, et al. Physical function and self-rated health status as predictors of mortality: results from longitudinal analysis in the ilSIRENTE study. BMC Geriatr. 2008;8:34.

69. Langlois JA, Maggi S, Harris T, Simonsick EM, Ferrucci L, Pavan M, et al. Self-report of difficulty in performing functional activities identifies a broad range of disability in old age. J Am Geriatr Soc. 1996 Dec;44(12):1421–1428.

70. Sayers SP, Jette AM, Haley SM, Heeren TC, Guralnik JM, Fielding RA. Validation of the Late-Life Function and Disability Instrument. J Am Geriatr Soc. 2004 Sep;52(9):1554–1559.

71. Denkinger MD, Igl W, Coll-Planas L, Bleicher J, Nikolaus T, Jamour M. Evaluation of the short form of the late-life function and disability instrument in geriatric inpatients-validity, responsiveness, and sensitivity to change. J Am Geriatr Soc. 2009 Feb;57(2):309–314.

72. Jette AM, Haley SM. Contemporary measurement techniques for rehabilitation outcomes assessment. J Rehabil Med. 2005 Nov;37(6):339–345.

73. Haley SM, Ni P, Hambleton RK, Slavin MD, Jette AM. Computer adaptive testing improved accuracy and precision of scores over random item selection in a physical functioning item bank. J Clin Epidemiol. 2006 Nov;59(11):1174–1182.

74. Rose M, Bjorner JB, Becker J, Fries JF, Ware JE. Evaluation of a preliminary physical function item bank supported the expected advantages of the Patient-Reported Outcomes Measurement Information System (PROMIS). J Clin Epidemiol. 2008 Jan;61(1):17–33.

75. Jette AM, Haley SM, Ni P, Olarsch S, Moed R. Creating a computer adaptive test version of the late-life function and disability instrument. J Gerontol A Biol Sci Med Sci. 2008 Nov;63(11):1246–1256.

76. Davenport L, Brown FF, Fein G, Van Dyke C. A fifteen-item modification of the Fuld Object-Memory Evaluation: preliminary data from healthy middle-aged adults. Arch Clin Neuropsychol. 1988;3(4):345–349.

77. de Morton NA, Berlowitz DJ, Keating JL. A systematic review of mobility instruments and their measurement properties for older acute medical patients. Health Qual Life Outcomes. 2008;6:44.

78. de Morton NA, Lane K. Validity and reliability of the de Morton Mobility Index in the sub-acute hospital setting in a geriatric evaluation and management population. J Rehabil Med. Nov;42(10):956–961.

79. Rejeski WJ, Ip EH, Marsh AP, Barnard RT. Development and validation of a video-animated tool for assessing mobility. J Gerontol A Biol Sci Med Sci. Jun;65(6):664–671.

CHAPTER 18

Exercise Interventions to Improve Sarcopenia

Mark D. Peterson
Department of Physical Medicine and Rehabilitation
University of Michigan, Ann Arbor, MI, USA

José A. Serra-Rexach
Chair Geriatric Department, University Hospital Gregorio Marañón,
Complutense University, Madrid, Spain

'Nobody really lives long enough to die of old age. We die from accidents, and most of all, disuse.'

—Walter Bortz, M.D.

INTRODUCTION

Although the term sarcopenia has taken on various definitions since the original use by Rosenberg [1], over the past decade it has evolved into an equivocal designation of vulnerability to weakness, disability, and diminished independence among aging adults. Indeed, decreases in muscle tissue quantity and quality may begin to occur prior to the fourth decade [2] and gradually worsens through the later stages of adulthood. However, these age-related changes in morphological and functional characteristics of skeletal muscle are often accompanied by other comorbid conditions which may cluster and serve to worsen the severity of sarcopenia. In particular, various cardiometabolic factors such as chronic inflammation and oxidative stress [3], insulin resistance [4], skeletal muscle fibrosis [5], myosteatosis (i.e. intra- and intermuscular adipose tissue infiltration), reduced mitochondrial area density and function [6–8], and increased overall fat mass (i.e. "sarcopenic obesity") [9–11], are known to be coincident with, caused by, or exacerbated through the trajectory of aging and sarcopenia. Thus, despite the ongoing debate and conjecture regarding its classification as a disease state versus the ubiquitous process of normal aging, sarcopenia represents a *very* complex phenotype with a multifactorial etiology.

Sarcopenia, First Edition. Edited by Alfonso J. Cruz-Jentoft and John E. Morley.
© 2012 John Wiley & Sons, Ltd. Published 2012 by John Wiley & Sons, Ltd.

Central to the pathophysiology of sarcopenia and related comorbidity, physical *inactivity* is consistently recognized as a predominant and perennial "cause" [12]. Thus, since sarcopenia is robustly associated with weakness, frailty and mobility disability [13,14], failure to prevent its progression with behavioral interventions including strategic physical activity (PA), exercise, and lifestyle modification may significantly impede optimal quality of life [15,16] and lead to early mortality [17–19].

DEFINITION OF TERMS

Several potent behavioral factors are recognized to independently contribute to onset and progression of sarcopenia and related comorbidity, including obesity, physical inactivity, smoking, and malnutrition. Of these factors, physical inactivity is perhaps the most detrimental for propagating impairment of function throughout late adulthood, and along with insufficient dietary provisions, is the risk component that has received the most research attention for treating age-related atrophy and weakness. Indeed, ample evidence exists to confirm a robust, independent association between sedentary behavior and disease, disability and shortened lifespan among older adults [20]. Despite this rather simplistic and predictable trajectory of age-related *decline*, substantial debate persists regarding the optimal strategy to slow or reverse the downward spiral of muscle tissue integrity and function. At the center of this debate, there is currently no consensus recommendation for PA and exercise among older adults with sarcopenia.

Concerns of elevated risk associated with activity for this population have prompted a minimalistic paradigm, and a general trend of non-progressive, yet 'safe' activity suggestions. However, and as an important point of clarification, 'activity participation' should not be interpreted as merely the inverse of 'inactivity.' Rather, in order to appreciate the extent to which various lifestyles, PA and exercise-strategies contribute value to the spectrum of health and physical fitness among older adults with sarcopenia, the unique attributes of each must be distinguished. Although maintenance or increases in leisure time PA is known to support preservation of function and longevity [20], there are also well-recognized health benefits associated with structured and progressive exercise. Thus, for the purpose of this chapter, a clear distinction is made between (a) lifestyle strategies to reduce sedentary behavior and related chronic health risks, (b) PA strategies that confer preservation of function and basic cardiometabolic health, and (c) structured exercise strategies that are intended to induce specific physiologic and morphologic adaptations.

Sedentary behavior (SB)

SB may be defined as time spent sitting or lying down [21], and is known to increase with age [22]. This modifiable risk factor has received significant attention as a robust predictor of chronic disease and mortality among adults [23,24], and moreover, is acknowledged to accelerate sarcopenia [25]. Importantly, SB should not be regarded as synonymous with extremely low PA levels, as these factors are each *independently* associated with diabetogenic and atherogenic profiles [23,24,26]. SB is generally defined as a range of behaviors that coincides with an energy expenditure less than or equal to 1.5x resting energy expenditure [27]. In using this definition, it is actually plausible to have a potentiated risk profile if someone is both physically inactive and also engages in extended bouts of SB.

Conversely, it is also possible to become deficient in only one, as these behaviors represent two viable targets of intervention. Although decrements in muscle mass and function have been considered the primary contributing factors of functional deficits among aging adults [28], it is conceivable that such changes are also the principal drivers of increased SB in this population. Thus, it is logical to presume that sarcopenia precedes functional deficit, but it is also quite likely that SB itself may lead to sarcopenia and weakness. Generally, both weakness and obesity precipitate SB, which ultimately results in a diminished volume and frequency of stimulus to the cardiometabolic and neuromuscular systems. Although sarcopenia is considered a readily preventable and treatable condition, it is rarely diagnosed at early-onset, and in turn may lead to decreases in functional capacity, and gradual yet significant muscle wasting over time. Clearly, the associated outcomes of functional deficit and chronic SB may also serve as a contributing risk factor for other chronic disease processes (e.g. the metabolic syndrome [29]). This circular cause and consequence of events has made the treatment of age-related comorbid conditions an exceedingly difficult directive; however, a simplistic and yet central preventive strategy from a clinical context is to encourage a lifestyle characterized by increasingly fragmented SB.

Physical activity (PA)

PA is an umbrella term loosely defined by the Institute of Medicine as body movements that are produced through contraction of skeletal muscles, that increase energy expenditure. Thus, baseline activity is operationalized as the smallest increments of body movements that increase energy above SB (e.g. standing, slow walking, lifting very light objects, etc.) [30]. Consistent with this definition, individuals who do only baseline activity are not sedentary, per se, but are *still* considered to be inactive. It is well known that older populations are less active than young adults, and this trend is coincident with various secondary effects of aging (i.e. those resulting from environment, behaviors and/or disease). Conversely, and from a holistic perspective, regular PA involvement is associated with significant attenuation of these secondary consequences, and thus can serve to mediate longevity. Towards that end, recent evidence reveals that increasing or maintaining PA is related to greater survival in older adults, even among those with obesity or functional limitations [20]. Thus, health-enhancing PA may be defined as any body movement that is distinct from baseline activity, and that is expected to add benefit for *enhanced* health. In 2007, the American College of Sports Medicine (ACSM) and American Heart Association (AHA) published joint PA and public health recommendations for older adults [31], in which specific modes and doses of activity were sanctioned to promote maintenance and/or improvement of health. In 2009 the ACSM extended those recommendations in a position stand to provide an overview of issues critical to both exercise and PA in the older adult population [32]. Consistent with the national report *Physical Activity Guidelines for Americans* [30], specific emphasis throughout each publication was placed on accumulation of daily PA volume as a general panacea for age-related comorbidities.

Indeed, regular PA is considered necessary for health maintenance, and is recommended to sustain a healthy body composition and/or body mass index (BMI), lipid/lipoprotein pro-file, glucose tolerance, blood pressure, ambulatory balance, and psychological well-being among older adults [31,32]. Lifestyle PA or leisure-time PA may be generally defined as aerobic in nature, and can take the form of any popular leisure activity (e.g. walking, gardening, biking, golf, etc.). In addition to avoiding SB, some lifestyle PA is certainly better than no activity at all, and for most outcomes there is a dose-response relationship between volume, frequency, and intensity of PA, and respective health benefit [32]. In an effort to provide quantifiable parameters of PA prescription, a focal point of the current guidelines [32] also includes recommendations of mode- and dose-dependent PA. Therefore, since the majority of older adults prefer short bouts of lower-intensity leisure activity [33], it is deemed necessary to operationalize, and provide rationale for inclusion of moderate- and vigorous-intensity PA. In remaining consistent with the ACSM/AHA nomenclature, moderate-intensity PA may be defined as PA that involves a moderate level of effort relative to an individual's aerobic capacity [31]. This type of PA is further characterized by noticeable increases in heart rate and respiration, and may be most easily performed using repetitive modalities such as brisk walking, biking, and aqua-based aerobic activity. Although baseline activity, lifestyle PA, and moderate-intensity PA are all very appropriate suggestions for many of the comorbidities associated with sarcopenia, none of these is particularly effective for preservation of skeletal muscle quantity or quality (i.e. strength/muscle mass).

Exercise is a type of PA that is associated with distinctive adaptations to a given physiological system, and is typically prescribed with the intent for weight loss, health, or physical fitness improvement. Whereas lifestyle PA can be accomplished at random and accumulate throughout the day, exercise is generally referred to as planned, structured, and repetitive. Further, whereas lifestyle PA may contribute to maintenance or improvements in global health and enhanced quality of life among older adults, only certain types of exercise are known to have profound benefits for sarcopenia-specific mechanisms and outcomes. In particular, tailored exercise is necessary for targeting components of health-related physical fitness, which include cardiorespiratory fitness, muscular strength and endurance, body composition, flexibility, and balance [34]. Each of these components either indirectly mediates risk of sarcopenic comorbidities, or is directly associated with reversal of sarcopenia itself. Table 18.1 offers the type of exercise needed to accommodate each of these health-related physical fitness outcomes, the mechanism(s) through which the adaptation occurs, and the nature of this contribution to directly or indirectly influence health and/or function.

BENEFITS OF PHYSICAL ACTIVITY AND AGING

Advancing age is associated with physiologic changes that result in reductions in functional capacity (decline in maximal aerobic capacity and skeletal muscle performance) and altered body composition (accumulation of body fat) [35]. Also physical activity volume and intensity decline with age [36].

Since the first paper of Morris in the early 1950s [37] there is huge scientific evidence about the benefits of physical activity [38,39]. However there is still scepticism between elderly, health professionals and policy makers, about the potency of exercise for disease prevention and treatment in the older generation, particularly in frail adults. Although PA can't stop the aging process, exercise can minimize the physiological effects of a SB and increase active life expectancy by limiting the development and progression of chronic disease and disabling conditions.

Aerobic exercise training can significantly increase VO_2 max, decrease heart rate at rest [40], reduce the artery stiffness [41], improve endothelial and baroreflex function, [42] increase vagal tone and increase maximal exercise stroke volume [43]. Resistance exercise training increases muscle strength, power and endurance [44–46] and has been

Table 18.1 Different types of exercise are needed to accommodate different health-related physical fitness outcomes

Type of Exercise	Health-Related Component of Physical Fitness	Example Modality Options	Mechanism(s) of Adaptation	Influence on Sarcopenia	Influence on Related Comorbidities
Moderate- and Vigorous PA: Aerobic Exercise	Cardiorespiratory Fitness, Body Composition, Muscular Endurance, Balance	Brisk Walking, Cycling, Jogging, Recumbent Stepping, Swimming and Aqua Aerobics, Hiking, Ellyptical Training, Group Aerobic Classes	*Central:* (1) Improved aerobic capacity (VO$_2$ max) through increases in cardiac output and stroke volume; and (2) decreased heart rate at rest and during exercise. *Peripheral:* (1) Increased capillarisation of type I muscle fibers (arteriovenous oxygen difference); (2) Increased mitochondrial size, density, and function (fatty acid oxidation); (3) Increased stores of metabolic energy (e.g. creatine phosphate, glycogen, triglycerides; and (4) increased aerobic enzyme activity (e.g. myokinase).	*Direct:* Significant improvement in muscle function (i.e. muscular endurance and fatigue resistance) *Indirect:* Modest improvement in balance, and thus reduction of slip-and-fall risk.	Improvement in all risk factors for cardiometabolic diseases, i.e. body composition (reduced adiposity), decreased blood pressure, improved insulin sensitivity, improved cholesterol/triglyceride profile, reduction in chronic inflammation.
Resistance Exercise	Muscular Strength and Endurance, Body Composition, Flexibility, and Balance	Free Weights, Selectorized Machines, Pneumatic Resistance Equipment, Body-Weight Movements (e.g. pushups, squats), Alternative Resistive Implements (e.g. Kettlebells, Medicine Balls, Elastic Bands)	*Morphological/Architectural:* (1) Increases in single fiber physiological cross-sectional area and whole muscle hypertrophy and thickness; (2) Increases in fascicle length (sarcomeres in series); and (3) Increases in pennation angle. *Neuromuscular:* (1) Increased force production capacity and rate of force development through greater recruitment capacity of Type II fiber and increased rate coding (motor unit discharge frequency); and (2) Improved neuromuscular efficiency through increased intra- and intermuscular coordination, and decreased antagonist coactivation.	*Direct:* Significant improvements in muscle size and function (i.e. hypertrophy, strength, power and endurance) *Indirect:* Significant improvements in balance and flexibility. Modest improvements in cardiorespiratory fitness, particularly for previously sedentary older adults.	(1) Decreases risk of slip-and-fall accident; (2) Improvement in glucose homeostasis and insulin sensitivity; (3) Increases in bone-mineral density and tendon strength; and (4) Improvement in mobility.

Stretching/Range of Motion Exercise	Flexibility, Balance	Static Stretching, Passive Stretching, Dynamic Range-of-Motion Exercise, Tai-Chi, Yoga , Pilates, Active-Isolated Stretching	(1) Decreased stiffness of musculotendinous unit; (2) Decreased passive resistive force; (3) Increased stretch tolerance.	None	(1) Improvement in mobility, and (2) Decreased risk of slip-and-fall accidents.
Balance Exercises	Balance	Single-Leg Stance Exercises, Lateral Weight-Shift Exercises, Unstable Surface Walking and Isometric Poses	(1) Small increases in strength capacity of ankle, knee, hip, and spinal stabilizer muscles, and (2) Improved proprioception and kinestetic awareness.	None	Decreased risk of slip-and-fall accidents.

shown to favourably impact walking, chair stand, and balance activities. Both, aerobic and resistance training play a role in the prevention and management of arthritis, cancer, chronic obstructive pulmonary disease, chronic renal failure, cognitive impairment, congestive heart failure, coronary artery disease, depression, disability, hypertension, obesity, osteoporosis, peripheral vascular disease, stroke and type 2 diabetes [32].

Flexibility refers to the ability to move a joint through a complete range of motion (ROM). With age there is a decline in the ROM that could affect mobility and physical independence [47]. Flexibility or stretching exercise refers to exercise that lengthens muscles to increase a joint's capacity to move through a full ROM. Balance training are exercises that help maintain stability during daily activities [48,49]. Flexibility and balance exercises are indicated in elderly people at high risk for falling and mobility problems.

Response to exercise

The physiological, cardiovascular and neuromuscular adjustments to exercise of healthy sedentary older adults are qualitatively similar to those of young adults [50,51]. Although improvements tend to be less in older versus young people, the relative increases in many variables, including VO_2, submaximal metabolic responses, exercise tolerance, muscle strength, endurance, and size are generally similar.

Optimization of body composition

The patterns of change in body composition seen in usual aging include increased adipose mass, decreased skeletal muscle mass and decreased bone mass, that may negatively impact metabolic, cardiovascular and musculoskeletal function [52]. Physically active older adults compared to sedentary adults have less total and abdominal body fat, a greater muscle mass in the limbs and higher bone mineral density [53].

Decrease the risk of developing many chronic diseases

The relative risk of developing many chronic diseases (cardiovascular disease, type 2 diabetes, hypertension, obesity and certain cancers), the prevalence of degenerative musculoskeletal conditions (osteoporosis, arthritis, sarcopenia) and disability increases with advancing age [31,32,39].

Regular PA reduces the risk of developing numerous chronic conditions (coronary artery disease, congestive heart failure, hypertension, type 2 diabetes, osteoporosis, obesity, colon cancer, breast cancer, chronic renal failure, stroke, anxiety, depression) and geriatric syndromes (cognitive impairment, frailty, disability, mobility impairments, falls, urinary stress incontinence, sarcopenia, insomnia). The mechanisms of the preventive exercise effect are varied and not completely known, and include: decreased body weight, maintenance of muscles and tendons strength, decreased estrogens levels, decreased blood pressure, decreased LDL cholesterol, decreased insulin resistance and hyperinsulinemia.

Treatment of chronic diseases

Traditional medical approaches usually don't address disuse and deconditioning accompanying some chronic disease (congestive heart failure, chronic obstructive pulmonary disease, intermittent claudication, and chronic renal failure), which may be responsible for much of their associated disability. Moreover, PA is a main therapeutic intervention for the treatment and management of many chronic diseases including coronary heart disease, hypertension, peripheral vascular disease, type 2 diabetes, obesity, hypercholesterolemia, osteoporosis, osteoarthritis, chronic obstructive pulmonary disease, depression and anxiety, dementia, pain, congestive heart failure, syncope, stroke, back pain and constipation [31,32,39].

Exercise may also lower the risk for recurrences of disease such as cardiovascular disease. Resistance exercises that improve skeletal muscle mass in patients with congestive heart failure counteracts the catabolic effects of cytokines [54]. Quadriceps exercises in patients with arthritis improve joint stability and may add benefits to analgesics [55]. Also exercise may counteract undesirable side effects of medications such as myopathy and osteopenia in patients receiving corticosteroid treatment [56].

Decrease falls and injuries

More than one-third of community-living older adults fall each year. Approximately 10% of falls result in a major injury such as a fracture, serious soft tissue injury, or traumatic brain injury. Falls are not only associated with morbidity and mortality, but are also linked to poorer overall functioning and early admission to long-term care facilities [57].

PA reduces risk of falls and injuries from falls [58] even amongst the oldest elderly population [46]. Effective approaches include multidimensional risk factor assessment tied to targeted interventions, exercise programmes (balance, strength and endurance training), and environmental assessment and modification. Exercise programmes can clearly improve strength, endurance and body mechanics, and several controlled trials have shown significant reduction in falls [59–61].

Decrease disability

Epidemiological studies have demonstrated a dose-response pattern for PA that is associated with a lower risk of physical limitations [62]. Additionally, many small studies have reported the benefits of PA on physical capacity and precursors of physical disability (increasing muscle strength, aerobic capacity and bone density) [63], even in frail elderly persons [64,65].

Physically active adults are more likely to survive to age 80 or beyond and have approximately 50% greater risk of dying with disability compared to their sedentary counterparts [66]. There is a clear overlap between the risk factors for disability and the consequences of inactivity: Decreased exercise capacity, gait instability and impaired lower extremity function and mobility characterized both populations. Older people with severe physical impairments generally have a great need for assistance in activities of daily living [67].

Improves psychological health

Physically active older people have a more positive psychological attitude and a lower prevalence and incidence of depressive symptoms. Exercise can improve psychological health and well-being including anxiety, depression, overall well-being, and quality of life [68]. There is strong evidence that high-intensity resistance exercise training is effective in the treatment of clinical depression [69]. Both aerobic and resistance exercise produce clinical improvements in depressed elderly, with response rates ranging from 25% to 88%. Most well-controlled exercise training studies result in significant improvements in both physical fitness and self efficacy for physical activity in older adults [70].

Mental and social health

Regular physical activity is associated with better mental health and social integration. Both cross-sectional and prospective cohort studies have linked participation in regular PA with a reduced risk for dementia or cognitive decline in older adults [71–73]. The mechanism for this relationship is not well understood; it has been suggested that enhanced blood flow, increased brain volume, elevations in brain-derived neurotrophic factor, and improvements in neurotransmitter systems and IGF-1 function may occur in response to behavioral and aerobic training [74]. Also it is well demonstrated that exercise training increases fitness, physical function, cognitive function, and positive behavior in people with dementia and related cognitive impairments [75].

Increase life expectancy

There is clear evidence of an inverse relationship between the volume of PA in a lifetime and all-cause mortality rates in both men and women and older and younger people [76]. Volumes of energy expenditure from doing exercise of at least 1000 Kcal/week reduce mortality by 30%; volumes closer to 2000 Kcal/week reduce the risk by 50%. Also older adults with chronic diseases experience a long-term beneficial mortality effect from participation in exercise programs [77]. It is important to know that despite the increasing likelihood of comorbidity, frailty, dependence, and ever-shortening life expectancy, remaining and even starting to be physically active increases the likelihood of living longer and staying functionally independent [78]. Regular PA increases life expectancy through its influence on chronic diseases development and treatment and also limits the impact of secondary aging through restoration of functional capacity in previously sedentary older adults.

Improve quality of life (QOL)

QOL is a psychological construct, which has commonly been defined as a conscious judgment of the satisfaction an individual has with respect to his/her own life. In a review of the literature that has examined the relationship between physical activity and QOL in old age, Rejeski and Mihalko [79] conclude that PA seems to be positively associated with many but not all domains of QOL. When PA is associated with significant increases in self-efficacy, improvements in health related QOL are most likely to occur [80].

TYPES OF EXERCISE

Aerobic Exercise (AE)

AE is a form of structured PA characterized by rhythmic and repetitive movements of large muscles, for sustained periods. AE is thus any continuous PA that depends primarily on the use of oxygen to meet energy demands through aerobic metabolism, and that is structured and intended to generate improvements in cardiorespiratory fitness, body composition, and/or cardiometabolic health. Since aerobic metabolism is needed for a continuum of physiologic processes spanning from basic energy needs at rest, to elite endurance-sport performance, specific cut-offs have been derived for apparently healthy adults to distinguish between *very light intensity* aerobic exercise ($<30\%$ VO_2R or HRR), *light intensity* aerobic exercise (30% to 39% VO_2R or HRR), *moderate intensity* aerobic exercise (40% to 59% VO_2R or HRR), *vigorous intensity* aerobic exercise (60% to 89% VO_2R or HRR), and *near-maximal to maximal intensity* aerobic exercise ($\geq90\%$ VO_2R or HRR) [81]. Despite these cut-offs, there is no accepted 'threshold' or minimum level of intensity that is needed for cardiorespiratory fitness. Indeed, most research has demonstrated that improvement in cardiorespiratory fitness (i.e. improvement in VO_2 max) is highly contingent upon initial fitness capacity, such that more highly fit individuals require greater relative intensities [82]. However, since the primary focus of aerobic activity and exercise for older adults has been to encourage initial participation and sustainable PA involvement, very little emphasis has been devoted to recommending specific exercise dosages for fitness improvement. Rather, current ACSM/AHA guidelines suggest that aerobic PA for older adults be prescribed to 'promote and maintain health,' and in accordance with a 0-to-10 rating scale of perceived physical exertion (RPE) for moderate-intensity (5 to 6 out of 10) and vigorous-intensity (7 to 8 out of 10) exercise [31,32]. Moreover, in order to meet the criterion definition of 'aerobic exercise,' aerobic PA must be performed at a *minimum* of moderate-intensity (i.e. 40% to 59% VO_2R or HRR; or 5-6 RPE out of 10), and continuously for a sufficient duration of time (≥10 minutes) [31,32,81].

Notwithstanding the value of AE for health promotion and cardiorespiratory fitness among older adults, its impact on sarcopenia is generally recognized as an indirect mediator of chronic comorbidities. Considering that sedentary older adults are at risk for simultaneous reduction in lean body mass and gradual increases in adiposity [9–11], presence of normal BMIs may actually conceal the extent of cardiometabolic risk, i.e. 'normal weight obesity' [83,84]. Further, considering the increased prevalence of the metabolic syndrome and type 2 diabetes among older adults [85–87], public health and clinical efforts must continue to bolster support for regular aerobic activity as a means to circumvent undue chronic health risk and early mortality in this population. The positive benefits of AE on cardiometabolic health are multifaceted, and can be explained by three phenomena [88]. During the acute phase, a single bout of exercise can significantly increase whole-body glucose disposal and thus, temporarily attenuate hyperglycemia. For several hours after the bout of exercise, insulin sensitivity is increased. Lastly and most importantly, repeated bouts of AE leads to a chronic adaptive-response, and is characterized by enhanced cardiorespiratory fitness and global improvements in insulin action [89,90]. AE is also effective for improving blood pressure and lipid profiles, decreasing visceral adiposity, enhancing fatty acid oxidation, increasing mitochondrial function and content, and attenuating the proinflammatory state [91–93].

Resistance Exercise (RE)

RE is a form of structured PA that is generally defined as exercise through which muscles must work against, or resist the force of an applied load. Structured RE relies on anaerobic metabolism to meet energy demands, and is typically prescribed with the intent to improve muscular strength and endurance, or to induce skeletal muscle hypertrophy. Since muscle weakness and atrophy are predictive of functional deficit, disability, and early all-cause mortality among older adults [14,94–96], RE may be considered the primary preventive or treatment strategy in the battle against sarcopenia. However, at present only 27% of the population [U.S.] is estimated to participate in leisure time RE, and these rates are dramatically less for individuals over the age of 50 years [97]. Moreover, although the effectiveness of RE for older adults has been deemed to be supported by the highest category of evidence (i.e. 'Evidence Category A.') [32], the overall reported value of RE for strength and hypertrophy among aging persons is inconsistent across investigations. Debate concerning the appropriateness of RE among older individuals has cultivated questions regarding general efficacy and safety for this population, particularly as applies to progression of training. There are very few published accounts that have examined the overall benefit of RE in aging persons while considering a continuum of dosage schemes, treatment durations, and/or age ranges on longitudinal adaptation. As a result, current PA recommendations for older adults include guidelines for RE [31,32], albeit at minimal dosages and not specific to sarcopenia treatment/prevention.

The extent of sarcopenia and weakness is widely variable among older adults, which is suggested to be attributable to the peak in mass and strength attained earlier in life [98] (Figure 18.1). Thus, even though significant adaptation is possible in the 'oldest old' [99], it may be expected that the benefits of early intervention will translate to preservation of long-term health and independence. Previous studies have documented a disproportionate decline of strength and muscle mass, which suggests that these age-related phenomena are somewhat independent [100,101]. Further, there is a robust association between strength deficit and diminished functional capacity [102,103], and although the rate of decline is largely an individual phenomenon [104], further decrement may be mitigated with early diagnosis and RE participation [105]. Several investigations have reported that after even short durations of RE, protein synthesis rate and neuromuscular adaptive-responses among elderly adults were similar to that of young subjects, despite a much lower pre-exercise rate [106–109].

The guidelines for RE are very different between young and middle-aged healthy adults [110,111], and those sanctioned for elderly populations [31,32,112]. Most notably, and in spite of a significant body of literature to support the safety and effectiveness of higher-dose training, current recommendations for older adults do not endorse progression to accommodate long-term adaptation. Considering that an entire ACSM Position Stand has been devoted to *Progression models in resistance training for healthy adults* [110], there is still much work to be done in determining optimal RE strategies for older adults with sarcopenia. Towards that end, recent evidence from two meta-analyses [44,113] has revealed that RE is effective for eliciting significant strength adaptation and increases in lean body mass among older adults, and that there is a robust dose-response relationship such that volume and intensity are strongly associated with adaptation. These findings reflect and support the viability of progression in RE dosage to accommodate a hierarchical muscular adaptive-response to training. Progressive RE should thus be encouraged among healthy adults, regardless of age, to minimize degenerative muscular morphology and dysfunction.

Volume of RE may be defined as the total number of sets performed per unit of time (i.e. not including warm-up sets). There has been substantial debate concerning the appropriate operational definition of training volume within the literature, which has made this a

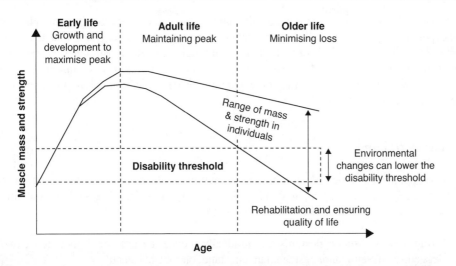

Figure 18.1   Sarcopenia may depend on the peak in mass and strength attained earlier in life. Adapted from: Sayer AA, Syddall H, Martin H, Patel H, Baylis D, Cooper C: The developmental origins of sarcopenia. *J Nutr Health Aging* 2008; 12(7): 427–32.

difficult parameter to control in research. A widely accepted definition for this is volume load (VL), which takes into account the total number of performed sets, repetitions and weight (kg) lifted (i.e. (total repetitions [no.] x external load [kg]); however, since most published RE studies for older adults do not include VL as a prescription entity, it is difficult to draw conclusions regarding the dose-response relationship. Therefore, total number of sets performed may be considered an appropriate surrogate index of the absolute volume of physiologic stress, through which RE can be prescribed. Training **frequency** is defined as the occurrence, per unit of time (e.g. calendar week) that a full-body RE regimen is completed. In many instances, published interventions that incorporated higher-volume training are partitioned to accommodate greater overall time requirements. As an example, full body training may be divided into two upper- and two lower-body training sessions per week (four total sessions). Thus, even though training has manifested over four days, the frequency of training is two days (i.e. the full-body was trained twice, in a given week). **Intensity** of training is commonly defined as the percentage of maximal ability for a given exercise (i.e. one-repetition maximum [1RM]). Although this operational definition for intensity provides a more objective, quantifiable unit than training fatigue or rating of perceived exertion, current recommendations for older adults still rely on a 0-to-10 RPE for moderate-intensity (5 to 6 out of 10) and vigorous-intensity (7 to 8 out of 10) RE [31,32]. Alternatively, intensity of RE may be modified based on a targeted number of repetitions, or by increasing loading within a prescribed repetition-maximum range (e.g. 8-12 RM) [110]. Since it is often challenging or unsafe to ascertain a true 1RM among older adults, using these latter methods to assign intensity is likely the most feasible, effective strategy.

Flexibility exercises

Flexibility, the ability to move a joint through a complete range of motion (ROM), declines with age. Limited ROM in the joints, especially hip, knee, and ankle increase the risk of falls and contribute to age-related gait changes that could affect mobility and physical independence [114]. Flexibility or stretching exercise refers to exercise that lengthens muscles to increase a joint's capacity to move through a full ROM. Stretches can be static (assume position, hold stretch, then relax); dynamic (fluid motion [e.g., tai chi]); active (balance while holding stretch, then moving [e.g., yoga]); or a combination (proprioceptive neuromuscular facilitation).

Balance training

Elderly people are at high risk for falling and mobility problems. Balance training consists of exercises that help maintain stability during daily activities. The ACSM guidelines recommend activities that include the following [32]:

1. Progressively difficult postures that gradually reduce the base of support (e.g., two-legged stand, semi tandem stand, tandem stand, one-legged stand).
2. Dynamic movements that perturb the centre of gravity (e.g., tandem walk, backward walking, sideways walking, heel walking, toe walking circle turns, standing from a sitting position, walking on compliant surface such as foam mattresses, maintaining balance on moving vehicles such as bus or train).
3. Stressing postural muscle groups (e.g., heel stands, toe stands).
4. Reducing sensory input (e.g., standing with eyes closed).

EXERCISE INTERVENTIONS AND SARCOPENIA

General recommendations

The promotion of PA in older adults should avoid ageism. Some older adults can achieve high levels of PA, while others not. Several areas should be emphasized in promoting PA in older adults [31,32,39]:

- Consider some issues like personal preferences, cultural norms, exercise history, readiness, motivation, self-discipline and short and long term goals and logistics.
- The plan should be tailored according to chronic conditions and activity limitations, risk for falls, individual abilities and fitness. Muscle strengthening activities and/or balance training may need to precede aerobic training activities among very frail individuals.
- Identify specific objectives and tasks. Care should be taken to identify, how, when, and where each activity will be performed. For example 'Take a 10-minute walk, three times a day, every day of the week. Choose a speed that allows you to talk but that is moderately hard work. The distance is not important, but make sure to walk for the entire 10 minutes.'
- Initiate activity at modest duration and intensity and progress gradually to minimize the risk of injury. Many months of activity at less than recommended levels is appropriate for very deconditioned older adults as they increase activity in a stepwise manner. In addition, activity plans need to be re-evaluated when there are changes in health status.
- Before and after PA there are necessary warm-up and cool-down activities at a slower speed or lower intensity. These exercises allow a gradual increase or decrease in heart

rate and breathing. A warm-up with aerobic activity usually consists of short intervals of low-intensity movement (e.g., walking for 5 minutes).

- Sensory impairments, such as hearing loss, can make it difficult to instruct older adults. Therefore, speaking loudly and slowly, using visual aids, and demonstrating exercises are all techniques that help older adults become active.

Lifestyle modifications

It is extremely important to encourage older adults to lead regularly active lifestyles, and to limit sedentary activities such as watching television and computer use. Self-transportation (walking, bicycling), taking stairs instead of elevators, parking further from entrances, going shopping, doing housework are all to be recommended.

Aerobic exercise

The emphasis behind ACSM/AHA recommendations [31,32] for older adults is centered on general health promotion, and thus the principal suggestions are related to accumulating habitual aerobic PA and exercise. According to these guidelines, older adults are encouraged to accumulate 30-60 minutes of moderate intensity PA per day (150–300 minutes per week), or at least 20–30 min per day (75–150 min per week) of vigorous intensity. Specifically, continuous or intermittent moderate intensity (40% to 59% VO_2R or HRR; or 5–6 RPE out of 10) to vigorous intensity (60% to 89% VO_2R or HRR; or 7–8 RPE out of 10) AE should be performed with the explicit goals of improved cardiorespiratory fitness. Exercise should be performed at least three days/week, but preferably five or more, with no more than two consecutive days between bouts. Sessions should be a minimum of 10 minutes for intermittent AE, and intended to reach energy expenditure goals of a minimum of 100–250 kcal per session. Gradual progression in duration and intensity may be effective for sarcopenic-obese older adults, and/or for further improvement in cardiorespiratory fitness capacity beyond the baseline requirements for health. However, caution is warranted since progressing sedentary older adults too quickly may exacerbate untoward responses such as musculoskeletal injury. Activities such as brisk walking, swimming, and recumbent cycling/stepping are usually well tolerated by older individuals; however, unless otherwise specified by a primary care physician or cardiologist, individuals may also progress to other modalities such as jogging, hiking, rowing, and stair-climbing.

Resistance Exercise (RE)

The current guidelines also call for RE to be performed two or more nonconsecutive days per week, using a single set of 8–10 exercises for the whole body, and at a moderate (5–6 RPE out of 10) to vigorous (7–8 RPE out of 10) level of effort that allows 8–12 repetitions [31,32]. Although there is indeed sufficient evidence to support the short term efficacy of light- to moderate-intensity RE for strength improvement among older adults [46], there is also ample evidence to confirm the viability of *progressive* RE for improving strength and muscle mass over the long term [45]. As is generally accepted for any novice trainees, prescription of RE should include a 'familiarization' period, in which very low dosage training (i.e. minimal sets and intensity) takes place one to two times per week. Following the familiarization, it may be expected that older adults with sarcopenia can benefit from gradual increases in training dosage to accommodate improvements in strength and muscle hypertrophy. Additional suggestions pertaining to progression in RE include [1] gradual increases in intensity from moderate (i.e. 50–70% of 1-RM [12–15 RM]; or 5–6 RPE out of 10) to vigorous (i.e. 70–85% of 1-RM [6–10RM]; or 7–8 RPE out of 10), [2] gradual increases in the number of sets from a single set-, to as many as three or four sets per muscle group, [3] gradual decreases in the number of repetitions performed (i.e. to coincide with progressively heavier loading), from 12–15 repetitions per set, to approximately 6–10 repetitions per set, and [4] progression in mode from primarily body weight or machine-based resistance exercise to machine plus free-weight resistance exercise.

Due to the disproportionate degree of muscle atrophy and strength decline of the lower limb musculature during aging [115], an RE intervention model for positive effects on lower-extremity strength is recommended to provide enhancement of overall functional capacity. Indeed, lower-extremity weakness in older adults is a primary independent contributor to reduced walking speed [116], decreased lower extremity performance and functional impairment [14,94], falls [117,118], physical disability [119,120], and frailty [121]. RE has also been associated with improvements in various cardiometabolic risk factors in the absence of weight loss, including [1] decreased LDL-cholesterol [122,123], decreased triglycerides [122], reductions in blood pressure [104], and increases in HDL-cholesterol [123]. Several studies have also documented the superiority of RE over traditional AE for glycemic control and insulin sensitivity among type 2 diabetic adults [124]. Therefore, with careful planning, the application of RE among older adults with sarcopenia is not only feasible for eliciting significant adaptation in both force production capacity and muscular hypertrophy, but is also effective for reducing risk of many sarcopenia-related comorbidities. Increased public health and clinical efforts are needed to encourage the provision of this mode of physical activity.

Flexibility

There are a small number of studies that have documented the effects of flexibility exercises in older populations. There is some evidence that flexibility can be increased in the major joints by these exercises; however, how much and what types of flexibility exercises are most effective have not been completely established [32]. The ACSM recommendations states that flexibility exercise should be done at least two days per week, ten minutes per day at a moderate intensity [5,6] on a scale of 0 to 10 and including exercise for the neck, shoulder, elbow, wrist, hip, knee and ankle [32].

Balance

There are no specific recommendations regarding specific frequency, intensity, or type of balance exercises for older adults. Preferably, older adults at risk of falls should do balance training three or more days a week. The exercises can increase in difficulty by progressing from holding onto a stable support (like furniture) while doing the exercises to doing them without support.

Safety

Many older adults initiating physical activity fear the risk of a cardiac event or a musculoskeletal injury. Fears can be mitigated with adequate supervision and education. General recommendations for safety, particularly in the initial stages of exercise, include exercising with supervision, carrying a cell phone to facilitate calling for emergency help, and adhering to an activity level that is comfortable and in which breathing is normal.

There are some absolute contraindications like recent changes in ECG, acute myocardial infarction, unstable angina, uncontrolled arrhythmias, acute heart failure, severe conduction disease and acute non-cardiac diseases that may be exacerbated by exercise (infection, renal failure, tirotoxicosis).

Many caregivers recommend that an exercise stress test precede exercise activity, especially for sedentary older adults, but not all clinicians feel that this is necessary, especially for patients they deem generally stable based upon clinical examination.

If injury occurs, interrupt activity and resume at a lower intensity level. Muscle soreness is common and frequently is innocuous and transient and can be modified with reduced training intensity, cold compresses, and sufficient time and patience to allow spontaneous healing to occur.

It is necessary to wear proper footwear and clothing, and adhere to good nutrition and liquid intake and adequate sleep. Exercise machines have advantages for older, especially frail, as the range of motion is easier to control. Chair and bed based exercise should be considered as a starting point and used by frail patients.

REFERENCES

1. Rosenberg I. Summary comments. Am J Clin Nutr 1989;50:1231–1233.
2. Lexell J. Ageing and human muscle: observations from Sweden. Can J Appl Physiol 1993;18:2–18.
3. Chung HY, Cesari M, Anton S, Marzetti E, Giovannini S, Seo AY, Carter C, et al. Molecular inflammation: underpinnings of aging and age-related diseases. Ageing Res Rev 2009;8:18–30.
4. Srikanthan P, Hevener A, Karlamangla A. Sarcopenia Exacerbates Obesity-Associated Insulin Resistance and Dysglycemia: Findings from the National Health and Nutrition Examination Survey III. PloS One 2010;5:e10805. doi:10810.11371/journal.pone.0010805.
5. Goldspink G, Fernandes K, Williams PE, Wells DJ. Age-related changes in collagen gene expression in the muscles of mdx dystrophic and normal mice. Neuromuscul Disord 1994;4:183–191.
6. Crane JD, Devries MC, Safdar A, Hamadeh MJ, Tarnopolsky MA. The effect of aging on human skeletal muscle mitochondrial and intramyocellular lipid ultrastructure. J Gerontol A Biol Sci Med Sci 2010;65:119–128.
7. Short KR, Bigelow ML, Kahl J, Singh R, Coenen-Schimke J, Raghavakaimal S, Nair KS. Decline in skeletal muscle mitochondrial function with aging in humans. Proc Natl Acad Sci U S A 2005;102:5618–5623.

8. Petersen KF, Befroy D, Dufour S, Dziura J, Ariyan C, Rothman DL, DiPietro L, et al. Mitochondrial dysfunction in the elderly: possible role in insulin resistance. Science 2003;300:1140–1142.

9. Schrager MA, Metter EJ, Simonsick E, Ble A, Bandinelli S, Lauretani F, Ferrucci L. Sarcopenic obesity and inflammation in the InCHIANTI study. J Appl Physiol 2007;102:919–925.

10. Delmonico MJ, Harris TB, Visser M, Park SW, Conroy MB, Velasquez-Mieyer P, Boudreau R, et al. Longitudinal study of muscle strength, quality, and adipose tissue infiltration. Am J Clin Nutr 2009;90:1579–1585.

11. Thornell LE. Sarcopenic obesity: satellite cells in the aging muscle. Curr Opin Clin Nutr Metab Care 2011;14:22–27.

12. Fielding RA, Vellas B, Evans WJ, Bhasin S, Morley JE, Newman AB, Abellan van Kan G, et al. Sarcopenia: an undiagnosed condition in older adults. Current consensus definition: prevalence, etiology, and consequences. International working group on sarcopenia. J Am Med Dir Assoc 2011;12:249–256.

13. Bauer JM, Sieber CC. Sarcopenia and frailty: a clinician's controversial point of view. Exp Gerontol 2008;43:674–678.

14. Janssen I, Heymsfield SB, Ross R. Low relative skeletal muscle mass (sarcopenia) in older persons is associated with functional impairment and physical disability. J Am Geriatr Soc 2002;50:889–896.

15. Cruz-Jentoft AJ, Baeyens JP, Bauer JM, Boirie Y, Cederholm T, Landi F, Martin FC, et al. Sarcopenia: European consensus on definition and diagnosis: Report of the European Working Group on Sarcopenia in Older People. Age Ageing 2010;39:412–423.

16. Morley JE, Abbatecola AM, Argiles JM, Baracos V, Bauer J, Bhasin S, Cederholm T, et al. Sarcopenia with limited mobility: an international consensus. J Am Med Dir Assoc 2011;12:403–409.

17. Cesari M, Pahor M, Lauretani F, Zamboni V, Bandinelli S, Bernabei R, Guralnik JM, et al. Skeletal muscle and mortality results from the InCHIANTI Study. J Gerontol A Biol Sci Med Sci 2009;64:377–384.

18. Metter EJ, Talbot LA, Schrager M, Conwit R. Skeletal muscle strength as a predictor of all-cause mortality in healthy men. J Gerontol A Biol Sci Med Sci 2002;57:B359–365.

19. Newman AB, Kupelian V, Visser M, Simonsick EM, Goodpaster BH, Kritchevsky SB, Tylavsky FA, et al. Strength, but not muscle mass, is associated with mortality in the health, aging and body composition study cohort. J Gerontol A Biol Sci Med Sci 2006;61:72–77.

20. Balboa-Castillo T, Guallar-Castillon P, Leon-Munoz LM, Graciani A, Lopez-Garcia E, Rodriguez-Artalejo F. Physical activity and mortality related to obesity and functional status in older adults in Spain. Am J Prev Med 2011;40:39–46.

21. Chastin SF, Ferriolli E, Stephens NA, Fearon KC, Greig C. Relationship between sedentary behaviour, physical activity, muscle quality and body composition in healthy older adults. Age Ageing 2011.

22. Matthews CE, Chen KY, Freedson PS, Buchowski MS, Beech BM, Pate RR, Troiano RP. Amount of time spent in sedentary behaviors in the United States, 2003–2004. Am J Epidemiol 2008;167:875–881.

23. Katzmarzyk PT, Church TS, Craig CL, Bouchard C. Sitting time and mortality from all causes, cardiovascular disease, and cancer. Med Sci Sports Exerc 2009;41:998–1005.

24. Hamilton MT, Hamilton DG, Zderic TW. Role of low energy expenditure and sitting in obesity, metabolic syndrome, type 2 diabetes, and cardiovascular disease. Diabetes 2007;56:2655–2667.

25. Kortebein P, Symons TB, Ferrando A, Paddon-Jones D, Ronsen O, Protas E, Conger S, et al. Functional impact of 10 days of bed rest in healthy older adults. J Gerontol A Biol Sci Med Sci 2008;63:1076–1081.

26. Healy GN, Dunstan DW, Salmon J, Shaw JE, Zimmet PZ, Owen N. Television time and continuous metabolic risk in physically active adults. Med Sci Sports Exerc 2008;40:639–645.

27. Owen N, Leslie E, Salmon J, Fotheringham MJ. Environmental determinants of physical activity and sedentary behavior. Exerc Sport Sci Rev 2000;28:153–158.

28. Mayhew DL, Kim JS, Cross JM, Ferrando AA, Bamman MM. Translational signaling responses preceding resistance training-mediated myofiber hypertrophy in young and old humans. J Appl Physiol 2009;107:1655–1662.

29. Gardiner PA, Healy GN, Eakin EG, Clark BK, Dunstan DW, Shaw JE, Zimmet PZ, et al. Associations between television viewing time and overall sitting time with the metabolic syndrome in older men and women: the Australian Diabetes, Obesity and Lifestyle study. J Am Geriatr Soc 2011;59:788–796.

30. DHHS. 2008 Physical Activity Guidelines for Americans. Rockville (MD): U.S. Department of Health and Human Services.; 2008.

31. Nelson ME, Rejeski WJ, Blair SN, Duncan PW, Judge JO, King AC, Macera CA, et al. Physical activity and public health in older adults: recommendation from the American College of Sports Medicine and the American Heart Association. Circulation 2007;116:1094–1105.

32. Chodzko-Zajko WJ, Proctor DN, Fiatarone Singh MA, Minson CT, Nigg CR, Salem GJ, Skinner JS. American College of Sports Medicine position stand. Exercise and physical activity for older adults. Med Sci Sports Exerc 2009;41:1510–1530.

33. Rafferty AP, Reeves MJ, McGee HB, Pivarnik JM. Physical activity patterns among walkers and compliance with public health recommendations. Med Sci Sports Exerc 2002;34:1255–1261.

34. Bouchard C, Blair SN, Haskell WL. Physical activity and health. 2nd Ed. Champaign, IL: Human Kinetics, 2007.

35. Holloszy JO. The biology of aging. Mayo Clin Proc 2000 Jan:S3–8; discussion S8–9.

36. Westerterp KR. Daily physical activity, aging and body composition. J Nutr Health Aging 2000;4:239–242.

37. Morris JN, Heady JA, Raffle PA, Roberts CG, Parks JW. Coronary heart-disease and physical activity of work. Lancet 1953;265:1053–1057; contd.

38. McDermott AY, Mernitz H. Exercise and older patients: prescribing guidelines. Am Fam Physician 2006;74:437–444.

39. Fiatarone M. Exercise comes of age: rationale and recommendations for a geriatric exercise prescription. J Gerontol 2002;57A:M262-M282.

40. Huang G, Shi X, Davis-Brezette JA, Osness WH. Resting heart rate changes after endurance training in older adults: a meta-analysis. Med Sci Sports Exerc 2005;37:1381–1386.

41. Tanaka H, Dinenno FA, Monahan KD, Clevenger CM, DeSouza CA, Seals DR. Aging, habitual exercise, and dynamic arterial compliance. Circulation 2000;102:1270–1275.

42. DeSouza CA, Shapiro LF, Clevenger CM, Dinenno FA, Monahan KD, Tanaka H, Seals DR. Regular aerobic exercise prevents and restores age-related declines in endothelium-dependent vasodilation in healthy men. Circulation 2000;102:1351–1357.

43. Okazaki K, Iwasaki K, Prasad A, Palmer MD, Martini ER, Fu Q, Arbab-Zadeh A, et al. Dose-response relationship of endurance training for autonomic circulatory control in healthy seniors. J Appl Physiol 2005;99:1041–1049.

44. Peterson M, Rhea M, Sen A, Gordon P. Resistance Exercise for Muscular Strength in Older Adults: A Meta-Analysis. Ageing Res Rev 2010;9:226–237.

45. Peterson MD, Gordon PM. Resistance exercise for the aging adult: clinical implications and prescription guidelines. Am J Med 2011;124:194–198.

46. Serra-Rexach JA, Bustamante-Ara N, Hierro Villaran M, Gonzalez Gil P, Sanz Ibanez MJ, Blanco Sanz N, Ortega Santamaria V, et al. Short-term, light- to moderate-intensity exercise training improves leg muscle strength in the oldest old: a randomized controlled trial. J Am Geriatr Soc 2011;59:594–602.

47. Singh MA. Exercise and aging. Clin Geriatr Med 2004;20:201–221.

48. Tinetti ME, Baker DI, McAvay G, Claus EB, Garrett P, Gottschalk M, Koch ML, et al. A multifactorial intervention to reduce the risk of falling among elderly people living in the community. N Engl J Med 1994;331:821–827.

49. Day L, Fildes B, Gordon I, Fitzharris M, Flamer H, Lord S. Randomised factorial trial of falls prevention among older people living in their own homes. Bmj 2002;325:128.

50. Seals DR, Hagberg JM, Hurley BF, Ehsani AA, Holloszy JO. Endurance training in older men and women. I. Cardiovascular responses to exercise. J Appl Physiol 1984;57:1024–1029.

51. Seals DR, Hurley BF, Schultz J, Hagberg JM. Endurance training in older men and women II. Blood lactate response to submaximal exercise. J Appl Physiol 1984;57:1030–1033.

52. Hughes VA, Frontera WR, Wood M, Evans WJ, Dallal GE, Roubenoff R, Fiatarone Singh MA. Longitudinal muscle strength changes in older adults: influence of muscle mass, physical activity, and health. J Gerontol A Biol Sci Med Sci 2001;56:B209–217.

53. Going S, Williams D, Lohman T. Aging and body composition: biological changes and methodological issues. Exerc Sport Sci Rev 1995;23:411–458.

54. Williams MA, Stewart KJ. Impact of strength and resistance training on cardiovascular disease risk factors and outcomes in older adults. Clin Geriatr Med 2009;25:703–714, ix.

55. Jadelis K, Miller ME, Ettinger WH, Jr., Messier SP. Strength, balance, and the modifying effects of obesity and knee pain: results from the Observational Arthritis Study in Seniors (oasis). J Am Geriatr Soc 2001;49:884–891.

56. Braith RW, Welsch MA, Mills RM, Jr., Keller JW, Pollock ML. Resistance exercise prevents glucocorticoid-induced myopathy in heart transplant recipients. Med Sci Sports Exerc 1998;30:483–489.

57. Tinetti ME, Kumar C. The patient who falls: 'It's always a trade-off'. JAMA 2010;303:258–266.

58. Sherrington C, Whitney JC, Lord SR, Herbert RD, Cumming RG, Close JC. Effective exercise for the prevention of falls: a systematic review and meta-analysis. J Am Geriatr Soc 2008;56:2234–2243.

59. Rubenstein LZ. Falls in older people: epidemiology, risk factors and strategies for prevention. Age Ageing 2006;35 Suppl 2:ii37–ii41.

60. Rubenstein LZ, Josephson KR. Falls and their prevention in elderly people: what does the evidence show? Med Clin North Am 2006;90:807–824.

61. Michael YL, Whitlock EP, Lin JS, Fu R, O'Connor EA, Gold R. Primary care-relevant interventions to prevent falling in older adults: a systematic evidence review for the U.S. Preventive Services Task Force. Ann Intern Med; 153:815–825.

62. Manini TM, Pahor M. Physical activity and maintaining physical function in older adults. Br J Sports Med 2009;43:28–31.

63. Latham NK, Bennett DA, Stretton CM, Anderson CS. Systematic review of progressive resistance strength training in older adults. J Gerontol A Biol Sci Med Sci 2004;59:48–61.

64. Fiatarone MA, Marks EC, Ryan ND, Meredith CN, Lipsitz LA, Evans WJ. High-intensity strength training in nonagenarians. Effects on skeletal muscle. Jama 1990;263:3029–3034.

65. Fiatarone MA, O'Neill EF, Ryan ND, Clements KM, Solares GR, Nelson ME, Roberts SB, et al. Exercise training and nutritional supplementation for physical frailty in very elderly people. N Engl J Med 1994;330:1769–1775.

66. Leveille SG, Guralnik JM, Ferrucci L, Langlois JA. Aging successfully until death in old age: opportunities for increasing active life expectancy. Am J Epidemiol 1999;149:654–664.

67. Littbrand H, Lundin-Olsson L, Gustafson Y, Rosendahl E. The effect of a high-intensity functional exercise program on activities of daily living: a randomized controlled trial in residential care facilities. J Am Geriatr Soc 2009;57:1741–1749.

68. Netz Y, Wu MJ, Becker BJ, Tenenbaum G. Physical activity and psychological well-being in advanced age: a meta-analysis of intervention studies. Psychol Aging 2005;20:272–284.

69. Mather AS, Rodriguez C, Guthrie MF, McHarg AM, Reid IC, McMurdo ME. Effects of exercise on depressive symptoms in older adults with poorly responsive depressive disorder: randomised controlled trial. Br J Psychiatry 2002;180:411–415.

70. McAuley E, Shaffer SM, Rudolph D. Affective responses to acute exercise in elderly impaired males: the moderating effects of self-efficacy and age. Int J Aging Hum Dev 1995;41:13–27.

71. Marquis S, Moore MM, Howieson DB, Sexton G, Payami H, Kaye JA, Camicioli R. Independent predictors of cognitive decline in healthy elderly persons. Arch Neurol 2002;59:601–606.

72. Tabbarah M, Crimmins EM, Seeman TE. The relationship between cognitive and physical performance: MacArthur Studies of Successful Aging. J Gerontol A Biol Sci Med Sci 2002;57:M228–235.

73. Yaffe K, Barnes D, Nevitt M, Lui LY, Covinsky K. A prospective study of physical activity and cognitive decline in elderly women: women who walk. Arch Intern Med 2001;161:1703–1708.

74. Kramer AF, Erickson KI, Colcombe SJ. Exercise, cognition, and the aging brain. J Appl Physiol 2006;101:1237–1242.

75. Heyn P, Abreu BC, Ottenbacher KJ. The effects of exercise training on elderly persons with cognitive impairment and dementia: a meta-analysis. Arch Phys Med Rehabil 2004;85:1694–1704.

76. Lee IM, Skerrett PJ. Physical activity and all-cause mortality: what is the dose-response relation? Med Sci Sports Exerc 2001;33:S459–471; discussion S493–454.

77. Morey MC, Pieper CF, Crowley GM, Sullivan RJ, Puglisi CM. Exercise adherence and 10-year mortality in chronically ill older adults. J Am Geriatr Soc 2002;50:1929–1933.

78. Stessman J, Hammerman-Rozenberg R, Cohen A, Ein-Mor E, Jacobs JM. Physical activity, function, and longevity among the very old. Arch Intern Med 2009;169:1476–1483.

79. Rejeski WJ, Mihalko SL. Physical activity and quality of life in older adults. J Gerontol A Biol Sci Med Sci 2001;56 Spec No 2:23–35.

80. McAuley E, Blissmer B, Marquez DX, Jerome GJ, Kramer AF, Katula J. Social relations, physical activity, and well-being in older adults. Prev Med 2000;31:608–617.

81. Garber CE, Blissmer B, Deschenes MR, Franklin BA, Lamonte MJ, Lee IM, Nieman DC, et al. American College of Sports Medicine position stand. Quantity and quality of exercise for developing and maintaining cardiorespiratory, musculoskeletal, and neuromotor fitness in apparently healthy adults: guidance for prescribing exercise. Med Sci Sports Exerc 2011;43:1334–1359.

82. Swain DP, Franklin BA. VO(2) reserve and the minimal intensity for improving cardiorespiratory fitness. Med Sci Sports Exerc 2002;34:152–157.

83. Romero-Corral A, Somers VK, Sierra-Johnson J, Korenfeld Y, Boarin S, Korinek J, Jensen MD, et al. Normal weight obesity: a risk factor for cardiometabolic dysregulation and cardiovascular mortality. Eur Heart J 2010;31:737–746.

84. Marques-Vidal P, Pecoud A, Hayoz D, Paccaud F, Mooser V, Waeber G, Vollenweider P. Normal weight obesity: relationship with lipids, glycaemic status, liver enzymes and inflammation. Nutr Metab Cardiovasc Dis 2010;20:669–675.

85. Ford ES, Li C, Zhao G. Prevalence and correlates of metabolic syndrome based on a harmonious definition among adults in the US. J Diabetes 2010;2:180–193.

86. Cowie CC, Rust KF, Ford ES, Eberhardt MS, Byrd-Holt DD, Li C, Williams DE, et al. Full accounting of diabetes and pre-diabetes in the U.S. population in 1988–1994 and 2005–2006. Diabetes Care 2009;32:287–294.

87. CDC. National diabetes fact sheet: national estimates and general information on diabetes and prediabetes in the United States, 2011. Atlanta, GA.: Department of Health and Human Services, Centers for Disease Control and Prevention.; 2011.

88. Richter EA, Derave W, Wojtaszewski JF. Glucose, exercise and insulin: emerging concepts. J Physiol 2001;535:313–322.

89. Nassis GP, Papantakou K, Skenderi K, Triandafillopoulou M, Kavouras SA, Yannakoulia M, Chrousos GP, et al. Aerobic exercise training improves insulin sensitivity without changes in body weight, body fat, adiponectin, and inflammatory markers in overweight and obese girls. Metabolism 2005;54:1472–1479.

90. Dela F, Larsen JJ, Mikines KJ, Ploug T, Petersen LN, Galbo H. Insulin-stimulated muscle glucose clearance in patients with NIDDM. Effects of one-legged physical training. Diabetes 1995;44:1010–1020.

91. Pedersen BK. The anti-inflammatory effect of exercise: its role in diabetes and cardiovascular disease control. Essays Biochem 2006;42:105–117.

92. Exercise and type 2 diabetes: American College of Sports Medicine and the American Diabetes Association: joint position statement. Exercise and type 2 diabetes. Med Sci Sports Exerc 2010;42:2282–2303.

93. Donnelly JE, Blair SN, Jakicic JM, Manore MM, Rankin JW, Smith BK. American College of Sports Medicine Position Stand. Appropriate physical activity intervention strategies for weight loss and prevention of weight regain for adults. Med Sci Sports Exerc 2009;41:459–471.

94. Visser M, Kritchevsky SB, Goodpaster BH, Newman AB, Nevitt M, Stamm E, Harris TB. Leg muscle mass and composition in relation to lower extremity performance in men and women aged 70 to 79: the health, aging and body composition study. J Am Geriatr Soc 2002;50:897–904.

95. Ruiz JR, Sui X, Lobelo F, Morrow JR, Jr., Jackson AW, Sjostrom M, Blair SN. Association between muscular strength and mortality in men: prospective cohort study. Bmj 2008;337:a439.

96. Artero EG, Lee DC, Ruiz JR, Sui X, Ortega FB, Church TS, Lavie CJ, et al. A prospective study of muscular strength and all-cause mortality in men with hypertension. J Am Coll Cardiol 2011;57:1831–1837.

97. CDC. QuickStats: Percentage of Adults Aged ≥18 Years Who Engaged in Leisure-Time Strengthening Activities,* by Age Group and Sex — National Health Interview Survey, United States, 2008; 2009.

98. Sayer AA, Syddall H, Martin H, Patel H, Baylis D, Cooper C. The developmental origins of sarcopenia. J Nutr Health Aging 2008;12:427–432.

99. Kryger AI, Andersen JL. Resistance training in the oldest old: consequences for muscle strength, fiber types, fiber size, and MHC isoforms. Scand J Med Sci Sports 2007;17:422–430.

100. Lynch NA, Metter EJ, Lindle RS, Fozard JL, Tobin JD, Roy TA, Fleg JL, et al. Muscle quality. I. Age-associated differences between arm and leg muscle groups. J Appl Physiol 1999;86:188–194.

101. Young A, Stokes M, Crowe M. The size and strength of the quadriceps muscles of old and young men. Clin Physiol 1985;5:145–154.

102. Bassey EJ, Harries UJ. Normal values for handgrip strength in 920 men and women aged over 65 years, and longitudinal changes over 4 years in 620 survivors. Clin Sci (Lond) 1993;84:331–337.

103. Ferrucci L, Guralnik JM, Pahor M, Corti MC, Havlik RJ. Hospital diagnoses, Medicare charges, and nursing home admissions in the year when older persons become severely disabled. Jama 1997;277:728–734.

104. Kelley GA, Kelley KS. Progressive resistance exercise and resting blood pressure : A meta-analysis of randomized controlled trials. Hypertension 2000;35:838–843.

105. Huber G. The Effect of Resistance training on disablement outcomes: a meta-analysis [Dissertation]. Chicago, IL: University of Illinois; 2005.

106. Holviala JH, Sallinen JM, Kraemer WJ, Alen MJ, Hakkinen KK. Effects of strength training on muscle strength characteristics, functional capabilities, and balance in middle-aged and older women. J Strength Cond Res 2006;20:336–344.

107. Newton RU, Hakkinen K, Hakkinen A, McCormick M, Volek J, Kraemer WJ. Mixed-methods resistance training increases power and strength of young and older men. Med Sci Sports Exerc 2002;34:1367–1375.

108. Roth SM, Ivey FM, Martel GF, Lemmer JT, Hurlbut DE, Siegel EL, Metter EJ, et al. Muscle size responses to strength training in young and older men and women. J Am Geriatr Soc 2001;49:1428–1433.

109. Yarasheski KE, Zachwieja JJ, Bier DM. Acute effects of resistance exercise on muscle protein synthesis rate in young and elderly men and women. Am J Physiol 1993;265:E210–214.

110. ACSM. American College of Sports Medicine position stand. Progression models in resistance training for healthy adults. Med Sci Sports Exerc 2009;41:687–708.

111. Kraemer WJ, Adams K, Cafarelli E, Dudley GA, Dooly C, Feigenbaum MS, Fleck SJ, et al. American College of Sports Medicine position stand. Progression models in resistance training for healthy adults. Med Sci Sports Exerc 2002;34:364–380.

112. ACSM. American College of Sports Medicine Position Stand. The recommended quantity and quality of exercise for developing and maintaining cardiorespiratory and muscular fitness, and flexibility in healthy adults. Med Sci Sports Exerc 1998;30:975–991.

113. Peterson M, Sen A, Gordon P. Influence of Resistance Exercise on Lean Body Mass in Aging Adults: A Meta-Analysis. Med Sci Sports Exerc 2011;43:249–258.

114. Harada ND, Chiu V, King AC, Stewart AL. An evaluation of three self-report physical activity instruments for older adults. Med Sci Sports Exerc 2001;33:962–970.

115. Doherty TJ. Invited review: Aging and sarcopenia. J Appl Physiol 2003;95:1717–1727.

116. Kelley GA, Kelley KS, Tran ZV. Exercise and bone mineral density in men: a meta-analysis. J Appl Physiol 2000;88:1730–1736.

117. Kelley GA, Kelley KS. Efficacy of resistance exercise on lumbar spine and femoral neck bone mineral density in premenopausal women: a meta-analysis of individual patient data. J Womens Health (Larchmt) 2004;13:293–300.

118. Roig M, O'Brien K, Kirk G, Murray R, McKinnon P, Shadgan B, Reid WD. The effects of eccentric versus concentric resistance training on muscle strength and mass in healthy adults: a systematic review with meta-analysis. Br J Sports Med 2009;43:556–568.

119. Baumgartner RN, Koehler KM, Gallagher D, Romero L, Heymsfield SB, Ross RR, Garry PJ, et al. Epidemiology of sarcopenia among the elderly in New Mexico. Am J Epidemiol 1998;147:755–763.

120. Janssen I, Baumgartner RN, Ross R, Rosenberg IH, Roubenoff R. Skeletal muscle cutpoints associated with elevated physical disability risk in older men and women. Am J Epidemiol 2004;159:413–421.

121. Orr R, Raymond J, Fiatarone Singh M. Efficacy of progressive resistance training on balance performance in older adults : a systematic review of randomized controlled trials. Sports Med 2008;38:317–343.

122. Goldberg L, Elliot DL, Schutz RW, Kloster FE. Changes in lipid and lipoprotein levels after weight training. JAMA 1984;252:504–506.

123. Hurley BF, Hagberg JM, Goldberg AP, Seals DR, Ehsani AA, Brennan RE, Holloszy JO. Resistive training can reduce coronary risk factors without altering VO2max or percent body fat. Med Sci Sports Exerc 1988;20:150–154.

124. Cauza E, Hanusch-Enserer U, Strasser B, Kostner K, Dunky A, Haber P. Strength and endurance training lead to different post exercise glucose profiles in diabetic participants using a continuous subcutaneous glucose monitoring system. Eur J Clin Invest 2005;35:745–751.

CHAPTER 19

Nutritional Approaches to Treating Sarcopenia

Douglas Paddon-Jones

Department of Nutrition and Metabolism, University of Texas Medical Branch, Texas, USA

Luc van Loon

Department of Human Movement Sciences Maastricht University Medical Centre, PO Box 616, 6200 MD Maastricht, The Netherlands

INTRODUCTION

Sarcopenia is a progressive, insidious process characterized by 3-8% reduction in muscle mass per decade after the age of 30 years. Recent collaborative efforts and innovative basic and translational research continues to improve our understanding of the mechanisms contributing to sarcopenia and refine treatment and prevention strategies [1,2]. However, despite our advances, the increasing incidence of sarcopenic muscle loss in older adults highlights the continued failure of one or more facets of the evidence-based care continuum. These may be summarized as:

(i) A failure to successfully adopt or implement management or treatment strategies.
(ii) A failure to communicate promising clinical trial results and strategies to key groups, such as older adults, care-givers, health care professionals and industry groups.
(iii) An inherent failure in the design, applicability or translation of clinical research studies.

The goal of this chapter is to explore the obstacles and opportunities for treating sarcopenia using a nutrition-focused approach. While it is clear that sarcopenia is the result of a complex interplay of various factors, in all cases, an adequate nutritional framework is the fundamental prerequisite for maintaining muscle mass, strength and ultimately functional capacity.

In addition to recent efforts that have provided much needed consensus statements on the definition, diagnosis and morphology of sarcopenia, clinicians and scientists have access

Sarcopenia, First Edition. Edited by Alfonso J. Cruz-Jentoft and John E. Morley.
© 2012 John Wiley & Sons, Ltd. Published 2012 by John Wiley & Sons, Ltd.

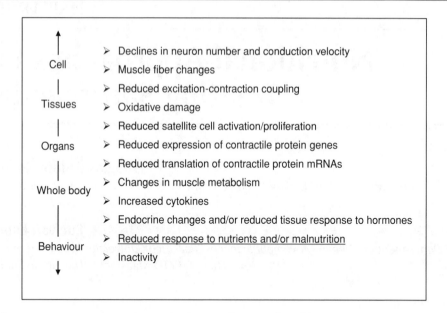

Figure 19.1 Sarcopenia is the result of a complex interplay of factors, however, an adequate nutritional framework is the fundamental prerequisite for maintaining muscle anabolism, mass and functional capacity.

to an increasing variety of strategies and interventions to prevent and treat sarcopenia (also *see* Chapters 4, 18, 20 and 21). This includes data and strategies derived from research focusing on protein metabolism and cell signaling, physical inactivity and bed rest and age-related changes in the anabolic response to protein ingestion [3–6] (Figure 19.1). In this chapter, we will highlight the strengths and weaknesses of current dietary practices and interventions and review the efficacy and potential translation of recent basic science and clinical research trials (Figure 19.2).

ADEQUACY OF CURRENT DIETARY PROTEIN RECOMMENDATIONS FOR OLDER ADULTS

While there is little doubt that older adults are at increased risk of food insecurity and protein-energy malnutrition [7], the adequacy of the recommended dietary allowance (RDA) for protein continues to be a topic of debate [8–13]. Several groups have suggested that the current RDA for protein, while fulfilling the criteria as the 'minimal daily average dietary intake level that meets the nutritional requirements of nearly all healthy individuals', does not promote optimal health or protect elders from sarcopenic muscle loss [10,14–16]. For example, while the Health ABC study data set demonstrated the expected negative correlation between protein intake and muscle mass (i.e., on average, older adults with a lower protein intake have lower muscle mass), the relationship could still be observed in populations who met the RDA for protein [17].

The current protein recommendation for all adults 19 years and older ($0.8\,g\cdot kg^{-1}\cdot d^{-1}$) was established by the Institute of Medicine (IOM) and based primarily on limited short-duration

Food	Serving size	Protein (g)
Lean beef	4 oz	30
Chicken breast	4 oz	30
Salmon	4 oz	25
Tuna in water	3.5 oz can	18
Eggs	2 whole	12
Milk 1%	8 oz	8
Yogurt low-fat	6 oz	6
Greek yogurt low-fat	6 oz	14
Cheddar cheese	1 oz	7
Almonds	1 oz, 23 nuts	6
Peanut butter	2 TBSP	8
Quinoa cooked	1/2 cup	4
Tofu	4 oz	8
Latte coffee medium	16 oz	8

Figure 19.2   A basic understanding of the protein content of a variety of foods is an important aspect of ensuring protein and energy needs are met and not grossly exceeded or under represented.

nitrogen balance studies in young adults [18,19]. While the RDA does not discriminate by age, it is clear that older adults tend to have a lower energy intake and, as such, consume less protein than their younger counterparts. Studies estimate that approximately one third of adults over the age of 50 fail to meet the RDA for protein while approximately 10% of older women fail to meet even the Estimated Average Requirement (EAR) for protein $(0.66 \text{ g·kg}^{-1}\text{·d}^{-1})$ [10,16]. The EAR represents a total daily protein intake of less than 40 g for a 65 kg adult.

While the EAR and RDA for protein have erroneously been viewed as desirable averages and upper-limit targets for protein consumption [9,10], the IOM's Acceptable Macronutrient Distribution Range (AMDR) provides a broader recommendation and permits greater flexibility with meal planning and consideration of individual needs. The AMDR for protein represents 10%-35% of an individual's total daily energy intake and is defined as 'the range of intake for a particular energy source (i.e., protein) that is associated with reduced risk of chronic disease while providing intakes of essential nutrients'. Unfortunately, the prescriptive usefulness of the AMDR is diminished by the magnitude of the 'acceptable' range and generous quantity of protein represented by the upper end of the range (Figure 19.3).

In this chapter, we argue that while a modest increase in dietary protein beyond the RDA may be beneficial for some older adults (perhaps $1.0\text{-}1.3 \text{ g·kg}^{-1}\text{·d}^{-1}$), there is a greater need to specifically examine the quality and quantity of protein consumed with each meal [20]. In broad terms, we propose that individuals should consume a moderate amount of high quality protein with each meal. For a reference 75 kg individual, an intake of 25–30 g of protein/meal for three daily meals represents a daily protein consumption of $1.0\text{-}1.2 \text{ g·kg·d}^{-1}$. This recommendation focuses on the potential longer-term benefits of achieving appropriate increases in protein synthesis following each meal period. By establishing a 'meal- driven, recommended protein intake', the argument over total daily protein

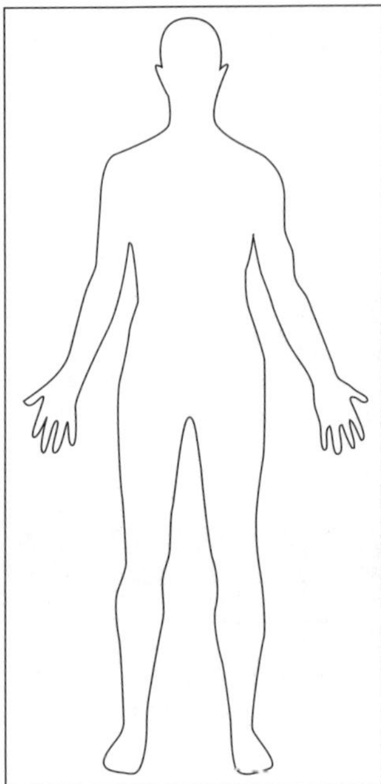

Acceptable Macronutrient Distribution Range?			
	RDA	AMDR 10%	AMDR 35%
Young sedentary female (20 yrs, 60 kg, 1.6 m)	0.8	0.81	3.08
Older sedentary female (70 yrs, 50 kg, 1.6 m)	0.8	0.68	2.40
Older active female (70 yrs, 50 kg, 1.6 m)	0.8	0.73	2.57
Young active female (20 yrs, 80 kg, 1.75 m)	0.8	0.94	3.30
Older sedentary male (70 yrs, 70 kg, 1.75 m)	0.8	0.73	2.57

Figure 19.3 While the RDA for all adults is 0.8 g protein/kg bodyweight/day, the AMDR is influenced by age, sex and body size. For some groups, the lower end of the AMDR (10% protein) falls below the RDA, while the majority of the AMDR is heavily skewed towards higher protein intakes.

intake is largely avoided and the focus shifted to an approach that emphasizes repeated maximal stimulation of skeletal muscle anabolic pathways throughout the day.

THE EFFECT OF AGE ON PROTEIN ANABOLISM IN RESPONSE TO MEALS

Stable isotope methodology and the related assessment of translation initiation and cell signaling via muscle biopsy tissue sampling is the current gold standard technique for assessing acute changes in *in vivo* protein anabolism in response to nutrient ingestion (Figure 19.4). In older populations, numerous acute stable isotope/metabolism studies have explored the mechanistic response to a single meal or supplement [5,6,21–25].

Most metabolic studies examining the effects of nutrient ingestion on muscle protein anabolism focus on two physiological periods; the postabsorptive/fasting period and the postprandial period. It seems clear that there is minimal, if any, reduction in fasting muscle protein synthesis with age. However, it should be noted that even a tiny decrease in protein net balance, which cannot be detected by observing a single point in time, could quite easily contribute to significant lean tissue loss over several years.

Compared to the postabsorptive period, potential age-related changes in anabolic resistance to nutrient ingestion have drawn considerably more attention. Nevertheless, the majority of studies agree that a moderate-to-large serving of protein or amino acids

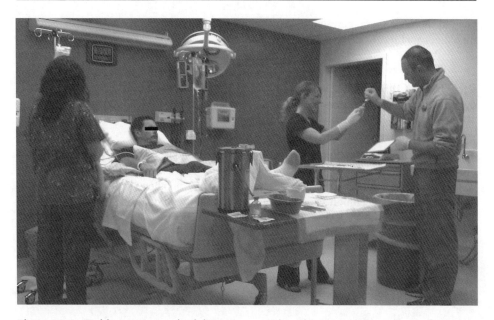

Figure 19.4 Stable isotope methodology can provide a direct assessment of muscle protein anabolism in healthy and clinical populations. (*A full color version of this figure appears in the color plate section.*)

increases muscle protein synthesis or markers of anabolism similarly in both young and older adults [21,22,26–32]. On face value, this is good news for older adults as it appears that aging does not necessarily impair the ability to mount an anabolic response to a protein-rich meal. There is, however, increasing evidence that an age-related disparity does exist in some common meal-related situations. For example, older adults appear to experience a less robust anabolic response to meals containing a lower protein content or even a mix of protein and carbohydrate [3,33]. While there is no evidence that co-ingestion of protein and fat negatively effects protein anabolism [24,34], ingestion of an amino acid–glucose mixture may not stimulate muscle protein synthesis as effectively in older as compared to younger adults [35].

Any reduction in the ability of mixed-nutrient meals to stimulate protein anabolism in older adults is troubling, largely due to the fact that it has obvious negative consequences. Unlike changes in fasting muscle protein anabolism, the response to meals is much more variable and either a small constant reduction (e.g., every meal) or frequent larger decrement (e.g., skipped breakfast) in the capacity for meal-driven protein anabolism could easily account for the gradual loss of muscle mass characteristic of sarcopenia.

In a laboratory setting, studies that examine age-related changes in protein metabolism following ingestion of a single macronutrient or menu item (e.g., amino acids, whey protein, beef, milk or soy) can provide a great deal of useful mechanistic data [36–39], however they generally fail to capture a realistic meal-like scenario where a variety of nutrients are consumed together. There is clearly a need to adopt a more translational research approach to current acute/mechanistic feeding studies. In order to affect policy change and ultimately improve the nutrition recommendations and dietary strategies given to older adults, we need to capture a more representative metabolic picture of the chronic interaction between mixed-nutrient meals, protein anabolism and aging.

PROTEIN QUANTITY AND QUALITY

Type of protein

There is considerable debate concerning the anabolic potential and health benefits of various protein types. Marketing and advertising claims would have us believe there are astonishing benefits to be had by choosing one type of protein over another. While some claims are clearly overstated, meaningful comparisons are often difficult due to the fact that:

(i) Acute research studies demonstrating the superiority of one type of protein over another have questionable long-term relevance.
(ii) Isolating the longer term health consequences of a single type/group of protein is often confounded by the fact that most adults consume a wide variety of different types of protein in their habitual diets.

When recommendations are made, they are typically quite broad. In terms of animal vs. plant-based proteins, for example, the 2010 Dietary Guidelines for Americans noted that animal products provided a greater quantity and quality of protein compared with plant-based sources. However, they also acknowledged that 'plant-based diets are able to meet protein requirements for essential amino acids...' [40]. In a research setting, it is clear that products such as whey protein or essential amino acids can acutely and robustly increase protein synthesis in young and older adults [21,22,29,30,32,41]. Supplement driven increases in the order of 50–100% or more above postabsorptive rates of protein synthesis are common. Nevertheless, when a reductionist approach is used to compare carefully constructed and controlled meals, there does appear to be subtle inherent differences in the ability of different protein sources to promote muscle protein synthesis. These differences are typically attributed to two key factors:

(i) Amino acid composition of the protein.
(ii) Digestion and absorption kinetics.

The essential amino acid content and composition of a protein is perhaps the most important determinant of its anabolic potential [21,30,39,42]. Nevertheless, there are limited data actively comparing the efficacy of different amino acid formulations. Indeed, many amino acid mixtures used in research studies were initially designed to simply mimic the amino acid profile of human skeletal muscle or common supplements such as whey protein [21,43,44]. While the presence of nonessential amino acids does not appear to provide a direct stimulatory effect [26,37,45], the essential amino acids and the branch chain amino acid leucine in particular, plays a pivotal role in translation initiation and is the focus of a considerable amount of ongoing research (see section 5.1)(46).

The digestion rate of ingested protein and its subsequent amino acid absorption in the gut is an independent regulating factor of postprandial protein anabolism [45]. Dietary protein digestion and/or absorption determines the appearance rate of dietary amino acids in the circulation, thereby driving the postprandial increase in muscle protein synthesis rate. Though impairments in protein digestion and absorption kinetics do not seem evident in older adults [47], it has become clear that changing the digestion and absorption kinetics of a protein can further increase post-prandial muscle protein retention [39,48]. The latter seems to be of particular relevance to the aging adult, as it had previously been shown that ingestion of more rapidly digestible dairy protein (*e.g., whey protein*) results in greater post-prandial protein retention when compared to the ingestion of more slowly digestible protein (*e.g., intact casein protein*) in older [45,49] but not younger adults [45,50]. This concept of fast versus slow protein may also be of relevance to the anabolic response following ingestion of mixed-nutrient meals. Supplements such as whey protein and essential amino acid mixtures appear in the plasma within 15 minutes of ingestion and could be regarded as 'fast' proteins. Conversely, proteins from most regular food sources (beef, chicken, dairy products etc.) generally take considerably longer to appear and could be considered 'slow' proteins. Therefore, we need to establish the impact of different types of protein within the matrix of a mixed meal.

A number of recent stable isotope studies have sought to expand on earlier free-form EAA studies by quantifying the ability of protein-rich foods (*e.g., milk, beef, eggs*) to stimulate protein anabolism. While many of these studies continue to focus on a younger population [37,63], they represent an important step forward as they more closely reflect responses to actual dietary practices and hence provide information on how meal choices may influence accrual and regulation of muscle mass. While a nutrition-derived increase in muscle protein anabolism is certainly advantageous and desirable, in the context of a typical meal that contains a variety of proteins and macronutrients, subtle inherent differences in the ability of individual protein sources to stimulate muscle protein anabolism are likely to be marginal. Nevertheless, the key point is that, irrespective of the source, meals should contain an appropriate amount of high quality protein.

Protein quantity and distribution across meals

While older adults are clearly at increased risk of sarcopenia and negative health consequences associated with insufficient protein or energy consumption [8,51,52], many also face challenges associated with nutrient excess and obesity [53–55]. For young and older adults alike, a modest increase in dietary protein consumption beyond the recommended dietary allowance of 0.8 g protein·kg^{-1}·d^{-1} may offer benefits associated with increased muscle protein accretion, satiety, thermogenesis and energy expenditure [56–59]. However, there is a clear balancing act in play as poor menu choices and a lack of portion control can easily result in excessive energy intake and accretion of body fat. Further, while there is no evidence that a moderate increase in dietary protein intake beyond the RDA poses a health risk, higher protein intakes (*e.g., 2.0 g protein/kg/day*) in older populations or those with existing renal disease could contribute to an increase in glomerular filtration rate (GFR) of hyperfiltration [25,60].

The relationship between protein and energy intake and muscle anabolism is further complicated by the fact that many individuals consume the majority of their daily protein during the evening meal [61]. The distribution of protein across three or more daily meals is seldom discussed. For a 75 kg individual, the RDA represents 60 g protein/day, or when

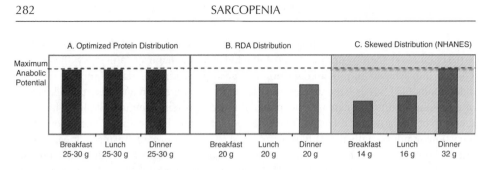

Figure 19.5   The distribution of protein over the course of a day may play an important role in the regulation of protein anabolism and ultimately muscle mass and function.

distributed evenly across three meals, 20 g protein/meal. A 20 g serving of most animal or plant-based proteins contains 5-8 g of essential amino acids. Simple calculations like this highlight an important concept. While we are lacking the data to recommend a specific dose or amount of protein that should be consumed per meal, a growing body of evidence suggests that aging is associated with an inability of skeletal muscle to respond to low doses of essential amino acids (< approx. 8 g), whereas moderate to higher doses (> approx. 10 g) are capable of stimulating muscle protein synthesis to a similar extent as the young [22,62].

How much protein is enough? Examining the effect of the quantity of a protein rich food on muscle protein anabolism in young and older adults, researchers recently demonstrated that a large single 340 g (12 oz) serving of lean beef (90 g protein, 36 g essential amino acids) did not elicit a greater anabolic response than a more moderate 113 g (4 oz) portion (30 g protein; 12 g essential amino acids). While the relationship between the amount of protein ingested and the subsequent increase in muscle protein anabolism may be influenced by a myriad of factors including: i) physical activity (*habitual and acute*), ii) health status, iii) daily energy requirements and iv) body size and composition, these data support the logical assertion that there is an upper limit on the amount of protein consumed in a single meal that can be used to promote muscle anabolism.

Although there is no magic number, it is likely that somewhere in the neighborhood of 30 g of high quality protein per meal is necessary to maximally stimulate skeletal muscle protein synthesis in healthy older adults. Figure 19.5 provides a pictorial example of the proposed relationship between the amount of protein ingested per meal and the resultant anabolic response. The influence of factors such as physical activity notwithstanding, it is clear that the distribution of protein depicted in Figure 19.5A, would result in a greater 24 h net protein balance than the protein distribution patterns depicted in panels B and C.

Moving forward, there is clearly a need for longer-term feeding trials to determine if ingestion of a moderate amount of high-quality protein at each meal could be a beneficial strategy to reduce sarcopenic muscle loss in the elderly. While useful for providing mechanistic insight or proof of concept, we must not lose sight of the fact that many of the positive responses observed in acute metabolic studies do not always translate to meaningful longer-term outcomes such as greater muscle mass, strength functional capacity or health [64].

EXERCISE AND NUTRITION

The synergistic effect of physical activity, exercise and nutrition

In addition to protein intake, physical activity is the key modifiable means of stimulating muscle protein synthesis [65]. A single bout of exercise stimulates both muscle protein synthesis and breakdown rate, albeit the latter to a lesser extent, thereby improving protein balance [66]. However, in the absence of substrate availability (i.e. food ingestion), muscle protein balance will remain negative. Protein and/or amino acid ingestion following exercise positively influences the balance between protein synthesis and breakdown, resulting in net muscle protein accretion [67]. Recent work has shown the importance of physical activity to drive the post-prandial muscle protein synthetic response to protein ingestion in both young and elderly adults [68]. By using specifically produced intrinsically labeled dietary protein it was shown that substantially more of the ingested protein is used for de novo muscle protein synthesis when 30 min of physical activity are performed prior to food intake. The latter clearly shows that nutritional requirements should always be assessed in light of the habitual physical activity level.

Prolonged resistance type exercise training can effectively increase muscle mass and strength in many older populations [70,71,73–80]. However, unlike younger individuals, the chronic additive or synergistic effects of protein supplementation and resistance type exercise training on muscle mass and function in older adults remain less clear [6,72]. Further, despite general acceptance of its efficacy, the volume or intensity threshold of resistance training needed to protect skeletal muscle mass and function during aging is not fully understood. Many studies have successfully employed relatively high intensity resistance exercise training programs [78,81]. However, in frail elders or compromised patient populations, high intensity exercise interventions may be medically contraindicated or simply not feasible. Nonetheless, any exercise or habitual physical activity is preferred over no activity at all. Even relatively low intensity, short duration bouts of physical activity such as weight bearing or walking may confer some benefit. A recent NASA-supported bed rest study demonstrated that as little as 1 h·d^{-1} on a specially designed human centrifuge (producing 2.5x gravity at the feet) was sufficient to maintain muscle protein synthesis [82] and attenuate muscle performance decrements in the knee extensors and plantar flexors [83].

Exercise and the timing of protein ingestion

The issue of optimizing muscle protein anabolism by manipulating the timing of protein/amino acid ingestion and resistance exercise continues to attract considerable academic and athletic attention [26,27]. In general, cell signaling and stable isotope studies suggest that an acute bout of resistance exercise temporarily inhibits protein synthesis via increased AMP-activated protein kinase (AMPK) activation and reduced phosphorylation of 4E-BP1 and other key regulators of translation initiation [12,26,28]. However, approximately 60 minutes post-exercise, the capacity for maximal muscle protein synthesis is restored and ultimately increased via the activation of protein kinase B, mTOR, S6K1 and eEF2 [29]. Consequently, increasing plasma and intracellular amino acid availability during this

Meal	Appearance in plasma	Timing to correspond with peak anabolic window
Whey Protein Amino Acids	10-20 minutes	Consume 0-60 minutes post exercise
Intact Proteins (beef, fish etc.)	120+ minutes	Consume approx.. 90 minutes before exercise

Figure 19.6   The relative timing of protein ingestion and exercise to optimize the potential for muscle protein anabolism. *Note, the timing relates only to muscle protein anabolism and does not take into account practical issues such as exercise performance, satiety, gastric comfort, hunger or coingestion of other nutrients.

rebound/recovery period appears to offer the greatest anabolic advantage. However, care must be taken not to be misled by the nuances of controlled research studies. Specifically, it is important to consider that the majority of studies have characterized the protein/exercise timing response using rapidly digested protein or amino acids. Freeform amino acids and whey protein can appear in the circulation within 15 minutes of ingestion [8,9]. In contrast, intact proteins, such as lean beef, may take up to 100 minutes to peak in the plasma [10]. Consequently, in terms of the plasma amino acid precursor supply and ultimately the protein synthetic response, consuming a slowly digested protein-rich mixed meal 60 minutes prior to exercise, may be the physiological equivalent of ingesting a rapidly digested protein source 30-60 minutes post-exercise (Figure 19.6).

In addition to timing considerations to promote maximal muscle protein accretion, care should be given to practical considerations. For example, consuming a large protein rich meal prior to some types of exercise may be tolerated by some individuals but impractical or uncomfortable for others. Therefore, recommendation on the most anabolically advantageous timing of meals and exercise must also be tempered by practical considerations such as satiety and gastric comfort.

DIETARY SUPPLEMENTATION AS AN ADJUNCT TREATMENT FOR SARCOPENIA

Justification for the use of dietary supplement to treat or prevent sarcopenia centers on the assumption that they will improve net muscle protein synthesis above that afforded by regular meals alone. Further, the additional energy/nutrient content of a supplement should not interfere with or compromise the normal anabolic response to protein consumed as part of daily meals [84]. Numerous attempts have been made to reduce the loss of muscle mass and strength in older adults by providing a simple protein or amino acid supplementation [85]. In some cases, protein-energy supplementation has been shown to be effective. However, other trials, particularly those involving acutely ill or frail patient populations, have been rather unsuccessful [11–13]. In some instances protein supplementation increases satiety and simply replaces voluntary ingestion of regular menu items (i.e., the 'supplement' becomes a 'replacement') [84,86]. In other situations, cost, availability and conditions such as dysphagia or impaired kidney function may limit the use or efficacy of supplementation. In such instances, maximizing protein anabolism while minimizing the amount or volume of a supplement would be advantageous. Several research groups are currently looking into the ability of the other macronutrients and nutritional compounds to further augment the post-prandial muscle protein anabolic response to meal ingestion (vitamin D, vitamin B, omega fatty acids, creatine, leucine etc.). Ultimately however, while supplements can play an important role in some situations for the majority of older adults, the first step in developing an effective treatment or prevention strategy for sarcopenia should be to include a moderate serving of protein of high biological value during each meal.

Leucine and branched chain amino acid supplementation

The branched chain amino acid leucine has well documented effects on translation initiation and muscle protein synthesis [38,41,87,88]. Notably, leucine is a potent activator of the mammalian target of rapamycin (mTOR) nutrient and energy-sensing signaling pathway in skeletal muscle. Increased insulin availability increases muscle protein synthesis by enhancing phosphorylation of Akt/PKB (an upstream regulator of mTOR), whereas increased leucine availability promotes the phosphorylation and activation of the downstream effectors of mTOR, 4E-BP1 and S6K1 [4,89]. With increasing age, muscle appears to become resistant to the stimulatory effects of normal post-prandial concentrations of leucine [87]. While such a deficit could contribute to reduced muscle protein anabolism and a loss of muscle mass, recent acute studies in both animals [87,90,91] and humans [92–94] suggest that the addition of a small amount of leucine to regular mixed nutrient meals may improve or normalize muscle protein synthesis in aging muscle. Specifically, Rieu et al. [91] reported that in older rats, muscle protein synthesis following a normal mixed nutrient meal, was blunted compared to younger animals. However, the addition of supplemental leucine to the meal restored muscle protein synthesis to youthful levels in the older rats [91]. In a follow-up study in older humans, the addition of leucine to a mixed nutrient meal also resulted in a significant increase in muscle protein synthesis (0.053 ± 0.009 %/h vs. 0.083 ± 0.008 %/h, $p<0.05$) [92]. Consequently, leucine has been proposed as a promising pharmaconutrient in the prevention and treatment of sarcopenia [46]. Though there are numerous applications for the proposed benefits of leucine in health and disease, recent long-term nutritional intervention studies do not confirm the clinical efficacy of leucine as a pharmaconutrient in well nourished, healthy older adults [95,96].

PRIORITY AREAS FOR TARGETED NUTRITION INTERVENTIONS

Bed rest and physical inactivity

Adults over the age of 65 years account for 40% of all hospital admissions and are more likely than younger adults to be physically incapacitated or placed on bed rest for an extended period of time [97–99]. Physical inactivity alone contributes to a host of poor outcomes including: impaired insulin action, loss of muscle and bone mass, fatigue, impaired motor control and functional capacity and increased morbidity and mortality [28,100–102]. In a recent 10 day bed rest study in older adults [103], researchers noted an approximate 3-fold greater loss of lean leg muscle mass compared to younger adults confined to bed for

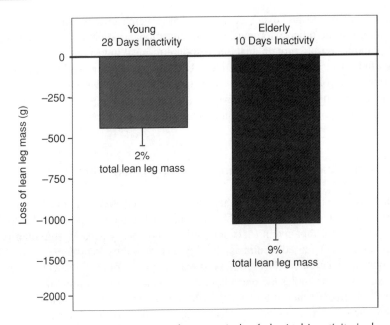

Figure 19.7 The loss of lean body mass during periods of physical inactivity is dramatically greater in older individuals.

28 days (Figure 19.7) [27]. These losses occurred despite the provision of diets meeting or exceeding the RDA for protein ($0.8 \text{ g·kg·day}^{-1}$) [27,104].

Pre-existing sarcopenia may also contribute to the disparate loss of muscle mass and function experienced by older adults following a period of physical inactivity. For example, in the United States, approximately 71% of men and 42% of women over the age of 65 years, can already be characterized as moderately sarcopenic based on skeletal muscle index [SMI = muscle mass (kg)/height (m^2); males: 8.51–10.75; females: 5.76–6.75] [105]. Further, 17% and 11% of older men and women, respectively, are severely sarcopenic (males: SMI < 8.51; females SMI < 5.76). Severe sarcopenia is associated with a 79% greater likelihood of disability [105]. Thus, with advancing age, it becomes increasingly likely that even relatively brief periods of bed rest or physical inactivity (<7 days) could seriously impact muscle strength and functional capacity and necessitate considerable rehabilitation efforts [106–108].

In the absence of illness or injury, muscle loss during bed rest appears to be driven primarily by a blunted protein synthetic response to mixed nutrient meals, or 'anabolic resistance' [82,104,109,110]. However, as noted in Chapter 10 (Cachexia and Sarcopenia), the consequences of reduced physical activity are amplified in many clinical situations where muscle protein breakdown/catabolism and turnover is greatly increased by concomitant inflammatory burden, malnutrition and lower immune function [111,112].

Nutritional support during bed rest

A large percentage of homebound and hospitalized elderly are protein-energy malnourished (PEM), consuming less than 0.7 g mixed protein·kg·d^{-1}, well below the recommended daily intake of $0.8 \ g \cdot kg \cdot d^{-1}$, which itself should be considered a minimal requirement [8,14,15]. In terms of interventions, there are compelling data supporting the health benefits of resistance exercise in many older populations [113–123]. Even simple weight bearing exercise, such as walking, can reduce the loss of function capacity associated with bed rest or hospitalization [124,125]. However, in many patient populations, the ability to move freely or exercise is compromised by physical disability, disease process and/or advanced frailty. Many inpatients spend as little as 5 $min \cdot day^{-1}$ walking [126,127] and a substantial proportion of hospitalized elders lack the ability to perform any weight-bearing activity [127].

Numerous passive interventional strategies including testosterone [128–132], growth hormone [133], and insulin-like growth factor-1 (IGF-1) (134) have been explored, yet the results have been mixed. Attempts to promote anabolism by simply increasing energy intake are desirable, but have generally proven unsuccessful, in part because of issues such as poor appetite, increased satiety, dentition problems, cost and accessibility [20,59,84].

Supplementation with products such as isolated amino acids or protein powders (whey, soy etc.) are a viable nutritional intervention for some older adults – a strategy that avoids some, but not all of the problems associated with simply increasing voluntary food intake. In the only study to date to examine the effects of amino acid supplementation in older adults during bed rest, subjects consumed 15 g of essential amino acids, three times/day between meals that provided the RDA for protein ($0.8 \ g \cdot kg \cdot d^{-1}$). After 10 days of bed rest, muscle protein synthesis was decreased 30% in controls but maintained in the supplementation group. Amino acid supplementation also protected some functional abilities such as floor transfer time and partially preserved stair ascent power [135]. It should be noted however, that three servings of 15 g of amino acids each day is a lot and while these data are encouraging, the successful translation to a less controlled, real-world population is uncertain.

Ideally, protein or amino acid supplementation should be implemented in concert with exercise as together they are more effective at attenuating the loss of muscle mass and strength than supplementation alone [136]. If exercise is performed without adequate nutritional support (i.e., protein/energy malnutrition or hypocaloric diet), losses in muscle mass and power are likely to persist [137].

CONCLUSION

An adequate nutritional framework is the fundamental prerequisite for maintaining muscle anabolism, mass and ultimately functional capacity. Rather than recommending a large, global increase in protein intake for all older adults, clinicians should stress the importance of maximizing the potential for muscle protein anabolism at each meal while being cognizant of total energy intake. We propose a dietary plan for older adults that includes a moderate amount of high quality protein with *each* meal. Wherever possible, meals should also be consumed in close proximity to exercise to enhance the anabolic response and allow a greater proportion of the ingested protein to be converted to skeletal muscle protein.

ACKNOWLEDGEMENTS

This work was supported by funding from the UTMB Claude D. Pepper Older Americans Independence Center # P30 AG024832, NIH grant T32HD007539, the National Cattlemens beef Association, the National Space Biomedical Research Institute grant NNJ08ZSA002N and 1UL1RR029876-01 from the National Center for Research Resources, National Institutes of Health.

REFERENCES

1. Fielding RA, Vellas B, Evans WJ, Bhasin S, Morley JE, Newman AB, et al. Sarcopenia: an undiagnosed condition in older adults. Current consensus definition: prevalence, etiology, and consequences. International working group on sarcopenia. J Am Med Dir Assoc. 2011;12(4):249–256.

2. Morley JE, Abbatecola AM, Argiles JM, Baracos V, Bauer J, Bhasin S, et al. Sarcopenia with limited mobility: an international consensus. J Am Med Dir Assoc. 2011;12(6):403–409.

3. Cuthbertson D, Smith K, Babraj J, Leese G, Waddell T, Atherton P, et al. Anabolic signaling deficits underlie amino acid resistance of wasting, aging muscle. Faseb J. 2005;19(3):422–424.

4. Fujita S, Dreyer HC, Drummond MJ, Glynn EL, Cadenas JG, Yoshizawa F, et al. Nutrient Signalling in the Regulation of Human Muscle Protein Synthesis. J Physiol. 2007.

5. Fujita S, Rasmussen BB, Cadenas J, Drummond MJ, Glynn EL, Sattler FR, et al. Aerobic Exercise Overcomes the Age-Related Insulin Resistance of Muscle Protein Metabolism by Improving Endothelial Function Uand Akt/mTOR signaling. Diabetes. 2007.

6. Campbell WW. Synergistic use of higher-protein diets or nutritional supplements with resistance training to counter sarcopenia. Nutr Rev. 2007;65(9):416–422.

7. Lee JS, Johnson MA, Brown A, Nord M. Food security of older adults requesting Older Americans Act Nutrition Program in Georgia can be validly measured using a short form of the U. S. Household Food Security Survey Module. J Nutr. 2011;141(7):1362–1368.

8. Campbell WW, Trappe TA, Wolfe RR, Evans WJ. The recommended dietary allowance for protein may not be adequate for older people to maintain skeletal muscle. J Gerontol A Biol Sci Med Sci. 2001;56(6):M373–80.

9. Wolfe RR. The underappreciated role of muscle in health and disease. Am J Clin Nutr. 2006;84(3):475–482.

10. Wolfe RR, Miller SL. The recommended dietary allowance of protein: a misunderstood concept. Jama. 2008;299(24):2891–2893.

11. Leidy HJ, Carnell NS, Mattes RD, Campbell WW. Higher protein intake preserves lean mass and satiety with weight loss in pre-obese and obese women. Obesity (Silver Spring). 2007;15(2):421–429.

12. Thalacker-Mercer AE, Fleet JC, Craig BA, Carnell NS, Campbell WW. Inadequate protein intake affects skeletal muscle transcript profiles in older humans. Am J Clin Nutr. 2007;85(5):1344–1352.

13. Millward DJ, Layman DK, Tome D, Schaafsma G. Protein quality assessment: impact of expanding understanding of protein and amino acid needs for optimal health. Am J Clin Nutr. 2008;87(5):1576S–81S.

14. Bunker VW, Lawson MS, Stansfield MF, Clayton BE. Nitrogen balance studies in apparently healthy elderly people and those who are housebound. Br J Nutr. 1987;57(2):211–221.

15. Pepersack T, Corretge M, Beyer I, Namias B, Andr S, Benoit F, et al. Examining the effect of intervention to nutritional problems of hospitalised elderly: a pilot project. J Nutr Health Aging. 2002;6(5):306–310.

16. Houston DK, Nicklas BJ, Ding J, Harris TB, Tylavsky FA, Newman AB, et al. Dietary protein intake is associated with lean mass change in older, community-dwelling adults: the Health, Aging, and Body Composition (Health ABC) Study. Am J Clin Nutr. 2008;87(1):150–155.

17. Houston DK, Nicklas BJ, Ding J, Harris TB, Tylavsky FA, Newman AB, et al. Dietary protein intake is associated with lean mass change in older, community-dwelling adults: the Health, Aging, and Body Composition (Health ABC) Study. Am J Clin Nutr. 2008;87(1):150–155.

18. Rand WM, Pellett PL, Young VR. Meta-analysis of nitrogen balance studies for estimating protein requirements in healthy adults. Am J Clin Nutr. 2003;77(1):109–127.

19. Trumbo P, Schlicker S, Yates AA, Poos M. Dietary reference intakes for energy, carbohydrate, fiber, fat, fatty acids, cholesterol, protein and amino acids. J Am Diet Assoc. 2002;102(11):1621–1630.

20. Paddon-Jones D, Rasmussen BB. Dietary protein recommendations and the prevention of sarcopenia. Current opinion in clinical nutrition and metabolic care. 2009;12(1):86–90.

21. Paddon-Jones D, Sheffield-Moore M, Katsanos CS, Zhang XJ, Wolfe RR. Differential stimulation of muscle protein synthesis in elderly humans following isocaloric ingestion of amino acids or whey protein. Exp Gerontol. 2006;41(2):215–219.

22. Paddon-Jones D, Sheffield-Moore M, Zhang XJ, Volpi E, Wolf SE, Aarsland A, et al. Amino acid ingestion improves muscle protein synthesis in the young and elderly. Am J Physiol Endocrinol Metab. 2004;286(3):E321–8.

23. Paddon-Jones D, Short KR, Campbell WW, Volpi E, Wolfe RR. Role of dietary protein in the sarcopenia of aging. Am J Clin Nutr. 2008;87(5):1562S–6S.

24. Symons TB, Schutzler SE, Cocke TL, Chinkes DL, Wolfe RR, Paddon-Jones D. Aging does not impair the anabolic response to a protein-rich meal. Am J Clin Nutr. 2007;86(2):451–456.

25. Walrand S, Short KR, Bigelow ML, Sweatt A, Hutson SM, Nair KS. Functional impact of high protein intake on healthy elderly people. Am J Physiol Endocrinol Metab. 2008.

26. Paddon-Jones D, Sheffield-Moore M, Aarsland A, Wolfe RR, Ferrando AA. Exogenous amino acids stimulate human muscle anabolism without interfering with the response to mixed meal ingestion. Am J Physiol Endocrinol Metab. 2005;288(4):E761–7.

27. Paddon-Jones D, Sheffield-Moore M, Urban RJ, Sanford AP, Aarsland A, Wolfe RR, et al. Essential amino acid and carbohydrate supplementation ameliorates muscle protein loss in humans during 28 days bedrest. The Journal of clinical endocrinology and metabolism. 2004;89(9):4351–4358.

28. Paddon-Jones D, Wolfe RR, Ferrando AA. Amino acid supplementation for reversing bed rest and steroid myopathies. J Nutr. 2005;135(7):1809S–12S.

29. Volpi E, Ferrando AA, Yeckel CW, Tipton KD, Wolfe RR. Exogenous amino acids stimulate net muscle protein synthesis in the elderly. J Clin Invest. 1998;101: 2000–2007.

30. Volpi E, Kobayashi H, Sheffield-Moore M, Mittendorfer B, Wolfe RR. Essential amino acids are primarily responsible for the amino acid stimulation of muscle protein anabolism in healthy elderly adults. Am J Clin Nutr. 2003;78(2):250–258.

31. Volpi E, Lucidi P, Cruciani G, Monacchia F, Reboldi G, Brunetti P, et al. Contribution of amino acids and insulin to protein anabolism during meal absorption. Diabetes. 1996;45: 1245–1252.

32. Volpi E, Mittendorfer B, Wolf SE, Wolfe RR. Oral amino acids stimulate muscle protein anabolism in the elderly despite higher first-pass splanchnic extraction. Am J Physiol Endocrinol Metab. 1999;277(40):E513–E20.

33. Volpi E, Mittendorfer B, Rasmussen BB, Wolfe RR. The response of muscle protein anabolism to combined hyperaminoacidemia and glucose-induced hyperinsulinemia is impaired in the elderly. The Journal of clinical endocrinology and metabolism. 2000;85(12):4481–4490.

34. Elliot TA, Cree MG, Sanford AP, Wolfe RR, Tipton KD. Milk ingestion stimulates net muscle protein synthesis following resistance exercise. Med Sci Sports Exerc. 2006;38(4):667–674.

35. Guillet C, Prod'homme M, Balage M, Gachon P, Giraudet C, Morin L, et al. Impaired anabolic response of muscle protein synthesis is associated with S6K1 dysregulation in elderly humans. Faseb J. 2004;18(13):1586–1587.

36. Symons TB, Schutzler SE, Cocke TL, Chinkes DL, Wolfe RR, Paddon-Jones D. Aging does not impair the anabolic response to a protein-rich meal. Am J Clin Nutr. 2007;86(2):451–456.

37. Wilkinson SB, Tarnopolsky MA, Macdonald MJ, Macdonald JR, Armstrong D, Phillips SM. Consumption of fluid skim milk promotes greater muscle protein accretion after resistance exercise than does consumption of an isonitrogenous and isoenergetic soy-protein beverage. Am J Clin Nutr. 2007;85(4):1031–1040.

38. Koopman R, Verdijk L, Manders RJ, Gijsen AP, Gorselink M, Pijpers E, et al. Co-ingestion of protein and leucine stimulates muscle protein synthesis rates to the same extent in young and elderly lean men. Am J Clin Nutr. 2006;84(3):623–632.

39. Pennings B, Boirie Y, Senden JM, Gijsen AP, Kuipers H, van Loon LJ. Whey protein stimulates postprandial muscle protein accretion more effectively than do casein and casein hydrolysate in older men. Am J Clin Nutr. 2011;93(5):997–1005.

40. Medicine Io. Dietary Reference Intakes for Energy, Carbohydrate, Fiber, Fat, Fatty Acids, Cholesterol, Protein and Amino Acids. Washington, DC: National Academy Press; 2010.

41. Katsanos CS, Kobayashi H, Sheffield-Moore M, Aarsland A, Wolfe RR. A high proportion of leucine is required for optimal stimulation of the rate of muscle protein synthesis by essential amino acids in the elderly. Am J Physiol Endocrinol Metab. 2006;291(2):E381–7.

42. Tipton KD, Gurki BE, Matin S, Wolfe RR. Nonessential amino acids are not necessary to stimulate net muscle protein synthesis in healthy volunteers. J Nutr Biochem. 1999;10: 89–95.

43. Paddon-Jones D, Sheffield-Moore M, Zhang XJ, Volpi E, Wolf SE, Aarsland A, et al. Amino acid ingestion improves muscle protein synthesis in the young and elderly. Am J Physiol Endocrinol Metab. 2004;286(3):E321–8.

44. Paddon-Jones D, Sheffield-Moore M, Aarsland A, Wolfe RR, Ferrando AA. Exogenous amino acids stimulate human muscle anabolism without interfering with the response to mixed meal ingestion. Am J Physiol Endocrinol Metab. 2005;288(4):E761–7.

45. Dangin M, Guillet C, Garcia-Rodenas C, Gachon P, Bouteloup-Demange C, Reiffers-Magnani K, et al. The rate of protein digestion affects protein gain differently during aging in humans. J Physiol. 2003;549(Pt 2):635–644.

46. Leenders M, van Loon LJ. Leucine as a pharmaconutrient to prevent and treat sarcopenia and type 2 diabetes. Nutr Rev. 2011;69(11):675–689.

47. Koopman R, Walrand S, Beelen M, Gijsen AP, Kies AK, Boirie Y, et al. Dietary protein digestion and absorption rates and the subsequent postprandial muscle protein synthetic response do not differ between young and elderly men. J Nutr. 2009;139(9):1707–1713.

48. Koopman R, Crombach N, Gijsen AP, Walrand S, Fauquant J, Kies AK, et al. Ingestion of a protein hydrolysate is accompanied by an accelerated in vivo digestion and absorption rate when compared with its intact protein. Am J Clin Nutr. 2009;90(1):106–115.

49. Boirie Y, Dangin M, Gachon P, Vasson MP, Maubois JL, Beaufrère B. Slow and fast dietary proteins differently modulate postprandial protein accretion. Proc Natl Acad Sci U S A. 1997;94(26):14930–14935.

50. Dangin M, Boirie Y, Guillet C, Beaufrère B. Influence of the protein digestion rate on protein turnover in young and elderly subjects. J Nutr. 2002;132(10):3228S–33S.

51. Janssen I, Shepard DS, Katzmarzyk PT, Roubenoff R. The healthcare costs of sarcopenia in the United States. J Am Geriatr Soc. 2004;52(1):80–85.

52. Evans W. Functional and metabolic consequences of sarcopenia. J Nutr. 1997;127(5 Suppl):998S–1003S.

53. Ello-Martin JA, Ledikwe JH, Rolls BJ. The influence of food portion size and energy density on energy intake: implications for weight management. Am J Clin Nutr. 2005;82(1 Suppl): 236S–41S.

54. Ledikwe JH, Ello-Martin JA, Rolls BJ. Portion sizes and the obesity epidemic. J Nutr. 2005;135(4):905–909.

55. Centers for Disease Control. U.S. Obesity Trends 1985–2006. http://www.cdc.gov/nccdphp/dnpa/obesity/trend/maps/2006.

56. Astrup A. The satiating power of protein–a key to obesity prevention? Am J Clin Nutr. 2005;82(1):1–2.

57. Westerterp-Plantenga MS. The significance of protein in food intake and body weight regulation. Curr Opin Clin Nutr Metab Care. 2003;6(6):635–638.

58. Westerterp-Plantenga MS, Lejeune MP, Nijs I, van Ooijen M, Kovacs EM. High protein intake sustains weight maintenance after body weight loss in humans. Int J Obes Relat Metab Disord. 2004;28(1):57–64.

59. Paddon-Jones D, Westman E, Mattes RD, Wolfe RR, Astrup A, Westerterp-Plantenga M. Protein, weight management, and satiety. Am J Clin Nutr. 2008;87(5):1558S–61S.

60. Knight EL, Stampfer MJ, Hankinson SE, Spiegelman D, Curhan GC. The impact of protein intake on renal function decline in women with normal renal function or mild renal insufficiency. Ann Intern Med. 2003;138(6):460–467.

61. Rousset S, Patureau Mirand P, Brandolini M, Martin JF, Boirie Y. Daily protein intakes and eating patterns in young and elderly French. Br J Nutr. 2003;90(6):1107–1115.

62. Katsanos CS, Kobayashi H, Sheffield-Moore M, Aarsland A, Wolfe RR. Aging is associated with diminished accretion of muscle proteins after the ingestion of a small bolus of essential amino acids. Am J Clin Nutr. 2005;82(5):1065–1073.

63. Hartman JW, Tang JE, Wilkinson SB, Tarnopolsky MA, Lawrence RL, Fullerton AV, et al. Consumption of fat-free fluid milk after resistance exercise promotes greater lean mass accretion than does consumption of soy or carbohydrate in young, novice, male weightlifters. Am J Clin Nutr. 2007;86(2):373–381.

64. Iglay HB, Apolzan JW, Gerrard DE, Eash JK, Anderson JC, Campbell WW. Moderately increased protein intake predominately from egg sources does not influence whole body, regional, or muscle composition responses to resistance training in older people. J Nutr Health Aging. 2009;13(2):108–114.

65. Phillips BE, Hill DS, Atherton PJ. Regulation of muscle protein synthesis in humans. Curr Opin Clin Nutr Metab Care. 2011.

66. Phillips SM, Tipton KD, Aarsland A, Wolf SE, Wolfe RR. Mixed muscle protein synthesis and breakdown after resistance exercise in humans. The American journal of physiology. 1997; 273(1 Pt 1):E99–107.

67. Borsheim E, Aarsland A, Wolfe RR. Effect of an amino acid, protein, and carbohydrate mixture on net muscle protein balance after resistance exercise. Int J Sport Nutr Exerc Metab. 2004;14(3):255–271.

68. Pennings B, Koopman R, Beelen M, Senden JM, Saris WH, van Loon LJ. Exercising before protein intake allows for greater use of dietary protein-derived amino acids for de novo muscle protein synthesis in both young and elderly men. Am J Clin Nutr. 2011;93(2):322–331.

69. Burd NA, West DW, Moore DR, Atherton PJ, Staples AW, Prior T, et al. Enhanced amino acid sensitivity of myofibrillar protein synthesis persists for up to 24 h after resistance exercise in young men. J Nutr. 2011;141(4):568–573.

70. Fiatarone MA, Marks EC, Ryan ND, Meredith CN, Lipsitz LA, Evans WJ. High-intensity strength training in nonagenarians. Effects on skeletal muscle. Jama. 1990;263(22):3029–3034.

71. Fiatarone MA, O'Neill EF, Ryan ND, Clements KM, Solares GR, Nelson ME, et al. Exercise training and nutritional supplementation for physical frailty in very elderly people. The New England journal of medicine. 1994;330(25):1769–1775.

72. Verdijk LB, Jonkers RA, Gleeson BG, Beelen M, Meijer K, Savelberg HH, et al. Protein supplementation before and after exercise does not further augment skeletal muscle hypertrophy after resistance training in elderly men. Am J Clin Nutr. 2009;89(2):608–616.

73. Beckers PJ, Denollet J, Possemiers NM, Wuyts FL, Vrints CJ, Conraads VM. Combined endurance-resistance training vs. endurance training in patients with chronic heart failure: a prospective randomized study. European heart journal. 2008;29(15):1858–1866.

74. Beyer N, Simonsen L, Bulow J, Lorenzen T, Jensen DV, Larsen L, et al. Old women with a recent fall history show improved muscle strength and function sustained for six months after finishing training. Aging clinical and experimental research. 2007;19(4):300–309.

75. Deley G, Kervio G, Van Hoecke J, Verges B, Grassi B, Casillas JM. Effects of a one-year exercise training program in adults over 70 years old: a study with a control group. Aging clinical and experimental research. 2007;19(4):310–315.

76. Fielding RA, LeBrasseur NK, Cuoco A, Bean J, Mizer K, Fiatarone Singh MA. High-velocity resistance training increases skeletal muscle peak power in older women. Journal of the American Geriatrics Society. 2002;50(4):655–662.

77. Henwood TR, Taaffe DR. Short-term resistance training and the older adult: the effect of varied programmes for the enhancement of muscle strength and functional performance. Clinical physiology and functional imaging. 2006;26(5):305–313.

78. Kryger AI, Andersen JL. Resistance training in the oldest old: consequences for muscle strength, fiber types, fiber size, and MHC isoforms. Scandinavian journal of medicine & science in sports. 2007;17(4):422–430.

79. Suetta C, Andersen JL, Dalgas U, Berget J, Koskinen S, Aagaard P, et al. Resistance training induces qualitative changes in muscle morphology, muscle architecture, and muscle function in elderly postoperative patients. J Appl Physiol. 2008;105(1):180–186.

80. Morse CI, Thom JM, Mian OS, Birch KM, Narici MV. Gastrocnemius specific force is increased in elderly males following a 12-month physical training programme. European journal of applied physiology. 2007;100(5):563–70.

81. Shackelford LC, LeBlanc AD, Driscoll TB, Evans HJ, Rianon NJ, Smith SM, et al. Resistance exercise as a countermeasure to disuse-induced bone loss. J Appl Physiol. 2004;97(1):119–129.

82. Symons TB, Sheffield-Moore M, Chinkes DL, Ferrando AA, Paddon-Jones D. Artificial gravity maintains skeletal muscle protein synthesis during 21 days of simulated microgravity. J Appl Physiol. 2009;107(1):34–38.

83. Caiozzo VJ, Haddad F, Lee S, Baker M, Paloski W, Baldwin KM. Artificial gravity as a countermeasure to microgravity: a pilot study examining the effects on knee extensor and plantar flexor muscle groups. J Appl Physiol. 2009;107(1):39–46.

84. Fiatarone Singh MA, Bernstein MA, Ryan AD, O'Neill EF, Clements KM, Evans WJ. The effect of oral nutritional supplements on habitual dietary quality and quantity in frail elders. J Nutr Health Aging. 2000;4(1):5–12.

85. Milne AC, Avenell A, Potter J. Meta-analysis: protein and energy supplementation in older people. Ann Intern Med. 2006;144(1):37–48.

86. Pupovac J, Anderson GH. Dietary peptides induce satiety via cholecystokinin-A and peripheral opioid receptors in rats. J Nutr. 2002;132(9):2775–2780.

87. Dardevet D, Sornet C, Balage M, Grizard J. Stimulation of in vitro rat muscle protein synthesis by leucine decreases with age. J Nutr. 2000;130(11):2630–2635.

88. Koopman R, Wagenmakers AJ, Manders RJ, Zorenc AH, Senden JM, Gorselink M, et al. Combined ingestion of protein and free leucine with carbohydrate increases postexercise muscle protein synthesis in vivo in male subjects. Am J Physiol Endocrinol Metab. 2005;288(4):E645–53.

89. Dreyer HC, Drummond MJ, Pennings B, Fujita S, Glynn EL, Chinkes DL, et al. Leucine-enriched essential amino acid and carbohydrate ingestion following resistance exercise enhances mTOR signaling and protein synthesis in human muscle. Am J Physiol Endocrinol Metab. 2008;294(2):E392–400.

90. Combaret L, Dardevet D, Rieu I, Pouch MN, Bechet D, Taillandier D, et al. A leucine-supplemented diet restores the defective postprandial inhibition of proteasome-dependent proteolysis in aged rat skeletal muscle. J Physiol. 2005;569(Pt 2):489–499.

91. Rieu I, Sornet C, Bayle G, Prugnaud J, Pouyet C, Balage M, et al. Leucine-supplemented meal feeding for ten days beneficially affects postprandial muscle protein synthesis in old rats. J Nutr. 2003;133(4):1198–1205.

92. Rieu I, Balage M, Sornet C, Giraudet C, Pujos E, Grizard J, et al. Leucine supplementation improves muscle protein synthesis in elderly men independently of hyperaminoacidaemia. J Physiol. 2006;575(Pt 1):305–315.

93. Layman DK. Role of leucine in protein metabolism during exercise and recovery. Can J Appl Physiol. 2002;27(6):646–663.

94. Layman DK, Walker DA. Potential importance of leucine in treatment of obesity and the metabolic syndrome. J Nutr. 2006;136(1 Suppl):319S–23S.

95. Verhoeven S, Vanschoonbeek K, Verdijk LB, Koopman R, Wodzig WK, Dendale P, et al. Long-term leucine supplementation does not increase muscle mass or strength in healthy elderly men. Am J Clin Nutr. 2009;89(5):1468–1475.

96. Leenders M, Verdijk LB, van der Hoeven L, van Kranenburg J, Hartgens F, Wodzig WK, et al. Prolonged leucine supplementation does not augment muscle mass or affect glycemic control in elderly type 2 diabetic men. J Nutr. 2011;141(6):1070–1076.

97. Kozak LJ, Owings MF, Hall MJ. National Hospital Discharge Survey: 2002 annual summary with detailed diagnosis and procedure data. Vital Health Stat 13. 2005;(158):1–199.

98. Wolfe RR, Miller SL, Miller KB. Optimal protein intake in the elderly. Clin Nutr. 2008;27(5):675–684.

99. Fisher SR, Goodwin JS, Protas EJ, Kuo YF, Graham JE, Ottenbacher KJ, et al. Ambulatory activity of older adults hospitalized with acute medical illness. J Am Geriatr Soc. 2011;59(1):91–95.

100. Urso ML, Clarkson PM, Price TB. Immobilization effects in young and older adults. Eur J Appl Physiol. 2006;96(5):564–571.

101. Urso ML, Scrimgeour AG, Chen YW, Thompson PD, Clarkson PM. Analysis of human skeletal muscle after 48 h immobilization reveals alterations in mRNA and protein for extracellular matrix components. J Appl Physiol. 2006;101(4):1136–1148.

102. Clark BC, Pierce JR, Manini TM, Ploutz-Snyder LL. Effect of prolonged unweighting of human skeletal muscle on neuromotor force control. Eur J Appl Physiol. 2007;100(1):53–62.

103. Kortebein P, Ferrando AA, Lombeida J, Wolfe RR, Evans WJ. Effect of 10 Days of Bed Rest on Skeletal Muscle in Healthy Older Adults. JAMA. 2007;297: 1772–1774.

104. Kortebein P, Ferrando A, Lombeida J, Wolfe R, Evans WJ. Effect of 10 days of bed rest on skeletal muscle in healthy older adults. Jama. 2007;297(16):1772–1774.

105. Janssen I. Influence of sarcopenia on the development of physical disability: the Cardiovascular Health Study. Journal of the American Geriatrics Society. 2006;54(1):56–62.

106. Covinsky KE, Palmer RM, Fortinsky RH, Counsell SR, Stewart AL, Kresevic D, et al. Loss of independence in activities of daily living in older adults hospitalized with medical illnesses: increased vulnerability with age. Journal of the American Geriatrics Society. 2003;51(4):451–458.

107. Hirsch CH, Sommers L, Olsen A, Mullen L, Winograd CH. The natural history of functional morbidity in hospitalized older patients. Journal of the American Geriatrics Society. 1990;38(12):1296–1303.

108. Visser M, Harris TB, Fox KM, Hawkes W, Hebel JR, Yahiro JY, et al. Change in muscle mass and muscle strength after a hip fracture: relationship to mobility recovery. The journals of gerontology. 2000;55(8):M434–40.

109. Paddon-Jones D, Sheffield-Moore M, Cree MG, Hewlings SJ, Aarsland A, Wolfe RR, et al. Atrophy and impaired muscle protein synthesis during prolonged inactivity and stress. The Journal of clinical endocrinology and metabolism. 2006;91(12):4836–4841.

110. Ferrando AA, Lane HW, Stuart CA, Davis-Street J, Wolfe RR. Prolonged bed rest decreases skeletal muscle and whole body protein synthesis. The American journal of physiology. 1996;270(4 Pt 1):E627–33.

111. Demling RH, DeSanti L. Involuntary weight loss and the nonhealing wound: the role of anabolic agents. Adv Wound Care. 1999;12(Suppl 1):1–14.

112. Constantin D, McCullough J, Mahajan RP, Greenhaff PL. Novel events in the molecular regulation of muscle mass in critically ill patients. J Physiol. 2011;589(Pt 15):3883–3895.

113. Fiatarone MA, O'Neill EF, Ryan ND, Clements KM, Solares GR, Nelson ME, et al. Exercise training and nutritional supplementation for physical frailty in very elderly people. N Engl J Med. 1994;330(25):1769–1775.

114. Frontera WR, Meredith CN, O'Reilly KP, Evans WJ. Strength training and determinants of VO2max in older men. J Appl Physiol. 1990;68(1):329–333.

115. Sheffield-Moore M, Paddon-Jones D, Sanford AP, Rosenblatt JI, Matlock AG, Cree MG, et al. Mixed muscle and hepatic-derived plasma protein metabolism is differentially regulated in older and younger men following resistance exercise. Am J Physiol Endocrinol Metab. 2005.

116. Dela F, Kjaer M. Resistance training, insulin sensitivity and muscle function in the elderly. Essays Biochem. 2006;42: 75–88.

117. Evans WJ. Reversing sarcopenia: how weight training can build strength and vitality. Geriatrics. 1996;51(5):46–47, 51–53; quiz 4.

118. Evans WJ. Effects of exercise on senescent muscle. Clin Orthop Relat Res. 2002 (403 Suppl):S211–20.

119. Fielding RA. The role of progressive resistance training and nutrition in the preservation of lean body mass in the elderly. J Am Coll Nutr. 1995;14(6):587–594.

120. Fielding RA. Effects of exercise training in the elderly: impact of progressive- resistance training on skeletal muscle and whole-body protein metabolism. Proc Nutr Soc. 1995;54(3):665–675.

121. Melov S, Tarnopolsky MA, Beckman K, Felkey K, Hubbard A. Resistance exercise reverses aging in human skeletal muscle. PLoS ONE. 2007;2: e465.

122. Parise G, Yarasheski KE. The utility of resistance exercise training and amino acid supplementation for reversing age-associated decrements in muscle protein mass and function. Curr Opin Clin Nutr Metab Care. 2000;3(6):489–495.

123. Taaffe DR. Sarcopenia–exercise as a treatment strategy. Aust Fam Physician. 2006;35(3): 130–134.

124. Dimeo F, Fetscher S, Lange W, Mertelsmann R, Keul J. Effects of aerobic exercise on the physical performance and incidence of treatment-related complications after high-dose chemotherapy. Blood. 1997;90(9):3390–3394.

125. Dimeo F, Stieglitz RD, Novelli-Fischer U, Fetscher S, Mertelsmann R, Keul J. Correlation between physical performance and fatigue in cancer patients. Ann Oncol. 1997;8(12):1251–1255.

126. Mahoney JE. Gender differences in hallway ambulation by older adults hospitalized for medical illness. Wmj. 1999;98(8):40–43.

127. Mahoney JE, Sager MA, Jalaluddin M. Use of an ambulation assistive device predicts functional decline associated with hospitalization. J Gerontol A Biol Sci Med Sci. 1999;54(2):M83–8.

128. Sheffield-Moore M, Paddon-Jones D, Casperson SL, Gilkison C, Volpi E, Wolf SE, et al. Androgen therapy induces muscle protein anabolism in older women. J Clin Endocrinol Metab. 2006;91(10):3844–3849.

129. Sheffield-Moore M, Urban RJ, Wolf SE, Jiang J, Catling DH, Herndon DN, et al. Short-term oxandrolone administration stimulates net muscle protein synthesis in young men. J Clin Endocrinol Metab. 1999;84(8):2705–2711.

130. Ferrando AA, Sheffield-Moore M, Yeckel CW, Gilkison C, Jiang J, Achacosa A, et al. Testosterone administration to older men improves muscle function: molecular and physiological mechanisms. Am J Physiol Endocrinol Metab. 2002;282(3):E601–7.

131. Snyder PJ, Peachey H, Hannoush P, Berlin JA, Loh L, Lenrow DA, et al. Effect of testosterone treatment on body composition and muscle strength in men over 65 years of age. J Clin Endocrinol Metab. 1999;84: 2647–2653.

132. Urban RJ, Bodenburg YH, Gilkison C, Foxworth J, Coggan AR, Wolfe RR, et al. Testosterone administration to elderly men increases skeletal muscle strength and protein synthesis. Am J Physiol (Endocrinol Metab). 1995;269(32):E820–E6.

133. Zachwieja JJ, Yarasheski KE. Does growth hormone therapy in conjunction with resistance exercise increase muscle force production and muscle mass in men and women aged 60 years or older? Phys Ther. 1999;79(1):76–82.

134. Butterfield GE, Thompson J, Rennie MJ, Marcus R, Hintz RL, Hoffman AR. Effect of rhGH and rhIGF-I treatment on protein utilization in elderly women. Am J Physiol. 1997;272(1 Pt 1): E94–9.

135. Ferrando AA, Paddon-Jones D, Hays NP, Kortebein P, Ronsen O, Williams RH, et al. EAA supplementation to increase nitrogen intake improves muscle function during bed rest in the elderly. Clinical nutrition (Edinburgh, Scotland). 2009.

136. Brooks N, Cloutier GJ, Cadena SM, Layne JE, Nelsen CA, Freed AM, et al. Resistance training and timed essential amino acids protect against the loss of muscle mass and strength during 28 days of bed rest and energy deficit. J Appl Physiol. 2008;105(1):241–248.

137. Trappe S, Costill D, Gallagher P, Creer A, Peters JR, Evans H, et al. Exercise in space: human skeletal muscle after 6 months aboard the International Space Station. J Appl Physiol. 2009;106(4):1159–1168.

CHAPTER 20

The Future of Drug Treatments

Francesco Landi and Graziano Onder

Department of Geriatrics, Catholic University of the Sacred Heart, Rome, Italy

Yves Rolland

INSERM 1027, University of Toulouse, Toulouse, France;
Gérontopôle of Toulouse, Toulouse, France

INTRODUCTION

The relationship between sarcopenia and negative outcomes has important implications regarding the therapeutic approaches. Lifestyle intervention (i.e. physical activity and nutrition) have shown to impact on sarcopenia. However, several drugs were suggested, with various levels of scientific evidence, to have an impact on muscle mass, strength and function. With growing understanding of the specific molecular pathways involved in the structural and functional modifications affecting the skeletal muscle during the aging process, many potential targets for pharmacological intervention to prevent and/or to treat sarcopenia have been suggested.

In this chapter we review the effect of three classes of drugs (cardiovascular, hormone and metabolic agents) on sarcopenia and muscular outcomes in older adults. For each class of medications, we describe the evidence from clinical studies and the biological plausibility.

CARDIOVASCULAR DRUGS

Angiotensin II Converting Enzyme inhibitors

In subjects with congestive heart failure (CHF), Angiotensin II Converting Enzyme inhibitors (ACE inhibitors) have been demonstrated to prevent morbidity, mortality and hospital admissions, and to reduce the decline in physical function and exercise capacity. The effects of ACE inhibitors on muscle function have been mainly attributed to positive cardiovascular effects. However, it has been hypothesized that ACE inhibitor-induced

Sarcopenia, First Edition. Edited by Alfonso J. Cruz-Jentoft and John E. Morley.

favorable effects may also be mediated by direct positive actions of these agents on the skeletal muscle [1].

Clinical experience

Firstly, the effect of ACE inhibitors on muscle strength was examined in an observational study among 641 older disabled women without CHF (mean age 79 years) [2]. In this group, continued ACE inhibitor users had a significantly lower average three-year decline in muscle strength (-1.0 kg) than either continued/intermittent users of other antihypertensive drugs (-3.7 kg; p = 0.016) or never users of antihypertensive drugs (-3.9 kg; p = 0.026).

The cross-sectional associations of antihypertensive medications use with lean body mass (LBM) was examined in a cross sectional study among 2,431 independent older adults [3]. Comparisons between groups demonstrated that lower extremity muscle mass was greater in users of ACE-inhibitors (Mean $\pm$ Standard Error 16.1 $\pm$ 0.2), as compared to either users of no drug (Mean $\pm$ SE: 15.9 $\pm$ 0.1, p vs ACE inhibitors 0.15) or users of other antihypertensive drugs (Mean $\pm$ SE: 15.7 $\pm$ 0.1, p vs ACE inhibitors = 0.001).

More recently, in a double-blind randomized controlled trial, 130 older adults (mean age 78.7 years) with functional impairment were randomly assigned to receive either perindopril or placebo for a period of 20 weeks [4]. Among 95 participants that completed the trial, the mean 6-minute walking test was significantly improved in the subjects receiving perindopril relative to the placebo group (mean between-group difference 31.4 m). However, in a prospective double blind trial, comparing the effects of treatment with enalapril versus nifedipine on physical performances in elderly subjects with hypertension, no significant differences in muscle strength, walking capacity or functional measures were observed [5]. Finally, in the Trial of Angiotensin-Converting Enzyme Inhibition and Novel Cardiovascular Risk Factors (TRAIN) study, no beneficial effect on physical performances was reported in the older subjects randomized in the ACE inhibitors group compared to the placebo group after six months of treatment [6].

Several genetic studies support the hypothesis that the ACE system may be involved in skeletal muscle function. Among elite athletes, the presence of the ACE II genotype seemed more common among long distance athletes, while the D allele was associated with power oriented performance in athletes such as short distance swimmers and sprinters [7]. A possible explanation for these findings derives from a genetic study by Zhang and colleagues, which showed that the ACE I allele is associated with an increased percentage of type I muscle fibers [8]. On the contrary, the D allele is associated with the expression of type II fibers which are less fatigue resistant and more efficient in power performance than type I isoforms. However, there is some contradictory evidence regarding the influence of the ACE gene on endurance and power performance among healthy young adults [9]. Among older adults no association between ACE gene and physical performance has been proved so far [10].

Further evidence is required before recommending ACE inhibitors to counter the effects of sarcopenia.

Mechanism of action

Potential mechanisms responsible for the beneficial effects of ACE inhibitors on skeletal muscle are summarized in Figure 20.1.

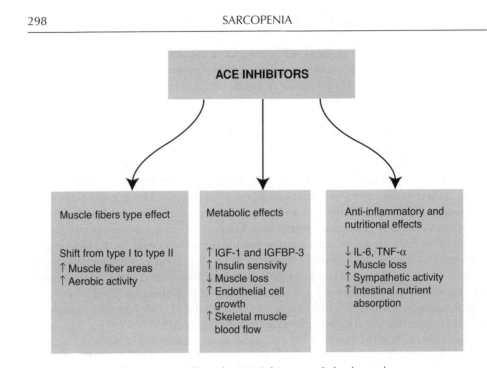

Figure 20.1   Effect of ACE inhibitors on skeletal muscke.

In patients with congestive heart failure enalapril and losartan were shown to determine a shift of the myosin-heavy chains of leg skeletal muscle gastrocnemius from type II toward type I fibers [11]. This result is in line with the study of Zhang and colleagues demonstrating that the ACE I allele (associated with low ACE activity) is associated with an increased percentage of type I muscle fibers, while the D allele (associated with high ACE activity) is associated with the expression of type II fibers [8].

The renin-angiotensin system may mediate the inflammatory response and therefore influence muscle function. Studies conducted *in vitro* have shown that angiotensin II increases IL-6 and TNF-α production in smooth vascular muscle [12]. Kranzhofer and colleagues confirmed this important function of angiotensin in triggering the inflammatory pathway and demonstrated that ACE inhibitors can suppress this angiotensin's pro-inflammatory activities [13]. The anti-inflammatory effect of ACE inhibitors has been confirmed in an observational study conducted among 161 subjects undergoing elective coronary artery bypass surgery. Subjects treated with ACE inhibitors had a significant lower increase in IL-6 concentration post-surgery compared with other participants [14].

ACE inhibitors may favorably impact on nutritional status by regulation of intestinal absorption on nutrients and may modulate appetite and physical activity by a direct effect on the central nervous system. Furthermore, some studies in animals have shown that ACE inhibitors treatment increased the natural angiogenesis and enhanced the collateral vessels development in the ischemic limb [15]. In addition, Zimmerman and colleagues demonstrated that the expression of vascular endothelial growth factor was augmented in cardiac tissue following treatment with ramipril [16].

Finally, the ACE inhibitors play an important role in the modulation of the GH/IGF-1 axis [17]. The insulin-like Growth Factor-1 (IGF-1) is known to be a potential contributor to sarcopenia. It has been hypothesized that ACE inhibitors may prevent the loss of muscle mass through modulation of the IGF-1 system. This effect may be related to the reduction of the autocrine IGF-1 system. The direct effect of ACE inhibitors on the IGF-1 system has been reported in two different large epidemiological cohort studies in older people. In the ilSIRENTE study [18] and in the InCHIANTI study [19], the older adults treated with the ACE inhibitors showed higher IGFBP-3 levels. On the other hand, over-expression of muscle-specific isoform of IGF-1 reduces the angiotensin II-induced muscle loss [17]. Taken together, these results suggest that medications that inhibit the conversion of angiotensin I to angiotensin II, such as ACE inhibitors, may delay or prevent muscle loss in older adults, possibly through modulation of the IGF-1 system.

Statins

The proteomic analysis performed in animals chronically treated with different hypolipidemic drugs, showed that either statin or fibrate administration is able to modify the expression of specific proteins essential for skeletal muscle function [20]. Based on this experimental evidence, the possible use of statin to treat sarcopenia has been hypothesized.

Clinical experience

The effect of statin on body composition has been tested in a clinical trial among 49 community dwelling subjects – 60 to 69 year-old men and women – who completed two weeks of nutrition education, followed by 12 weeks of high intensity resistance exercise training, with post-exercise protein supplementation [21]. This trial documented that serum cholesterol and statin treatment were independently associated with greater increases in lean body mass after training, suggesting that statin may improve muscle response to exercise program. Furthermore, in an observational study among 756 community-dwelling older adults, statin users over a one-year period performed modestly better than nonusers for timed chair stands test (−0.5 seconds; P = .04) [22].

However, it is important to highlight that statins have also been recognized to cause adverse effects on skeletal muscle mass. Statins may reduce aerobic exercise tolerance through impaired mitochondrial function, decreased mitochondrial content, and apoptotic pathways. In a longitudinal study performed in community-dwelling older adults, treatment with statin was associated with greater declines in strength and increases the risk of falls [23].

Mechanism of action

The potential positive effects of statins on skeletal muscle and physical performance are summarized in Figure 20.2.

Statins might affect muscle mass and function retarding the negative effects of atherosclerosis on blood vessels of skeletal muscle, ensuring a better perfusion and therefore preventing muscle wasting and reducing muscle weakness and/or fatigue. Statins also increase the production of nitric oxide in the endothelium, which has local vasodilatory properties.

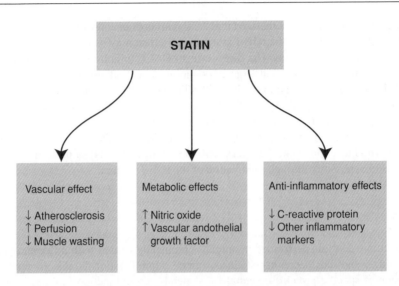

Figure 20.2 Effect of statin on skeletal muscle.

Furthermore, Bitto and colleagues have recently demonstrated that simvastatin improves the rate of wound healing in diabetic mice; this process seems to be mediated by increased vascular endothelial growth factor [24].

Statins may reduce inflammation, which, in turn is an important determinant of sarcopenia. Several studies have pointed out that treatment with statin reduces C-reactive protein and other inflammatory markers level independently of the effect on cholesterol [25]. This hypothesis is indirectly confirmed by the Heart Prevention Study (HPS) [26] and the JUPITER trial [27] which suggested that the reduction of cardiovascular events among pravastatin and rosuvastatin users is independent of baseline cholesterol levels.

The evidence that the use of statins reduces inflammation, together with the recognition of inflammation as an important determinant of muscle mass and function, appears to provide a rationale to hypothesize a direct effect of statins on sarcopenia. However, further studies are required to better define the effects of statins on skeletal muscle mass, strength, endurance, and performance [28].

HORMONE REPLACEMENT

Testosterone

Testosterone is secreted by the ovarian thecal cells in women and by the Leydig cells in men. Testosterone has been associated with higher muscle mass and muscle protein synthesis. It also appears to increase the number of satellite cells in both animals and humans studies, which are important for muscle cell function. In elderly men, epidemiologic studies support the relationship between declines in testosterone levels with age and loss of muscle mass and strength. As a consequence, hormone replacement has received considerable interest as a potential therapy for sarcopenia.

Clinical experience

Several randomized controlled studies have been conducted with testosterone showing a direct effect of this hormone on muscle mass and in several cases on muscle strength, particularly in men with testosterone deficits [28–31]. Studies of testosterone replacement therapy in men have shown varied results, depending on age of the subjects and on the plasmatic testosterone level before the treatment. A recent meta-analysis, including data from 11 randomized-clinical trials, suggested that testosterone treatment produced a moderate increase in muscle strength compared with placebo [32]. More recently, Srinivas-Shankar and colleagues documented in frail and intermediate frail older men that administration of 50 mg per day of transdermal testosterone for a period of 6 months resulted in a significant increase in lean body mass associated with increased knee extensor strength [33]. Testosterone supplementation showed better results in increasing muscle mass and function in frail older adults when it is combined with nutritional supplements in undernourished subjects [34] or with physical activity programs [35]. Overall, the effects of testosterone therapy in older subjects with normal level of testosterone have not been adequately studied. Furthermore, despite the positive effect of testosterone supplementation on muscle mass, a conclusive evidence of a direct effect of this treatment on disability and physical performance is still lacking.

When considering testosterone replacement therapy, the potential benefits of treatment must be weighed against the possible side effects. The Baltimore Longitudinal Study on Aging involving 781 subjects showed a direct correlation between prostate cancer and the testosterone levels. The likelihood of acquiring a high risk prostate cancer in men 65 years or older doubled for every 0.1 unit increase in free testosterone level [36]. This, along with other potential side effects of testosterone treatment, such as peripheral edema, gynecomastia, polycythemia, and sleep apnea, limits its use as a safe treatment for sarcopenia [37]. Recently, application of testosterone gel was associated with an increased risk of cardiovascular adverse events in older men with limitations in mobility and multimorbidity [38]. Therefore, at present, the most prudent course of action is to treat only older men with repeatedly low serum testosterone levels and symptoms and signs consistent with androgen deficiency.

Mechanism of action

Anabolic effects and effects on motor neurons have been suggested for the role of testosterone in muscle function (Figure 20.3).

Some data suggest that testosterone induces muscle fibers hypertrophy by acting at multiple steps in the pathways regulating muscle protein synthesis and breakdown. A study conducted in older men showed that testosterone administration promotes muscle anabolism by reducing protein breakdown [39]. Testosterone does not provide additional stimulation of muscle anabolism when combined with amino acid supplementation.

Testosterone administration is associated with an increase in the cross-sectional areas of both type I and II muscle fibers [40]. In young men, testosterone-induced gains in muscle size were associated with a significant increase in muscle fibers cross-sectional area and the cross-sectional areas of both types I and II fibers increased in proportion to testosterone concentrations [41]. The observation that differentiation of pluripotent cells is testosterone

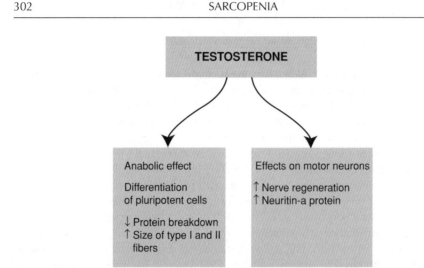

Figure 20.3 Effect of testosterone on skeletal muscle.

dependent gives a unifying explanation for the shared effects of testosterone on muscle and fat mass. In this respect, it is important to highlight that some studies demonstrated that testosterone controls and regulates the lineage determination in mesenchymal pluripotent cells, by promoting their commitment to the myogenic lineage and inhibiting their differentiation into the adipogenic lineage through an androgen receptor-mediated pathway.

Motor neurons have androgen receptors and are potential sites of testosterone action. The importance of androgens in motor neurons is confirmed by the fact that a particular mutation in the androgen receptor gene may cause a degenerative disorder known as Spinal and Bulbar Muscular Atrophy, which is characterized by death of motor neurons expressing high levels of androgen receptors, which are mainly located in the anterior horns of the spinal cord and in the bulbar region [42]. Finally, it has been shown that testosterone may enhance peripheral nerve regeneration following injury by stimulating the production of neuritin-a protein that is involved in the re-establishment of neuronal connectivity following traumatic damage to the central nervous system [43].

Estrogens and tibolone

Women experience an accelerated loss of muscle mass and strength after menopause [44]. Modifications in lifestyle habits (low level of physical activity) and hormonal changes may be the two main causes of both loss muscle mass and strength [44]. Some evidences demonstrating the association between hormonal replacement treatment and muscle mass and muscle strength have been documented. Nevertheless, disagreement still exists regarding the role of estrogen on skeletal muscle in women.

Clinical experience

Three of five clinical trials on estrogens showed a significant positive effect on muscle strength [45–47]; on the contrary, two other randomized controlled trials did not find any effect on muscle mass and strength [48,49]. Plausible explanations for these controversial results may be related to the duration of the observation period and the different mean age of participants; in this respect, it is important to highlight that older women included in these studies showed no effects related to treatment with estrogens.

The only clinical trial on tibolone, a synthetic steroid with oestrogenic, progestagenic and androgenic activity, showed a significant positive effect on muscle strength [50]. At the same time, tibolone seems to be associated with significant and positive effects on muscle mass [51]. In particular, tibolone increases fat-free mass and total body water content and reduces fat mass. Positive effects of tibolone were confirmed even if used in combination with estrogens. Only Hanggi and colleagues documented that tibolone treatment had no impact on muscle mass suggesting that this treatment may play a role only in fat distribution [52].

The effect of estrogens on body composition is more controversial, with studies suggesting that this drug can either increase lean body mass or decrease fat mass and other studies showing no effects [44].

Overall, only a few of the described clinical studies on estrogens and none on tibolone included older women. Considering also the well known side effects associated with use of these drugs, estrogens or tibolone treatment should not be recommended as a primary line of treatment for sarcopenia. Further researches are needed to better clarify the effects of these drugs on muscle mass and strength and their long term safety in older subjects.

Mechanism of action

Estrogen and tibolone may both react with intra-nuclear receptors in muscle fibers, and tibolone may also act by binding androgen receptors in muscle fibers and increase free testosterone and growth hormone. Tibolone was shown to directly increase serum IGF-1 levels [53] and also to increase the amount of free testosterone. Estrogen is converted to testosterone, which has an anabolic effect on muscle protein synthesis. Moreover, both sex hormones may suppress inflammatory cytokines that have catabolic effects on skeletal muscle.

Tibolone may have another positive effect on muscle strength, increasing the plasma levels of nitric oxide that mediates satellite cell activation [54]. In postmenopausal women, estrogen therapy results in a higher myogenic regulatory factor gene expression, a greater myogenic response to physical exercise, and a lower muscle damage after maximal exentric exercise [55]. Finally, estrogen replacement treatment has been reported to improve insulin response during a physical activity training programs [56].

Dehydroepiandrosterone

Dehydroepiandrosterone (DHEA) is a hormone precursor which is converted to testosterone/estrogen hormones at specific target tissues [57]. Since DHEA is a precursor in the biosynthesis of these hormones, DHEA supplementation in both males and females could potentially help in enhancing muscle mass and strength.

Clinical experience

The studies assessing the effects of DHEA supplementation in older adults are few, and the effects on muscle mass and function have been variable. Some studies conducted in aged men and women demonstrated that supplementation of DHEA increases the bone density, testosterone and estradiol levels, but has no effects on muscle size, strength, or function [57]. Kenny and colleagues conducted a randomized trial in 99 women (mean age 76.6 ± 6.0) to investigate the effects of DHEA combined with exercise on bone mass, muscle strength, and physical function [58]. It has been documented that DHEA supplementation improved lower extremity strength and function in older, frail women involved in an aerobic exercise program. Another study showed improvement in strength in a group of healthy older adults only after adding high-resistance training to DHEA supplementation [59]. Improvement in strength and function may require a combination of DHEA and exercise, although this result was not seen in all studies. More recently, Christiansen and colleagues investigated the effects of DHEA supplementation in women with adrenal failure [60]. After six months, treatment with DEHA had no effects on muscle mass, fat mass, and bone tissue; only a small increase in lean body mass was observed while a high frequency of side effects was documented. Researchers evaluating DHEA use in aging adults suggest that its effects should be evaluated over a longer period of time, and it might be more efficacious if the DHEA dosage administered resulted in circulating androgen levels exceeding those of young, healthy adults [57]. Finally, in a recent systematic review Baker and colleagues [61] showed that the benefit of DHEA on muscle strength and physical function in older adults remains inconclusive. DHEA does not appear to routinely benefit measures of physical function or performance. Some measures of muscle strength may improve, although consensus was not reached. Even though DHEA supplementation may give other benefits such as increased bone density and sex hormone levels, it has not yet been proven to counter sarcopenia.

Mechanism of action

In the inChianti study, Valenti and colleagues demonstrated that in men aged 60-79 years, circulating DHEA is an independent correlate of muscle strength and calf muscle area [62]. There are several mechanisms by which DHEA may influence muscle mass and strength, including the ability of skeletal muscle to convert DHEA to active androgens and increases in insulin-like growth factor-1. The importance of DHEA in older subjects is that almost all of the total androgens are derived from these adrenal precursor steroids [61]. Studies conducted in animal models have demonstrated that skeletal muscle contains specific enzymes able of converting circulating DHEA to testosterone and further to dehydrotestosterone, the androgen that acts on the local steroid receptors [63]. Moreover, DHEA supplementation increases IGF-1 levels that stimulates the proliferation and migration of myogenic or muscle precursor cells.

Growth hormone

Extensive interest has been devoted to study the effects of growth hormone (GH) on sarcopenia. Levels of GH are usually lower in the elderly subjects and the amplitude and frequency of pulsatile GH release are significantly reduced; thus it was hypothesized that GH would be useful in preventing the age-related muscle mass loss. However, despite the large number of studies which have assessed the effects of GH supplementation on muscle mass, strength, and physical performance, there is still an ongoing debate whether or not to use GH to prevent and/or to treat sarcopenia. Noteworthy, controversial findings have been reported in healthy or moderately frail, non-GH-deficient older adults following GH treatment.

Clinical experience

Many studies reported only marginal effects of GH supplementation. Brill and colleagues demonstrated that one month of GH supplementation improved balance and, in combination with testosterone, ameliorated physical function, but was unable to enhance muscle strength [64]. Papadakis and colleagues documented that among healthy subjects older than 69 years of age, GH treatment for 6 months increased muscle mass and decreased fat mass, without improving physical performance [65]. Blackman and colleagues found no significant effect on muscle strength among healthy older women after supplementation with GH and reported only a marginal significant increase of muscle strength in men treated with GH and testosterone [66]. For instance, some other studies reported an increase of muscle mass and strength in healthy older persons after GH supplementation [37,57]. More recently, in a group of older men, those who received the highest doses of combined supplementation of GH with testosterone for 4 months increased their muscle mass by at mean three kilograms and their muscle strength by 30%, while the mean fat mass decreased [67].

Most studies have documented that GH supplementation is ineffective in the elderly subjects, both considering muscle mass and muscle strength. Taaffe and colleagues showed that treatment with recombinant human GH to elderly men performing regularly an exercise program did not increase muscle mass or tissue IGF-1 expression [68]. Yarasheski and colleagues demonstrated in a small sample of sedentary men that resistance exercise training improved muscle strength and metabolism, but these improvements were not augmented when exercise training was combined with GH supplementation [69]. Similarly, Thompson and colleagues failed to show in moderately obese postmenopausal women any effect of GH supplementation on muscle strength [70]. Lange and colleagues conducted a randomized clinical trial examining the effects of GH alone, exercise alone and GH combined with exercise [71]. This trial showed that GH alone had no effect on muscle mass, strength, and power; the exercise induced improvements were not further augmented by GH supplementation.

These contrasting findings may be explained by methodological differences between the studies and by the small number of subjects enrolled. Numerous causes may explain the ineffectiveness of GH supplementation to improve muscle mass and strength, such as the failure of exogenous GH administration to mimic the pulsatile pattern of natural GH secretion or the induction of GH-related insulin resistance [37]. Furthermore, it is important to consider that the majority of the trials conducted on GH supplementation have reported a high incidence of adverse effects, such as fluid retention, soft tissue edema, orthostatic hypotension, diabetes, carpal tunnel syndrome, arthralgias, and gynecomastia. In conclusion, based on the current evidence, GH treatment should not be considered as a safe strategy to improve body composition and functionality in older individuals.

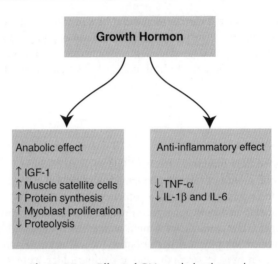

Figure 20.4   Effect of GH on skeletal muscle.

Mechanism of action

Two important mechanisms of action – anti-inflammatory and anabolic – have been suggested for the role of GH on skeletal muscle function (Figure 20.4).

The effect of GH on the muscle is mainly mediated by IGF-1. In response to GH, the liver and the skeletal muscle produces IGF-1 for systemic release. IGF-1 has hyperplastic and hypertrophic effects on the skeletal muscle. The hyperplastic effect results in the proliferation of muscle satellite cells, while the hypertrophic effect results in increased synthesis of contractile proteins. In addition, IGF-1 suppresses proteolysis, promotes the delivery of amino acids and glucose to myocytes, and stimulates myoblast proliferation and differentiation. Systemic IGF-1 administration enhances the rate of muscle functional recovery after injury and improves endurance and contractile muscle function.

Some studies have recently demonstrated that muscle expression of IGF-1 accelerates the regenerative process after injury modulating the inflammatory response and limiting the onset of fibrosis [72]. The IGF-1 expression significantly down-regulates pro-inflammatory cytokines, such as tumor necrosis factor (TNF)-alpha and interleukin (IL)-1beta. Administration of IGF-1 has been recently shown as a promising strategy to improve cardiac function and reduce infarct size after acute myocardial injury [73]. Mechanisms hypothesized for this effect include the reduction of inflammatory response (e.g., IL-6 and IL-1β) and the severity of cardiomyocyte apoptosis.

Ghrelin

Ghrelin is a peptide hormone secreted by the stomach in response to fasting. An enhanced ghrelin blood concentration results in an increased sensation of hunger and food intake. Considering that anorexia and malnutrition are important causes of sarcopenia, it has been hypothesized that ghrelin supplementation could be effective in preventing age-related muscle mass loss.

Clinical experience

Some promising effects of ghrelin supplementation have been recently reported [74]. In a sample of 25 subjects with chronic obstructive pulmonary disease, subcutaneous injections of a synthetic ghrelin analogue tended to increase the lean mass and the physical performances [74]. Furthermore, ghrelin concentrations have been reported to be strongly correlated with the amount of skeletal muscle mass [75]. However, very few clinical studies on synthetic ghrelin or ghrelin agonist treatment have been conducted in older subjects. In healthy older adults, without sarcopenia, two years of an oral ghrelin mimetic agent increased the GH and IGF-1 blood levels and muscle mass but without significant changes in strength or physical function [76].

Mechanism of action

Ghrelin stimulates the release of GH through an activation of the GH secretagogue-receptor (GHS-R 1a) present in the hypothalamus; moreover, ghrelin mimetic re-establish the pulsatile GH secretion in older adults. Subsequently, in older adults GH secretagogue or GH secretagogue-receptor agonist may be involved in the metabolism of muscle mass. This effect, partially related to melanocortin receptor antagonism that modulates food intake, has led to exploring ghrelin as a potential therapy to reduce wasting in cachexia and sarcopenia [74].

METABOLIC AGENTS

Creatine

Creatine plays an important role in protein and cellular metabolisms. The benefit of creatine supplementation on exercise performances has been reported in young adults and creatine has been recently proposed as a potential therapy for the prevention and management of sarcopenia [77].

Clinical experience

Several studies have assessed the effects of creatine supplementation in middle-aged and older adults with conflicting results. Brose and colleagues have shown a significant increase in muscle mass and muscle strength in older adults after a creatine supplementation combined with 14 weeks of resistance training [78]. Similarly, other studies have documented a significant increase in muscle mass after following 2-12 weeks of creatine supplementation and resistance training in older men [29]. In contrast to these findings, Rawson and colleagues found that one month of creatine supplementation did not enhance fat free mass,

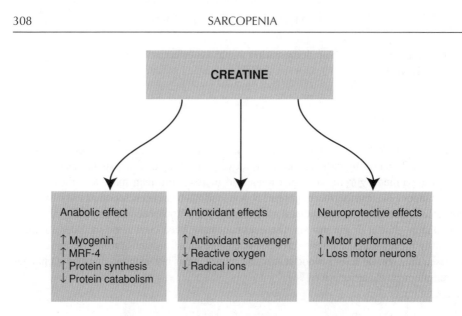

Figure 20.5   Effect of creatine on skeletal muscle.

total body mass, or upper extremity strength gains, yet it reduced leg fatigue [79]. Bermon and colleagues failed to find an increase in lower limb muscle mass after eight weeks of creatine supplementation and resistance training in older men and women [80]. In a group of 46 middle-aged to older adult men ([55–75] years), no differences were found in response to 6 months of resistance training with creatine supplementation [81]. In other studies, creatine supplementation in older males did not improve muscle mass or neuromuscular fatigue [28,29].

There is substantial controversy over whether creatine supplementation increases the benefits of resistance training alone in older subjects. Based on these conflicting results and considering that creatine may increase the risk of interstitial nephritis, creatine supplementation can not be recommended as routinely treatment for sarcopenia in older adults [29].

Mechanism of action

Anabolic, antioxidant and neuroprotective effects have been suggested for the role of creatine on muscle function (Figure 20.5).

It has been hypothesized that creatine increases the expression of myogenic transcription factors and facilitates the up-regulation of muscle specific-genes such as myogenin and myogenic regulatory factor-4 (MRF-4], thereby facilitating an increase in muscle mass and strength.

A study conducted in young healthy volunteers demonstrated that creatine supplementation during two weeks of leg immobilization followed by ten weeks of rehabilitation training significantly increased the expression of myogenic transcription factor MRF-4, which in turn was correlated with an increase in muscle cross-sectional area [82]. In another study, creatine supplementation combined with 12-weeks of resistance training significantly increased mRNA and protein expression of myogenin and MRF-4 [83]. Creatine may also increase the muscle-specific protein synthesis in skeletal muscle and/or decrease the rate of protein catabolism.

Some authors demonstrated that creatine has a role as antioxidant scavenger, mainly against radical ions. Creatine exerts a significant antioxidant activity, via a mechanism depending on direct scavenging of reactive oxygen and nitrogen species. This antioxidant role of creatine seems to lead also to a neuroprotective effect. In an animal model of amyotrophic lateral sclerosis, creatine was demonstrated to have a dose-dependent enhancement in motor performance and protect from loss of motor neurons.

Vitamin D

It is known that vitamin D plays an important role in bone and muscle metabolism. One of the characteristic clinical symptoms of vitamin D deficiency is the muscle weakness. Prevalence of low level of vitamin D has been documented to be high in older people [84]. For this reason, the nutritional recommendations for the management of sarcopenia proposed to evaluate plasma 25(OH) vitamin D level in all subjects at risk of sarcopenia and to supplement all persons with low values [77].

Clinical experience

Vitamin D has the potential to improve muscle strength. A recent systematic review of vitamin D and its impact on physical performance in older people showed conflicting evidence from cross-sectional studies, also demonstrated inconsistent cross-sectional associations between 25(OH) vitamin D level and muscle strength [85]. Recently, Kyoung Kim and colleagues found a strong inverse association between 25(OH) vitamin D level and sarcopenia in the older Korean population [86]. Prospective analyses of the Longitudinal Aging Study Amsterdam (LASA) have shown that 25(OH) vitamin D level is predictive of increased muscle mass and strength over three years [87]. In the Tasmanian Older Adult Cohort Study, a prospective study of community-dwelling older adults, the higher 25(OH) vitamin D is modestly but significantly associated with greater muscle mass, and also predictive of improved muscle strength in older adults [86].

In three different randomized controlled trials, vitamin D supplementation has been reported to increase muscle strength [88–90]. Furthermore, in adults age 65 years and older, the supplementation with 800 IU of vitamin D significantly improve by 4 to 11% lower extremity strength or function [91] after 2 to 12 months. The positive effects of vitamin D supplement on muscle mass and function has been hypothesized as the mechanism behind a fall reduction in older nursing home residents given vitamin D [37]. A recent meta-analysis has documented that 700 to 1000 IU per day of vitamin D reduces the risk of falling by 19% in older people [92]. More recently, Verschueren and colleagues documented in a randomized clinical study of 113 institutionalized elderly females aged over 70 years an increase by 6.4% in knee extensor strength after 6 months of vitamin D supplementation [93]. On the other hand, some studies failed to find significant benefits on physical function, falls risk or quality of life with vitamin D supplementation in subjects with vitamin D deficits [37,74]. The difference in muscle mass and strength response between studies may in part be attributed to differences in the dose of vitamin D used (with better outcomes seen when higher doses are used), the differences in measurement techniques (hand grip dynamometer versus leg press), age, and serum vitamin D level at baseline [28,29,37].

Taking into account the high prevalence of vitamin D deficiency (more than 70%) among institutionalized subjects, vitamin D supplementation has to be considered as a possible approach to prevent sarcopenia and to improve the effects of sarcopenia in terms of morbidity and mortality in this population. Vitamin D plasmatic levels should be measured in frail elderly people and in particular in institutionalized individuals. Vitamin D oral supplementation should be provided to subjects with vitamin D plasmatic levels lower than 40nmol/L [94]. The recommended daily intake of vitamin D is between 400 IU and 600 IU per day which may be insufficient to raise serum vitamin D levels to a desirable level of 75–100nmol/L [37]. Some studies have demonstrated that in order to achieve optimal levels of 25(OH) vitamin D, doses between 700 to 1000 IU would be needed [37]. In the United States, fortification of some foods – such as milk and orange juice – is mandatory, whereas in European countries only a few foods are fortified with vitamin D. However, the question of whether it should be obligatory for food products to be added with vitamin D remains controversial [37].

Mechanism of action

Several mechanisms of action have been suggested for the role of vitamin D on muscle function (Figure 20.6). The activation of the vitamin D receptors in skeletal muscle results in protein synthesis and subsequent muscle cell growth. Muscle anabolism decreases when vitamin D plasma level is low [28,74]. Low levels of vitamin D influences muscle protein turn-over through reduced insulin secretion and increase myofibrillar degradation [28]. Some authors have observed histological muscle atrophy – predominantly type II fibers – in the presence of vitamin D deficiency [95].

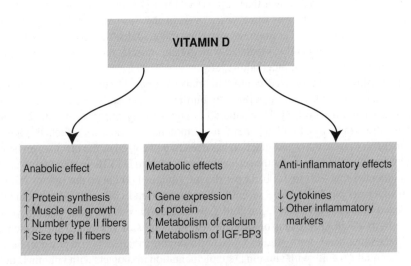

Figure 20.6   Effect of vitamin D on skeletal muscle.

Vitamin D supplementation for 3 months in a small, uncontrolled study resulted in significant increases in the relative number and size of type II muscle fibers in elderly women [96]. Similarly, it is observed that a supplementation of 1000 IU of vitamin D per day in elderly stroke survivors increased type II muscle fibers mean diameter by 2.5-fold over a two-year period [97].

Nuclear vitamin D receptors have various genetic polymorphisms which have been associated with muscle mass. Vitamin D and vitamin D receptors have a direct effect on both the metabolic processes and the transcriptional regulation of skeletal muscle. In combination with other factors, vitamin D linked with its nuclear receptor can modulate gene expression of proteins such as protein involved in the metabolism of calcium or insulin-like growth factor binding protein-3. Muscle function may also be influenced by vitamin D membrane receptors through the ability to modulate the membrane calcium channels of the muscle fibers.

Finally, recent researches indicate that vitamin D supplementation is associated with decreases in pro-inflammatory and increases in anti-inflammatory cytokines. Given that inflammation has been proposed as a cause of sarcopenia onset and progression, improved vitamin D status may prevent functional declines through lowering inflammation levels [98].

β-HYDROXY β-METHYLBUTYRATE

The β-hydroxy β-methylbutyrate (HMB) is an amino acid metabolite that occurs naturally in human muscle cells. Traditionally, HMB has been used by athletes to enhance performance and build muscle mass. Recent studies have focused on the use of HMB to preserve or rebuild muscle mass in populations in whom loss of lean body mass would increase risk for injury, disability, or mortality.

Clinical experience

HMB has been widely studied in healthy adults, alone and in combination with other amino acids, as an adjunct to exercise to help improve body composition and physical performance. Several studies support the effectiveness of HMB in decreasing delayed onset of muscle soreness and markers of muscle damage, increasing lean body mass without fat gain, increasing various markers of physical performance, including muscle mass and strength.

In elderly women, HMB in combination with arginine and lysine significantly increased protein synthesis and improved body composition, muscle strength, and functionality [99]. A randomized, double-blind, placebo-controlled study demonstrated that 12 weeks of HMB supplementation increased the rate of protein synthesis approximately of 20%, significantly improved the body composition and physical performance ('get-up-and-go' test performance improved 17% versus no change with placebo), and significantly enhanced the muscle strength (knee flexor and extensor force, and hand grip) [99]. In a randomized, double-blind, placebo-controlled study, Vukovich and colleagues evaluated the effects of adding 3 g of HMB per day (n = 14) or placebo (n = 17) to a 5-days/week program of weight training in healthy men and women (mean age 70 years) [100]. After 8 weeks, elderly adults taking HMB alone showed significant improvement from baseline in body composition compared with those who were taking placebo (change in lean body mass +0.8kg with HMB, –0.2kg with placebo) [100]. Furthermore, daily supplementation with the HMB nutrient mixture increased weight gain and lean body mass in cancer patients. Similarly, HMB in combination with arginine and glutamine significantly improved weight and muscle mass and provided immune benefits in patients with AIDS [101]. The HMB plus arginine and glutamine supplementation improved nitrogen balance in severely ill trauma patients, indicating increased protein synthesis. A randomized trial examined the effects of HMB supplementation on inflammation, protein metabolism, and pulmonary function in patients requiring mechanical ventilation for chronic obstructive pulmonary disease. After 7 days, patients who received HMB had significant reductions in C-reactive protein and in white blood cell counts from baseline [102]. In addition, 56% of subjects in the HMB group had improved pulmonary function compared with only 25% of the subjects in the control group. Overall, these data documented that HMB, alone or as part of an amino acid–nutrient mixture, has rebuilt lean body mass and has improved protein synthesis in elderly and critical care patients. These studies demonstrated a good safety profile for HMB supplementation and support a daily effective dose of 3 grams per day.

Mechanism of action

The HMB exerts its effects through protective, anticatabolic mechanisms and has been shown to directly influence protein synthesis. The HMB has been shown to stabilize the muscle cell membrane, to modulate protein degradation, and to up-regulate protein synthesis [103]. As a substrate for cholesterol synthesis in the muscle cell, HMB contributes to the strengthening of the cell membrane. In this way, HMB helps to stabilize the muscle cell membrane to keep the muscle cell intact. Furthermore, it selectively inhibits intracellular inflammation to attenuate protein degradation pathways. The HMB inhibits the activation of caspase-8, thereby preventing the down-regulation of protein synthesis and increasing inhibition of protein degradation initiated by nuclear factor kappa B (NFκB) [104]. Thus, by inhibiting caspase-8 activation on the cell membrane, HMB maintains protein synthesis and prevents additional protein degradation. In addition, the HMB increases protein synthesis directly by activating mTOR (the mammalian target of rapamycin), the intracellular protein that controls protein synthesis. It is the active leucine metabolite that consistently activates the mTOR signal pathway. Insulin-like growth factor-1 (IGF-1) is one of the growth factors that activates mTOR in muscle cells. The HMB also activates mTOR, and its effects are boosted by IGF-1. In this way, HMB may help overcome the age-related reduction in tissue response to endogenous growth hormones such as IGF-1 that contributes to sarcopenia [105].

OTHER POSSIBLE PHARMACOLOGIC APPROACHES

Selective Androgen Receptor Modulators

Synthetic androgen modulators such as Selective Androgen Receptor Modulators (SARMs) are potential alternatives to testosterone. SARMs have the same anabolic effect on muscle tissue as testosterone, without its undesirable side-effects of treatment obtained by improving the tissue selectivity of this drug. One single trial in healthy older men and women has been conducted with the SARM, ostarin. This study demonstrated that the 3 months treatment with ostarin increased muscle mass and stair climbing power [106]. These new drugs may expand the clinical application of androgens in sarcopenia as they enter the clinical phase research. In particular, one of the biggest potential advantages of SARMs is that these drugs might be safe to use in women. With improved tissue selectivity, SARMs that maintain the anabolic actions of androgens without causing the undesirable side effects associated with traditional androgen therapies would really expand the sarcopenia therapeutic options for androgen use in women.

Phyto-estrogen supplementation Isoflavones

A potential approach to prevent or to treat sarcopenia might be phyto-estrogen supplementation. Isoflavones are produced almost exclusively by the members of the leguminosae family and most of them act as phyto-estrogens. Some clinical studies investigated the effect of soy isoflavone supplementation on muscle mass and physical performance.

Aubertin-Leheudre and colleagues [107] demonstrated that a 70mg per day of soy isoflavone supplementation for a period of 24 weeks in obese-sarcopenic postmenopausal women was associated with a significant increase in fat free mass (+0.5 kg). In a randomized study conducted in postmenopausal women, Moeller and colleagues have shown that lean body mass increased to a greater extent in the isoflavone-rich group (+3.4%) than in the isoflavone-poor (+1%) or control (0%) groups [108]. More recently, Maesta and colleagues [109] evaluated the combined effect of soy protein [25 g] with resistance training on body composition in postmenopausal women. This study showed that soy protein combined with 16 weeks of resistance training did not result in greater increases in muscle mass compared to resistance training alone, suggesting that soy protein supplementation had no influence on muscle mass.

Phyto-estrogens may have a beneficial effect on muscle mass, possibly because of their affinity to estrogen receptor-α, which is found on muscle, or through their effects on reducing inflammation. One animal study demonstrated that chronic high soy protein diet was effective to reduce the activation of pathway involved in muscle protein degradation [110]. In particular, isoflavones supplements are found in soy products and exert its effects through a lipid-lowering effect, favour vasodilatation as well as arterial compliance and the regulation of fasting glucose and insulin levels [111]. Some isoflavones, in particular soy isoflavones, when studied in populations eating soy protein, have indicated that there is a lower incidence of breast cancer because of its role in influencing sex hormone metabolism and biological activity through intracellular enzymes, protein synthesis, growth factor actions, and angiogenesis [111].

Melanocortin-4 receptor antagonists

The melanocortin-4 receptor (MC4R) is a G-protein-coupled receptor that is expressed in the hypothalamus. It plays an important role in the regulation of food intake, energy expenditure and catabolism [28,74]. The central melanocortin system seems important in the pathogenesis of cachexia. Its effect on feeding behavior and the metabolic rate is mediated by MC4R.

In mice, stimulation of the MC4R has been demonstrated to decrease food-seeking behavior, to increase basal metabolic rate and to decrease lean body mass [74]. In humans, mutations of the MC4R resulted in severe obesity [112]. On the other hand, blockade of central melanocortin signaling increased both lean body mass and fat mass in a rat model of cardiac cachexia [113].

Inhibition of the melanocortin system either through antagonism or by an antibody against the MC4R has shown encouraging results in animal models of cachexia. A melanocortin 4 receptor antagonist was reported to have beneficial effect in attenuating body composition changes – such as sarcopenia – related to cachexia [74]. Clinical trials in humans should be reported soon.

Ornithine alpha-ketoglutarate

Ornithine alpha-ketoglutarate is a precursor of biologically active amino acids such as glutamine and arginine, and other active compounds that are important in the regulation of protein metabolism in skeletal muscle. Ornithine has a potent effect on the secretion of anabolic hormones, like insulin and growth hormones; furthermore, it is not only a precursor of active metabolites and hormones but important interactions exist between each component produced after ornithine supplementation [114].

Supplementation of total parenteral nutrition with ornithine alpha-ketoglutarate has been shown to maintain nitrogen balance and to reduce skeletal muscle protein breakdown after abdominal surgery [114]. Ornithine alpha-ketoglutarate has been demonstrated to improve nutritional status when given to elderly patients soon after discharge from hospital. In a study conducted on 370 free-living malnourished elderly subjects (mean age 80.0 ± 0.5 years), a significant beneficial effect on weight, body mass index and plasma albumin and transthyretin was noted after ornithine alpha-ketoglutarate supplementation compared to the control group receiving only a placebo [114].

Ornithine alpha-ketoglutarate by its various direct and indirect potential actions on protein metabolism could be a valuable candidate to limit muscle weakness in older subjects with sarcopenia. However, the possible effect of ornithine supplementation on muscle mass and strength has never been investigated in sarcopenic subjects without nutritional problems.

Leptin

The cytokine-like hormone leptin is an important factor linking food intake with energy expenditure and subsequently body composition. Leptin is an adipokin secreted by the adipose tissue that down-regulated satiety and the size of adipose tissue mass, but muscle is also a primary source of leptin, and serum leptin levels increase with increased muscle mass. Leptin has also been reported to regulate several physiological processes including skeletal muscle protein synthesis. Leptin receptors have been identified in human skeletal muscle, while their expression is elevated with disuse atrophy, and leptin-deficiency increases expression of the muscle-wasting protein myostatin [115].

Leptin-deficient mice are obese and display a reduced skeletal muscle mass [28]. Recently, Hamrick and colleagues demonstrated that leptin supplementation increased the relative mass of quadriceps muscle in aged mice as well as the fibers size of skeletal muscle fibers in the extensor digitorum longus [115]. These results are consistent with previous work in leptin-deficient ob/ob mice, where recombinant leptin therapy increased muscle mass in part by suppressing myostatin. Exogenous leptin is capable of inducing a significant anabolic response in skeletal muscle, as well as producing changes in the expression of specific miRNAs. While leptin supplementation plays an important role in metabolism of skeletal muscle of aged mice, leptin is able to regulate 37 miRNA gene expression, but to reverse only three dysregulated miRNAs in aged mice (miR-685, miR-142-3p, and miR-155), suggesting that other therapeutic approaches need to be investigated in order to target certain miRNAs identified in aged muscle [115].

In clinical practice, obese patients may not be the target population to benefit from leptin supplementation as they exhibit leptin resistance [28]. This leptin resistance appears to be due to hyper-triglyceridemia and as a consequence lowering triglycerides may overcome the leptin resistance. However, leptin may be a promising approach to prevent the muscle mass loss during bed rest, limb disuse, or cachexia.

Myostatin inhibition

Myostatin, also identified as growth differentiation factor-8, is a member of the transforming growth factor-β (TGF-β). It is expressed almost exclusively in skeletal muscle and it has an important role for the normal metabolism of muscle mass [74]. Myostatin inhibits myoblast proliferation and thus acts as a negative regulator of skeletal muscle mass [74]. Myostatin inhibition may, therefore, represent an interesting therapeutic approach to sarcopenia prevention and treatment. It was originally discovered when mutations of the myostatin gene were found to be associated with muscle hypertrophy [37].

Animals' studies demonstrated that antibody-directed myostatin inhibition improves muscle mass and function in ageing mice [74]. Recently, Murphy and colleagues reported a statistically significant increased muscle mass by 8 to 18%, muscle fiber size by 12% and muscle strength by 35% after 14 weeks of myostatin antibody treatment. At the same time, the arte of type II fibers increased by 114% and muscle fiber oxidative capacity improved by 39% [116]. These results also extend those observed in middle-aged (13–16 mo) mice, where 6-week treatment with a myostatin antagonist enhanced grip strength [117]. In animals and humans, mutations in the myostatin gene result in increased muscle mass. A single gene myostatin inhibitor enhances muscle mass and strength in the mouse. Antagonism of myostatin enhanced muscle tissue regeneration in aged mice.

Different approaches to inhibit the negative effects of myostatin on skeletal muscle are presently under development. Hormones such as follistatin – a myostatin binding protein – or drugs such as trichostatin-A can antagonize myostatin and are potential new drugs for sarcopenia treatment [118]. Inhibition of myostatin with follistatin may have potential therapeutic benefits on skeletal muscle. The effects of follistatin, originally named FSH-suppressing protein (FSP), are multiple. It induces muscle hypertrophy through satellite cell proliferation by inhibiting both myostatin and activin. Recombinant human antibodies to myostatin are currently tested in human suffering of muscular dystrophy. Phase II trials have been carried out in muscular dystrophy and preliminary results have shown that

MYO-29, a recombinant antibody to myostatin, had good safety and tolerability profile [119]. In the future, gene administration of myostatin-inhibitor-proteins may also to be an option to enhance muscle mass and strength. However, it has been reported that muscle tissue may be more susceptible to muscle and tendon injuries in mice with myostatin deficiency [37].

Agents which target the myostatin pathway may be useful in increasing muscle mass and, therefore, play an important role in muscle wasting disorders as well as age-related sarcopenia [37]. At present, no other conclusive data have been reported from human studies [74].

CONCLUSIONS

Some promising results of clinical studies suggest beneficial effects of several drug classes for the prevention and treatment of sarcopenia in older adults. As shown, these medications with various mechanisms may influence muscular outcomes which may contribute to age-related physical decline. However, despite being extremely exciting for the geriatric community, these results are not sufficiently strong to support routine use of these medications to prevent disability and functional impairment in older adults and further studies are needed to confirm the hypothesis that these drugs could provide an effective intervention to prevent physical decline in the elderly, leading to greater autonomy in this growing population.

REFERENCES

1. Onder G, Vedova CD, Pahor M. Effects of ACE inhibitors on skeletal muscle. Curr Pharm Des. 2006;12:2057–2064.
2. Onder G, Penninx BW, Balkrishnan R, Fried LP, Chaves PHM, Williamson JD, Carter C, Di Bari M, Guralnik JM, Pahor M. Relation between use of angiotensin-converting enzyme inhibitors and muscle strength and physical function in older women: an observational study. Lancet 2002;359:926–930.
3. Di Bari M, Franse LV, Onder G, Kritchevsky SB, Newman A, Harris TB, Williamson JD, Marchionni N, Pahor M. Antihypertensive medications and differences in muscle mass in older persons: the Health, Aging and Body Composition Study. J Am Geriatr Soc. 2004;52:961–966.
4. Sumukadas D, Witham MD, Struthers AD, McMurdo ME. Effect of perindopril on physical function in elderly people with functional impairment: a randomized controlled trial. CMAJ. 2007;177:867–874.
5. Bunout D, Barrera G, de la Maza MP, Leiva L, Backhouse C, Hirsch S. Effects of enalapril or nifedipine on muscle strength or functional capacity in elderly subjects. A double blind trial. J Renin Angiotensin Aldosterone Syst. 2009;10:77–84.
6. Cesari M, Pedone C, Incalzi RA, Pahor M. ACE-inhibition and physical function: results from the Trial of Angiotensin-Converting Enzyme Inhibition and Novel Cardiovascular Risk Factors (TRAIN) study. J Am Med Dir Assoc. 2010;11:26–32.
7. Rankinen T, Wolfarth B, Simoneau JA, Maier-Lenz D, Rauramaa R, Rivera MA, Boulay MR, Chagnon YC, Perusse L, Keul J, Bouchard C. No association between the angiotensin-converting enzyme ID polymorphism and elite endurance athlete status. J Appl Physiol. 2000;88:1571–1575.

8. Zhang B, Tanaka H, Shono N, Miura S, Kiyonaga A, Shindo M, Saku K. The I allele of the angiotensin-converting enzyme gene is associated with an increased percentage of slow-twitch type I fibers in human skeletal muscle. Clin Genet. 2003;63:139–144.

9. Pescatello LS, Kostek MA, Gordish-Dressman H, Thompson PD, Seip RL, Price TB, Angelopoulos TJ, Clarkson PM, Gordon PM, Moyna NM, Visich PS, Zoeller RF, Devaney JM, Hoffman EP. ACE ID genotype and the muscle strength and size response to unilateral resistance training. Med Sci Sports Exerc. 2006;38:1074–1081.

10. Kritchevsky SB, Nicklas BJ, Visser M, Simonsick EM, Newman AB, Harris TB, Penninx B, Satterfield S, Colbert L, Rubin SM, Pahor M. Angiotensin Converting Enzyme Insertion/Deletion genotype, exercise and physical decline: Evidence of a gene-environment interaction. J Am Geriatr Soc. 2004; 52:A29.

11. Vescovo G, Dalla Libera L, Serafini F, Leprotti C, Facchin L, Volterrani M, Ceconi C, Ambrosio GB. Improved exercise tolerance after losartan and enalapril in heart failure: correlation with changes in skeletal muscle myosin heavy chain composition. Circulation. 1998;98: 1742–1749.

12. Han Y, Runge MS, Brasier AR. Angiotensin II induces interleukin-6 transcription in vascular smooth muscle cells through pleiotropic activation of nuclear factor-kappa B transcription factors. Circ Res 1999;84:695–703.

13. Kranzhofer R, Schmidt J, Pfeiffer CA, Hagl S, Libby P, Kubler W. Angiotensin induces inflammatory activation of human vascular smooth muscle cells. Arterioscler Thromb Vasc Biol 1999;19:1623–1629.

14. Brull, D J, Sanders, J, Rumley, A, Lowe, G D, Humphries, S E, Montgomery, H E. Impact of angiotensin converting enzyme inhibition on post-coronary artery bypass interleukin 6 release. Heart 2002;87:252–255.

15. Takeshita S, Tomiyama H, Yokoyama N, Kawamura Y, Furukawa T, Ishigai Y, Shibano T, Isshiki T, Sato T. Angiotensin-converting enzyme inhibition improves defective angiogenesis in the ischemic limb of spontaneously hypertensive rats. Cardiovasc Res. 2001;52: 314–320.

16. Zimmermann R, Kastens J, Linz W, Wiemer G, Scholkens BA, Schaper J. Effect of long-term ACE inhibition on myocardial tissue in hypertensive stroke-prone rats. J Mol Cell Cardiol. 1999;31:1447–1456.

17. Giovannini S, Marzetti E, Borst SE, Leeuwenburgh C. Modulation of GH/IGF-1 axis: potential strategies to counteract sarcopenia in older adults. Mech Ageing Dev. 2008;129:593–601.

18. Onder G, Liperoti R, Russo A, et al. Use of ACE inhibitors is associated with elevated levels of IGFBP-3 among hypertensive older adults: results from the IISIRENTE study. Eur J Clin Pharmacol. 2007;63:389–395.

19. Maggio M, Ceda GP, Lauretani F, et al. Relation of angiotensin-converting enzyme inhibitor treatment to insulin-like growth factor-1 serum levels in subjects >65 years of age (the InCHIANTI study). Am J Cardiol. 2006;97:1525–1529.

20. Camerino GM, Pellegrino MA, Brocca L, Digennaro C, Camerino DC, Pierno S, Bottinelli R. Statin or fibrate chronic treatment modifies the proteomic profile of rat skeletal muscle. Biochem Pharmacol. 2011;81:1054–1064.

21. Riechman SE, Andrews RD, Maclean DA, Sheather S. Statins and dietary and serum cholesterol are associated with increased lean mass following resistance training. J Gerontol A Biol Sci Med Sci. 2007;62:1164–1171.

22. Agostini JV, Tinetti ME, Han L, McAvay G, Foody JM, Concato J. Effects of statin use on muscle strength, cognition, and depressive symptoms in older adults. J Am Geriatr Soc. 2007;55:420–425.

23. Armitage J, Bowman L, Collins R, Parish S, Tobert J. Effects of simvastatin 40 mg daily on muscle and liver adverse effects in a 5-year randomized placebo-controlled trial in 20,536 high-risk people. BMC Clin Pharmacol. 2009;9:6.

24. Bitto A, Minutoli L, Altavilla D, Polito F, Fiumara T, Marini H, Galeano M, Calò M, Lo Cascio P, Bonaiuto M, Migliorato A, Caputi AP, Squadrito F. Simvastatin enhances VEGF production and ameliorates impaired wound healing in experimental diabetes. Pharmacol Res. 2008;57:159–169.

25. Ridker PM, Rifai N, Clearfield M, Downs JR, Weis SE, Miles JS, Gotto AM Jr; Air Force/Texas Coronary Atherosclerosis Prevention Study Investigators. Measurement of C-reactive protein for the targeting of statin therapy in the primary prevention of acute coronary events. N Engl J Med. 2001;344:1959–1965.

26. Heart Protection Study Collaborative Group. MRC/BHF Heart Protection Study of cholesterol lowering with simvastatin in 20,536 high-risk individuals: a randomised placebo-controlled trial. Lancet. 2002;360:7–22.

27. Ridker PM, Danielson E, Fonseca FA, Genest J, Gotto AM Jr, Kastelein JJ, Koenig W, Libby P, Lorenzatti AJ, MacFadyen JG, Nordestgaard BG, Shepherd J, Willerson JT, Glynn RJ; JUPITER Study Group. Rosuvastatin to prevent vascular events in men and women with elevated C-reactive protein. N Engl J Med. 2008;359:2195–2207.

28. Rolland Y, Onder G, Morley JE, Gillette-Guyonet S, Abellan van Kan G, Vellas B. Current and future pharmacologic treatment of sarcopenia. Clin Geriatr Med. 2011;27:423–447.

29. Onder G, Della Vedova C, Landi F. Validated treatments and therapeutics prospectives regarding pharmacological products for sarcopenia. J Nutr Health Aging 2009;13:746–756.

30. Visvanathan R, Chapman I. Preventing sarcopaenia in older people. Maturitas 2010;66:383–388.

31. Emmelot-Vonk MH, Verhaar Hj, et al. Effect of Testosterone Supplementation on Functional Mobility, Cognition, and Other Parameters in Older Men: A Randomized Controlled Trial. JAMA 2008;299:39–52.

32. Ottenbacher KJ, Ottenbacher ME, Ottenbacher AJ, Acha AA, Ostir GV. Androgen treatment and muscle strength in elderly men: A meta-analysis. J Am Geriatr Soc. 2006;54:1666–1673.

33. Srinivas-Shankar U, Roberts SA, Connolly MJ, et al. Effects of testosterone on muscle strength, physical function, body composition, and quality of life in intermediate-frail and frail elderly men: a randomized, double-blind, placebo-controlled study. J Clin Endocrinol Metab. 2010;95(2):639–650.

34. Chapman IM, Visvanathan R, Hammond AJ, et al. Effect of testosterone and a nutritional supplement, alone and in combination, on hospital admissions in undernourished older men and women. Am J Clin Nutr. 2009;89:880–889.

35. Kenny AM, Boxer RS, Kleppinger A, Brindisi J, Feinn R, Burleson JA. Dehydroepiandrosterone combined with exercise improves muscle strength and physical function in frail older women. J Am Geriatr Soc. 2010;58:1707–1714.

36. Pierorazio PM, Ferrucci L, Kettermann AE, Metter EJ, Carter HB. Serum testosterone is associated with aggressive prostate cancer: results from the Baltimore longitudinal study of aging. J Urol 2008;179:150.

37. Burton LA, Sumukadas D. Optimal management of sarcopenia. Clin Interv Aging. 2010;5:217–228.

38. Basaria S, Coviello AD, Travison TG, et al. Adverse events associated with testosterone administration. N Engl J Med. 2010;363:109–122.

39. Ferrando AA, Sheffield-Moore M, Paddon-Jones D, Wolfe RR, Urban RJ. Differential anabolic effects of testosterone and amino acid feeding in older men. J Clin Endocrinol Metab. 2003;88:358–362.

40. Verdijk LB, Snijders T, Beelen M, Savelberg HH, Meijer K, Kuipers H, Van Loon LJ. Characteristics of muscle fiber type are predictive of skeletal muscle mass and strength in elderly men. J Am Geriatr Soc. 2010;58:2069–2075.

41. Sinha-Hikim I, Artaza J, Woodhouse L, Gonzalez-Cadavid N, Singh AB, Lee MI, Storer TW, Casaburi R, Shen R, Bhasin S. Testosterone-induced increase in muscle size in healthy young men is associated with muscle fiber hypertrophy. Am J Physiol Endocrinol Metab. 2002;283:E154–64.

42. Palazzolo I, Gliozzi A, Rusmini P, Sau D, Crippa V, Simonini F, Onesto E, Bolzoni E, Poletti A. The role of the polyglutamine tract in androgen receptor. J Steroid Biochem Mol Biol. 2008;108:245–253.

43. Fargo KN, Alexander TD, Tanzer L, Poletti A, Jones KJ. Androgen regulates neuritin mRNA levels in an in vivo model of steroid-enhanced peripheral nerve regeneration. J Neurotrauma. 2008;25:561–566.

44. Messier V, Rabasa-Lhoret R, Barbat-Artigas S, Elisha B, Karelis AD, Aubertin-Leheudre M. Menopause and sarcopenia: A potential role for sex hormones. Maturitas. 2011;68: 331–336.

45. Sipila S, Taaffe DR, Cheng S, Puolaka J, Toivanen J, Suominen H. Effects of hormone replacement therapy and high impact physical exercise on skeletal muscle in post-menopausal women: a randomized placebo-controlled study. Clin Sci 2001;101:147–157.

46. Heikkinen J, Kyllonen E, Kurtilla-Matero E, et al. HRT and exercise: effects on bone density, muscle strength and lipid metabolism. A placebo controlled 2 year prospective trial on two estrogen–progestin regimens in healthy postmenopausal women. Maturitas 1997;26: 139–149.

47. Skelton DA, Phillips K, Bruce SA, Naylor CH, Woledge RC. Hormone replacement therapy increases isometric muscle strength of adductor pollicis in post-menopausal women. Clin Sci 1999;96:357–364.

48. Ribom EL, Piehl-Aulin K, Ljunghall S, et al. Six months of hormone replacement therapy does not influence muscle strength in postmenopausal women. Sci Direct 2002;42:225–237.

49. Armstrong AL, Oborne J, Coupland CAC, et al. Effects of hormone replacement therapy on muscle performance and balance in post-menopausal women. Clin Sci 1996;91:685–690.

50. Meeuwsen IBAE, Samson MM, Duursma SA, Verhaar HJJ. Muscle strength and tibolone: a randomised, double blind placebo-controlled study. BJOG 2002;109:77–84.

51. Boyanov MA, Shinkov AD. Effects of tibolone on body composition in postmenopausal women: a 1 year follow up study. Maturitas 2005;51:363–369.

52. Hanggi W, Lippuner K, Jaeger P, et al. Differential impact of conventional oral or transdermal hormone replacement therapy or tibolone on body composition in postmenopausal women. Clin Endocrinol 1998;48:691–699.

53. Porcile A, Gallardo E, Duarte P, Aedo S. Differential effects on serum IGF-1 of tibolone (5 mg/day) vs. combined continuous estrogen/progestagen in post menopausal women. Rev Med Chil 2003;131:1151–1156.

54. Cicinelli E, Ignarro LJ, Galantino P, Pinto V, Barba B, Schonauer S. Effects of tibolone on plasma levels of nitric oxide in postmenopausal women. Fertil Steril 2002;78:464–468.

55. Dieli-Conwright CM, Spektor TM, Rice JC, Sattler FR, Schroeder ET. Hormone therapy attenuates exercise-induced skeletal muscle damage in postmenopausal women. J Appl Physiol. 2009;107:853–858.

56. Huffman KM, Slentz CA, Johnson JL, et al. Impact of hormone replacement therapy on exercise training-induced improvements in insulin action in sedentary overweight adults. Metabolism. 2008;57:888–895.

57. Jones TE, Stephenson KW, King JG, Knight KR, Marshall TL, Scott WB. Sarcopenia– mechanisms and treatments. J Geriatr Phys Ther. 2009;32:83–89.

58. Kenny AM, Boxer RS, Kleppinger A, Brindisi J, Feinn R, Burleson JA. Dehydroepiandrosterone combined with exercise improves muscle strength and physical function in frail older women. J Am Geriatr Soc 2010;58:1707–1714.

59. Villareal DT, Holloszy JO. DHEA enhances effects of weight training on muscle mass and strength in elderly women and men. Am J Physiol Endocrinol Metab 2006;291:E1003–E1008.

60. Christiansen JJ, Bruun JM, Christiansen JS, Jørgensen JO, Gravholt CH. Long-term DHEA substitution in female adrenocortical failure, body composition, muscle function, and bone metabolism: a randomized trial. Eur J Endocrinol 2011;165:293–300.

61. Baker WL, Karan S, Kenny AM. Effect of dehydroepiandrosterone on muscle strength and physical function in older adults: a systematic review. J Am Geriatr Soc 2011;59:997–1002.

62. Valenti G, Denti L, Maggio M, Ceda G, Volpato S, Bandinelli S, Ceresini G, Cappola A, Guralnik JM, Ferrucci L. Effect of DHEAS on skeletal muscle over the life span: the InCHIANTI study. J Gerontol A Biol Sci Med Sci 2004;59:466–472.

63. Sato K, Iemitsu M, Aizawa K et al. Testosterone and DHEA activate the glucose metabolism-related signaling pathway in skeletal muscle. Am J Physiol Endocrinol Metab 2008;294:E961–E968.

64. Brill KT, Weltman AL, Gentili A, Patrie JT, Fryburg DA, Hanks JB, Urban RJ, Veldhuis JD. Single and combined effects of growth hormone and testosterone administration on measures of body composition, physical performance, mood, sexual function, bone turnover, and muscle gene expression in healthy older men. J. Clin. Endocrinol. Metab. 2002;87:5649–5657.

65. Papadakis MA, Grady D, Black D, Tierney MJ, Gooding GA, Schambelan M, Grunfeld C. Growth hormone replacement in healthy older men improves body composition but not functional ability. Ann. Intern. Med. 1996;124:708–716.

66. Blackman MR, Sorkin JD, Munzer T, Bellantoni MF, Busby-Whitehead J, Stevens TE, Jayme J, O'Connor KG, Christmas C, Tobin JD, Stewart KJ, Cottrell E, Pabst KM, Harman SM. Growth hormone and sex steroid administration in healthy aged women and men: a randomized controlled trial. JAMA 2002;288:2282–2292.

67. Sattler FR, Castaneda-Sceppa C, Binder EF, et al. Testosterone and growth hormone improve body composition and muscle performance in older men. J Clin Endocrinol Metab 2009;94:1991–2001.

68. Taaffe DR, Pruitt L, Reim J, Hintz RL, Butterfield G, Hoffman AR, Marcus R. Effect of recombinant human growth hormone on the muscle strength response to resistance exercise in elderly men. J. Clin. Endocrinol. Metab. 1994;79:1361–1366.

69. Yarasheski KE, Zachwieja JJ, Campbell JA, Bier DM. Effect of growth hormone and resistance exercise on muscle growth and strength in older men. Am. J. Physiol. 1995;268:E268–E276.

70. Thompson JL, Butterfield GE, Gylfadottir UK, Yesavage J, Marcus R, Hintz RL, Pearman A, Hoffman AR. Effects of human growth hormone, insulinlike growth factor I, and diet and exercise on body composition of obese postmenopausal women. J. Clin. Endocrinol. Metab. 1998;83:1477–1484.

71. Lange KH, Andersen JL, Beyer N, Isaksson F, Larsson B, Rasmussen MH, Juul A, Bulow J, Kjaer M. GH administration changes myosin heavy chain isoforms in skeletal muscle but does not augment muscle strength or hypertrophy, either alone or combined with resistance exercise training in healthy elderly men. J. Clin. Endocrinol. Metab. 2002;87:513–523.

72. Carpenter V, Matthews K, Devlin G, Stuart S, Jensen J, Conaglen J, Jeanplong F, Goldspink P, Yang SY, Goldspink G, Bass J, McMahon C. Mechano-growth factor reduces loss of cardiac function in acute myocardial infarction. Heart Lung Circ. 2008;17:33–39.

73. Santini MP, Tsao L, Monassier L, Theodoropoulos C, Carter J, Lara-Pezzi E, Slonimsky E, Salimova E, Delafontaine P, Song YH, Bergmann M, Freund C, Suzuki K, Rosenthal N. Enhancing repair of the mammalian heart. Circ Res. 2007;100:1732–1740.

74. Kung T, Springer J, Doehner W, Anker SD, von Haehling S. Novel treatment approaches to cachexia and sarcopenia: highlights from the 5th Cachexia Conference. Expert Opin Investig Drugs. 2010;19:579–585.

75. Tai K, Visvanathan R, Hammond AJ, Wishart JM, Horowitz M, Chapman IM. Fasting ghrelin is related to skeletal muscle mass in healthy adults. Eur J Nutr. 2009;48(3):176–183.

76. Nass R, Pezzoli SS, Oliveri MC, et al. Effects of an oral ghrelin mimetic on body composition and clinical outcomes in healthy older adults: a randomized trial. Ann Intern Med 2008;149(9):601–611.

77. Morley JE, Argiles JM, Evans WJ, et al. Nutritional recommendations for the management of sarcopenia. J Am Med Dir Assoc. 2009;11:391–396.

78. Brose A, Parise G, Tarnopolsky MA. Creatine supplementation enhances isometric strength and body composition improvements following strength exercise training in older adults. J. Gerontol. Biol. Med. Sci. 2003, 58:11–19.

79. Rawson ES, Wehnert ML, Clarkson PM. Effects of 30 days of creatine ingestion in older men. Eur. J. Appl. Physiol. 1999, 80:139–144.

80. Bermon S, Venembre P, Sachet C, Valour S, Dolisi C. Effect of creatine monohydrate ingestion in sedentary and weight-trained older adults. Acta Physiologica Scand. 1998, 164; 147–115.

81. Eijnde BO, Van Leemputte M, Goris M, et al. Effects of creatine supplementation and exercise training on fitness in males 55 to 75 years old. J. Appl. Physiol. 2003, 95:818–828.

82. Francaux M, Poortmans JR. Effects of training and creatine supplement on muscle strength and body mass. Eur J Appl Physiol 1999;80:165–168.

83. Ingwall JS, Weiner CD, Morales MF, Stockdale FE. Specificity of creatine in the control of muscle protein synthesis. J Cell Physiol 1974, 63:145–151.

84. Morley JE. Vitamin d redux. J Am Med Dir Assoc. 2009;10:591–592.

85. Annweiler, C., Schott, A.M., Berrut, G. et al. Vitamin D related changes in physical performance: a systematic review. Journal of Nutrition, Health and Aging 2009;13:893–898.

86. Kim MK, Baek KH, Song KH, Kang MI, Park CY, Lee WY, Oh KW. Vitamin D Deficiency Is Associated with Sarcopenia in Older Koreans, Regardless of Obesity: The Fourth Korea National Health and Nutrition Examination Surveys (KNHANES IV) 2009. J Clin Endocrinol Metab. 2011, in press.

87. Visser, M., Deeg, D.J.H. & Lips, P. Low vitamin D and high parathyroid hormone levels as determinants of loss of muscle strength and muscle mass (sarcopenia): the Longitudinal Aging Study Amsterdam. Journal of Clinical Endocrinology and Metabolism 2003;88:5766–5772.

88. Bischoff HA, Stahelin HB, Dick W, et al. Effects of vitamin D and calcium supplementation on falls: a randomized controlled trial. J Bone Miner Res. 2003;18:343–351.

89. Pfeifer M, Begerow B, Minne HW, Suppan K, Fahrleitner-Pammer A, Dobnig H. Effects of a long-term vitamin D and calcium supplementation on falls and parameters of muscle function in community-dwelling older individuals. Osteoporos Int. 2009;20:315–322.

90. Moreira-Pfrimer LD, Pedrosa MA, Teixeira L, Lazaretti-Castro M. Treatment of vitamin D deficiency increases lower limb muscle strength in institutionalized older people independently of regular physical activity: a randomized double-blind controlled trial. Ann Nutr Metab. 2009;54:291–300.

91. Pfeifer M, Begerow B, Minne HW, Abrams C, Nachtigall D, Hansen C. Effects of a short-term vitamin D and calcium supplementation on body sway and secondary hyperparathyroidism in elderly women. J Bone Miner Res 2000;15:1113–1118.

92. Bischoff-Ferrari HA, Dawson-Hughes B, Staehelin HB, et al. Fall prevention with supplemental and active forms of vitamin D: a meta-analysis of randomised controlled trials. BMJ 2009;339:b3692.

93. Verschueren SM, Bogaerts A, Delecluse C, Claessens AL, Haentjens P, Vanderschueren D, Boonen S. The effects of whole-body vibration training and vitamin D supplementation on muscle strength, muscle mass, and bone density in institutionalized elderly women: a 6-month randomized, controlled trial. J Bone Miner Res 2011;26:42–49.

94. Landi F, Liperoti R, Fusco D, Mastropaolo S, Quattrociocchi D, Proia A, Russo A, Bernabei R, Onder G. Prevalence and Risk Factors of Sarcopenia Among Nursing Home Older Residents. J Gerontol A Biol Sci Med Sci 2011, in press.

95. Janssen HC, Samson MM, Verhaar HJ. Vitamin D deficiency, muscle function, and falls in elderly people. Am J Clin Nutr 2002;75:611–615.

96. Sorensen OH, Lund B, Saltin B, et al. Myopathy in bone loss of ageing: improvement by treatment with 1 alpha-hydroxycholecalciferol and calcium. Clin Sci (Lond) 1979;56:157–161.

97. Sato Y, Iwamoto J, Kanoko T, Satoh K. Low-dose vitamin D prevents muscular atrophy and reduces falls and hip fractures in women after stroke: a randomized controlled trial. Cerebrovasc Dis. 2005;20:187–192.

98. Scott D, Blizzard L, Fell J, Ding C, Winzenberg T, Jones G. A prospective study of the associations between 25-hydroxy-vitamin D, sarcopenia progression and physical activity in older adults. Clin Endocrinol 2010;73(5):581–587.

99. Flakoll P, Sharp R, Baier S, Levenhagen D, Carr C, Nissen S. Effect of β-hydroxy-β-methylbutyrate, arginine, and lysine supplementation on strength, functionality, body composition, and protein metabolism in elderly women. Nutrition 2004;20:445–451.

100. Vukovich MD, Stubbs NB, Bohlken RM. Body composition in 70-year old adults responds to dietary β-hydroxy-β-methylbutyrate similarly to that of young adults. J Nutr. 2001;131:2049–2052.

101. Clark RH, Feleke G, Din M, et al. Nutritional treatment for acquired immunodeficiency virus-associated wasting using β-hydroxy β-methybutyrate, glutamine, and arginine: a randomised, double-blind, placebo controlled study. J Parenter Enteral Nutr 2000;24:133–139.

102. Hsieh LC, Chien SL, Huang MS, Tseng HF, Chang CK. Anti-inflammatory and anticatabolic effects of short-term β-hydroxy-β-methylbutyrate supplementation on chronic obstructive pulmonary disease patients in intensive care unit. Asia Pac J Clin Nutr. 2006;15:544–550.

103. Eley HL, Russell ST, Tisdale MJ. Mechanism of attenuation of muscle protein degradation induced by tumor necrosis factor-a and angiotensin II by β-hydroxy-β-methylbutyrate. Am J Physiol Endocrinol Metab 2008;295:E1417-E1426.

104. Eley HL, Russell ST, Baxter JH, Mukerji P, Tisdale MJ. Signaling pathways initiated by β-hydroxy-β-methylbutyrate to attenuate the depression of protein synthesis in skeletal muscle in response to cachectic stimuli. Am J Physiol Endocrinol Metab 2007;293:E923-E931.

105. Paddon-Jones D, Short KR, Campbell WW, Volpi E, Wolfe RR. Role of dietary protein in the sarcopenia of aging. Am J Clin Nutr. 2008;87(suppl):1562S-1566S.

106. Morley JE. Developing novel therapeutic approaches to frailty. Curr Pharm Des 2009;15:3384–3395.

107. Aubertin-Leheudre M, Lord C, Khalil A, Dionne IJ. Six months of isoflavone supplement increases fat-free mass in obese-sarcopenic postmenopausal women: a randomized double-blind controlled trial. Eur J Clin Nutr 2007;61:1442–1444.

108. Moeller LE, Peterson CT, Hanson KB, et al. Isoflavone-rich soy protein prevents loss of hip lean mass but does not prevent the shift in regional fat distribution in perimenopausal women. Menopause 2003;10(4):322–331.

109. Maesta N, Nahas EA, Nahas-Neto J, et al. Effects of soy protein and resistance exercise on body composition and blood lipids in postmenopausal women. Maturitas 2007;56(4):350–358.

110. Nikawa T, Ikemoto M, Sakai T, Kano M, Kitano T, Kawahara T, Teshima S, Rokutan K, Kishi K. Effects of a soy protein diet on exercise-induced muscle protein catabolism in rats. Nutrition. 2002;18:490–495.

111. Candow DG, Chilibeck PD, Abeysekara S, Zello GA. Short-term heavy resistance training eliminates age-related deficits in muscle mass and strength in healthy older males. J Strength Cond Res. 2011;25:326–333.

112. Farooqi IS, Keogh JM, Yeo GS, Lank EJ, Cheetham T, O'Rahilly S. Clinical spectrum of obesity and mutations in the melanocortin 4 receptor gene. N Engl J Med 2003;348:1085–1095.

113. Scarlett JM, Bowe DD, Zhu X, Batra AK, Grant WF, Marks DL. Genetic and pharmacologic blockade of central melanocortin signaling attenuates cardiac cachexia in rodent models of heart failure. J Endocrinol 2010;206:121–130.

114. Walrand S. Ornithine alpha-ketoglutarate: could it be a new therapeutic option for sarcopenia? J Nutr Health Aging 2010;14(7):570–577.

115. Hamrick MW, Herberg S, Arounleut P, He HZ, Shiver A, Qi RQ, Zhou L, Isales CM, Mi QS. The adipokine leptin increases skeletal muscle mass and significantly alters skeletal muscle miRNA expression profile in aged mice. Biochem Biophys Res Commun 2010;400:379–383.

116. Murphy KT, Koopman R, Naim T, Léger B, Trieu J, Ibebunjo C, Lynch GS. Antibody-directed myostatin inhibition in 21-mo-old mice reveals novel roles for myostatin signaling in skeletal muscle structure and function. FASEB J 2010;24:4433–4442.

117. Siriett V., Salerno MS, Berry C, Nicholas G, Bower R, Kambadur R, Sharma M. Antagonism of myostatin enhances muscle regeneration during sarcopenia. Mol. Ther 2007;15:1463–1470.

118. Solomon AM, Bouloux PM. Modifying muscle mass - the endocrine perspective. J Endocrinol 2006;191:349–360.

119. Wagner KR. Phase II trial of MYO-29 in adult subjects with muscular dystrophy. Ann Neurol 2008;63:561–571.

CHAPTER 21

Sarcopenia: Is It Preventable?

Maurits Vandewoude

*Professor in Geriatric Medicine, Medical School, Geriatrics Department,
University of Antwerp, Antwerp, Belgium*

Ivan Bautmans

*Frailty in Ageing Research Department (FRIA), Vrije Universiteit Brussel,
Brussels, Belgium*

INTRODUCTION

Sarcopenia is a syndrome characterized by progressive and generalized loss of skeletal muscle mass and strength with a risk of adverse outcomes [1]. As befits an age-related trait, the process of sarcopenia is universal with age. Indeed most human physiologic systems regress with ageing, independently of substantial disease effects, at an average linear loss of 0.34–1.28% per year between the age of 30 and 70 [2]. Therefore, sarcopenia can be considered as the effect of ageing on muscle mass in every human being. This is true even for athletes who, although they continue to be physically active and perform at levels well above those of sedentary adults, demonstrate a decline in lean tissue with age [3]. Next to the intrinsic, age-related processes, a multitude of extrinsic and behavioral factors can aggravate the development and/or progression of sarcopenia; such as disuse and lack of physical activity, malnutrition, chronic inflammation and (co-)morbidity. The relative contribution of these factors can show important variability from person to person and, therefore, there is a huge variation in the loss of muscle mass and muscle strength between individuals. Some older people have a muscle mass that is comparable to that of younger adults, whereas other older adults have a muscle mass that is so low that it compromises their functional abilities. Sarcopenia, thus, can be thought of as both a process and an outcome.

AGE RELATED CHANGES IN BODY COMPOSITION

The age related changes in body composition develop very gradually. Muscle mass begins to decline at approximately 1% per year after the age of 30. Longitudinal changes in body composition show in men a tendency to gain fat and lean mass through their 40s,

Sarcopenia, First Edition. Edited by Alfonso J. Cruz-Jentoft and John E. Morley.
© 2012 John Wiley & Sons, Ltd. Published 2012 by John Wiley & Sons, Ltd.

followed by a trend toward weight loss, resulting in the loss of both compartments after age 60 [4]. Studies in women show consistent gains in fat across the age spectrum. Cross-sectional data suggest that whole body protein declines curvilinearly with age, such that there is an accelerated decline after 65 years of age [5]. Recently, it has been shown that there is an exponential increase in the loss of lean tissue in subjects older than 75 years compared to younger older people [6]. Initially, clinical relevance is very low, symptoms being absent. In later stages the loss of muscle mass has been shown to be associated with disability. However, the development of disability is a very complex area and is almost always multifactorial in these subjects. Whether sarcopenia becomes a clinically evident problem depends on many factors, including the starting level of muscle mass and the rate of its decline. There are several mechanisms that may be involved in the onset and progression of sarcopenia. These mechanisms involve, among others, protein synthesis, proteolysis, neuromuscular integrity and muscle fat content. In an individual with sarcopenia, several mechanisms may be involved, and relative contributions may vary over time. It would be interesting if the effects of aging *per se* could be separated from the effects of chronic disease or physical activity, which itself tends to decline with age.

PREVALENCE OF SARCOPENIA

The general trend in prevalence studies of sarcopenia is that in older cohorts prevalence rises both in men and women with an even higher prevalence in men. Several longitudinal studies indicate that muscle mass and size decrease by approximately 6% per decade in the average person beginning at approximately 45 years of age [7]. In the existing literature a wide variability in prevalence has been reported depending on the criteria used [8]. Some authors estimate the prevalence of sarcopenia at 5 to 13% in 60 to 70 year olds and 11 to 50% for the population aged 80 years or older [9–11]. However, it can be assumed that in a specific age cohort people who do not fulfill criteria for the diagnosis of sarcopenia also have lost muscle both in a qualitative and quantitative way. Indeed, they have been and still are exposed to the same pathophysiological mechanisms as those who actually fulfill the criteria for sarcopenia. So, it can be said that the prevalence of sarcopenia in the older adult population reaches a 100%. The diagnosis, however, based on cut-off values [12], such as two standard deviations below a reference value for age and gender adjusted young healthy adults, converts the continuous process of muscle mass loss into a categorical one with categories such as presarcopenia and sarcopenia [1]. This approach is designed for the identification of subjects with an already existing sarcopenia and presenting with a (risk for the development of) functional disability due to muscle weakness. As with other degenerative conditions, it is open to debate whether everybody will eventually develop sarcopenia up to a degree corresponding to the diagnostic criteria proposed.

PREVENTION

Preventing disability involves a wide range of interrelated programs, actions, and activities from different parties. It involves public health policy makers as well as health care practitioners (physicians, nurses, and allied health professionals) working at different levels. Preventive strategies are typically described as taking place at the primary, secondary,

Table 21.1 Level of prevention according to the condition of the patient (presenting with or without possibly sarcopenia related symptoms) and the evaluation of the practitioner (based on performance based evaluation)

		Sarcopenia signs Doctor	
		absent	present
Sarcopenia symptoms Patient	absent	Primary prevention	Secondary prevention
	present	Quaternary prevention	Tertiary prevention

tertiary and quaternary levels (Table 21.1). Next to the typical levels of prevention other preventive intervention classification systems have been proposed in the area of disease prevention by Gordon [13]. They consist of a three-tiered preventive intervention system with universal, selective, and indicated prevention levels (Table 21.2). This three step model overlaps partly with primary and secondary prevention from the more traditional model but it can help with supplying specific prevention strategies in the algorithm for the prevention of sarcopenia. The effectiveness of prevention programs, however, largely depends on the extent to which individuals take personal responsibility for their own health and are willing to follow the recommendations about nutrition and exercise.

Primary

Primary prevention includes actions to protect against disease and disability before they occur. Today, the most pressing health problems in developed countries are chronic diseases and conditions based on the increasing multimorbidity found in people growing older. This increasing multimorbidity is the cradle of the geriatric syndromes. Primary prevention of such syndromes is more challenging than primary prevention of well-defined diseases because it requires changing health behaviors. In the case of sarcopenia this includes the basic

Table 21.2 Preventive intervention system with universal, selective, and indicated prevention levels

Prevention	Target	Aim	Action
Universal	entire population	to prevent or delay sarcopenia	information and skills to prevent sarcopenia
Selective	groups whose risk of developing sarcopenia is above average	to prevent or delay sarcopenia	• information about nutritional supplements • websites for active seniors
Indicated	• to identify individuals who exhibit early signs of sarcopenia • identifiers may include low muscle functionality and increased falls	involves a screening process	specific and personal interventions in nutrition and exercise

activities of a healthy lifestyle such as good nutrition and hygiene and adequate exercise and rest. However, efforts to change deeply rooted and often culturally influenced patterns of behaviors, such as diet and physical inactivity, generally have been less successful than environmental health and immunization programs.

Secondary

The goal of secondary prevention is to identify and detect a disease or a condition in its earliest stages, before noticeable symptoms develop, when it is most likely to be treated successfully. With early detection and diagnosis, it may be possible to reverse a condition, slow its progression, prevent or minimize its complications, and limit ensuing disability.

Tertiary

Tertiary prevention programs aim to improve the quality of life for people already affected by a disease or condition by limiting complications and disabilities, reducing the severity and progression of the condition and providing rehabilitation to restore functionality and self-sufficiency.

Quaternary

This term describes the set of health activities that mitigate or avoid the consequences of unnecessary or excessive interventions in the health system.

Prevention strategy

In the strategy of dealing with sarcopenia, prevention should be distinguished from treatment. However, interventions will target similar underlying pathophysiological processes. The difference lies in the actual support and coaching of the individual. Therefore, an algorithm for management of the sarcopenia process should be developed to guide the actual interventions needed in different stages.

Sarcopenia as 'a condition' is a major cause of frailty and disability in older people, but as 'an active process' it is present in every person reaching adult life. Given the intrinsic, age-related character of sarcopenia, primary prevention, if possible, should start as early as the onset of the underlying process (i.e. at a young adult age); at higher ages, secondary and tertiary preventive strategies can be considered in order to avoid excessive progression of sarcopenia (see Table 21.1 for definition of prevention levels).

In the primary prevention strategy, people should be clearly informed about evidence-based approaches in order to preserve muscle mass and performance as long as possible. At the same time their awareness for (often commercial) non-evidence based anti-ageing treatments should be raised. When consulting PubMed (last search on September 26th 2011) for peer-reviewed publications with the keywords *SARCOPENIA AND PREVENTION*, 226 hits were found (188 hits when limited for reports on humans only). Based on the existing body of knowledge, physical exercise and nutrition seem to be the major elements in all levels of the prevention of sarcopenia.

In order to identify individuals for primary, secondary or higher prevention levels, low-cost, but sensitive assessment tools are necessary. The actual proposed screening algorithms are focused at identifying subjects corresponding to the *diagnostic* criteria for sarcopenia (i.e. T-score < -2 for muscle mass and/or strength). In fact, using these criteria, subjects presenting with an (increased risk for) sarcopenia-related disability can be identified. In this context, the European Working Group on Sarcopenia in Older People recently proposed a cut-off point of 0.8 m/s for gait speed for case-finding [1]. The International Working Group on Sarcopenia recommends gait speed < 1 m/s as cut-off point to refer subjects for further body-composition assessment in order to confirm the diagnosis of sarcopenia [9]. However, in order to identify subjects susceptible for primary and secondary prevention, the phase corresponding to decreased gait speed is probably too advanced, and suggests already an indication for tertiary prevention and/or treatment. Therefore, muscle performance assessment, using an easy and reliable method, and providing a score on a continuous scale, is probably more suitable to identify persons with sarcopenia-induced muscle weakness without presenting clinical signs of functional disability. Grip strength is easy to measure, and age-related changes in grip strength are well described [14] and run parallel to the strength losses in other muscle groups [15]. Therefore, grip strength is proposed here as a preferential screening tool for muscle strength in ageing. Because daily activities often require sustained intense muscle contractions (e.g. when bearing shopping bags), sarcopenia could incur a sense of fatigue in older persons. Therefore, muscle fatigue can be proposed as a supplementary factor in the screening for early signs of muscle weakness. Recently, a fatigue resistance test based on grip strength (expressed as the time for grip strength to decrease to 50% of its maximum during sustained contraction) as well as a simple equation to calculate grip work (0.75 x Fatigue Resistance x Maximal grip Strength) has been elaborated and validated. This resistance test could be easily integrated in the early assessment [16–20].

Here, we propose a clinical decision-making algorithm for the preventive management of subjects/patients in the stages before sarcopenia-induced disability becomes apparent (see Figure 21.1). Primary prevention targets all subjects of adult age, presenting grip strength corresponding to levels higher or within the gender-matched normal values that can be expected at a young age. Secondary prevention targets subjects that show lower grip strength, but still above the statistically defined cutoff-points (T-scores or $p < 0.05$ levels) [1,9,14,16] and without signs of sarcopenia-induced functional disability (as proposed in the 'diagnosis' of sarcopenia) [1,9].

PHYSICAL EXERCISE

Regular physical activity is one of the major elements in general health prevention. In order to obtain significant health benefits, 30 minutes of moderate physical activity on a daily basis is recommended [21]. Physical exercise can be prescribed in a wide variety of modalities, depending on the intensity (load or resistance, number of repetitions, number of series), duration, frequency and type (weight-lifting, walking or running, bicycling, etc.). Resistance training, preferentially at higher intensity, appears to be the most appropriate physical exercise modality in order to prevent loss of and/or improve muscle strength in older persons [22,23]. This type of training consists classically of three series of ten to twelve repetitions at 70 to 80% of the one repetition maximum [1 RM = the weight that can

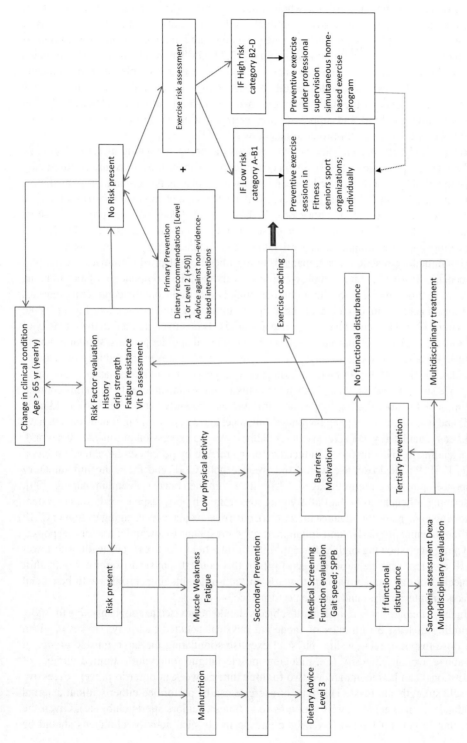

Figure 21.1 A clinical decision-making algorithm for the preventive management of sarcopenia.

be moved maximum once over the whole range of movement). A frequency of one to three exercise sessions per week leads to optimal results. With this training regimen excessive age-related strength loss can, at least partly, be countered and significant gains in muscle strength can be obtained within a short time [22,24,25]. The mechanisms through which physical activity maintains muscle mass and performance are complex and incompletely understood. Physical exercise (especially resistance exercise) stimulates muscular protein synthesis by activating the IGF1 signalling pathway (acting via AKT, mTOR and further downstream signalling), and suppresses protein degradation (via FOXO, and via repression of NF-κB and the ubiquitin-proteasome pathway) [26].

Interestingly, regular physical activity has also a strong regulating effect on systemic inflammatory processes [27,28]. In fact, ageing, even in healthy persons, is commonly accompanied by slightly elevated concentrations of circulating pro-inflammatory mediators (such as Interleukin[IL]-6 and Tumor Necrosis Factor-α), a phenomenon corresponding to a chronic low-grade inflammatory profile (CLIP) [29]. Older persons presenting more pronounced CLIP show indeed lower muscle mass and muscle strength [30,31]. Besides providing anabolic stimuli, it is well known that intensive physical training provokes an inflammatory reaction, accompanied by the liberation of pro-inflammatory cytokines (especially IL-6) [32] and complex changes in the cellular components of the immune system. In this context, IL-6 is thought to be mainly released from the contracting muscles and would act as a 'myokine', exerting a different function from that seen during e.g. acute infections [32]. The acute phase response to exercise is positively related to the intensity of the muscle work delivered. Recently, it has been shown that older persons, similar to young adults, are able to respond to physical stress by a significant exercise-induced increase of circulating IL-6 [33,34]. In fact, the exposure to (repetitive) mild stress has been shown to improve survival and longevity both at the cellular and organism level [35]. In this context, an improved wound healing by physical training, has recently been described in old mice [36] and in older humans [37]; the underlying mechanisms, possibly immune-related, have not been elucidated yet. Exercise can probably lower the expression of toll-like receptor 4, thus leading to lower infection-induced cytokine release by peripheral mononuclear blood cells [38]. Physical exercise would thus reduce both CLIP and the acute inflammatory response upon infection in the aged. CLIP fits within the concept of 'inflammaging' [39], describing a benefit to be had at a young age from a highly responsive immune system (showing good resistance against infections), but a disadvantage when aging by higher CLIP and sarcopenia. Similarly, 'anti-inflammaging' corresponds to low inflammatory responses at young age (showing higher susceptibility to infectious diseases), but leading to lower CLIP and less sarcopenia in old age [39]. In this context, physical exercise would shift subjects from an 'inflammaging' towards an 'anti-inflammaging' profile, with beneficial effects on muscle mass and muscle performance.

In the *primary prevention*, all adult subjects should be advised to adopt an active lifestyle, including at least 30 minutes of moderate physical activity each day. However, given the dose-response relationship, physical exercise stimulating the large muscle groups at an above average intensity (i.e. inducing muscle fatigue following a limited number of repetitions) can be recommended two to three times a week in order to prevent excessive muscle strength and mass. This type of exercise can be performed either without external guidance or in specific exercise settings (e.g. fitness, seniors sports club, etc). Given the fact that in general far too few people engage in physical activity, clinicians should be

Table 21.3   Health categories for risk stratification of complications during physical exercise in older persons (adapted from Bautmans et al. [45])

Health Category	Description*	Clinical examples
A	Completely healthy; no medication	
A1 A2	Completely healthy; using only preventive medication	Hormonal replacement therapy, aspirin, …
B	Functioning normally; presence of stabilised, non cardiovascular disease; absence of cardiovascular abnormalities	Treated hypothyroidism, stable diabetes, …
B1 B2	Functioning normally; using medication with cardiovascular effect, no overt cardiovascular disease other than normalized arterial hypertension	Arterial hypertension; β blocking agent, …
C	(History of) cardio-vascular pathology or abnormal ECG.	Bundle branch block; angina, CABG; …
D	Presenting signs of acute or active disease at the moment of examination.	Bronchospasm, swollen joints, influenza, …

aware of potential motivators and barriers for physical activity. It has been shown that in Western European countries such as Belgium, only one in two citizens attains a minimum of 2.5 hours of moderate physical activity per week [40], and that this proportion decreases to one in five at the age of 75 years and over. The same trend can be observed in other European [41] and non-European industrialized countries [42]. Moreover, from the age of 80 years and over, physical activity shows a sharp decrease. Motivators and barriers for physical activity have been described for different age-groups including children, middle-aged and older people [43], as well as for the oldest old [44]. When promoting physical activity in older persons, special attention should be paid to the health benefits of physical activity, to the subject's fears, individual preferences and social support, and to constraints related to the physical environment [44].

Secondary prevention targets subjects with lower muscle performance than on average expected at young adult age, but without showing evidence for sarcopenia-induced functional disability. For these subjects, the exercise recommendations are similar to those for subjects with normal muscle performance. However, special attention to the barriers for physical activity should be identified as well as other factors that can contribute to increased progression of sarcopenia (e.g. episodes of acute inflammation and/or sources of chronic inflammation). When patients show an increased risk for complications due to co-morbidity (e.g. chronic heart failure, painful joints, etc.) or medication use, higher levels of exercise supervision can be considered; such as adapted exercise classes or physical exercise under supervision of a physical therapist. Recently, a simple classification system has been proposed, which stratifies health categories corresponding to an increasing risk for complications during physical exercise (see Table 21.3), and which can be used by clinicians in the context of exercise prescription [8,45]. The classification system was primarily designed to allow the establishment of recommendations concerning the exercise schedule (type, duration and intensity) of older persons in the absence of direct medical supervision. Therefore, the classification system is rather conservative and it is easy to use for an individual considered at risk for complications. Roughly, participants in category A (completely healthy) will have no particular limitations for exercising; for those in category B1 (functioning normally, but presenting chronic non-cardiovascular disorders) the instructions will vary with the nature of the health problem; those in category B2 will only exercise at higher intensity (e.g. up to 80% of maximal heart rate or higher) when guided by an instructor qualified for training elderly persons; those in category C will only be allowed to exercise under supervision of an instructor and with medical guidance of the training program; those in category D will not exercise unless cleared by a physician.

NUTRITIONAL BASICS

Protein

Skeletal muscle mass is relatively constant during young to middle-aged adulthood, suggesting that there is an equilibrium between protein synthesis during absorptive states (i.e., postprandial, following feeding) that is balanced by the catabolism during fasting states. However, this equilibrium in healthy muscle between protein synthesis and breakdown is getting progressively disrupted with aging. In older people synthesis rate of mixed muscle proteins including myofibrillar and mitochondrial proteins decrease with 30% [46]. Muscle protein synthesis is stimulated by dietary intake of both essential and nonessential amino acids. There is a substantial body of research suggesting that over 80% of the stimulatory effect on protein synthesis observed after a meal can be attributed to amino acids [47]. In older people compared to younger individuals this stimulatory effect is being blunted but not absent. It can be overruled by increasing the amount of protein. In addition to their role in protein synthesis, amino acids also play a role in the regulation of protein breakdown [48]. Nitrogen balance studies in aging populations (56–80 years of age) have indicated greater protein needs for the elderly (1.14 g/kg/d) relative to the young (0.8 g/kg/d) [49]. The same research group, however, showed in a short-term nitrogen balance study that the requirement for total dietary protein was not different for healthy older adults than for younger adults and that the allowance estimate does not differ statistically from the RDA [50]. On the other hand, older individuals whose consumption levels approach the RDA are at greater risk for disease than those consuming more than 1.2 g/kg/d [51]. This provides critical information in terms of inadequate protein intake as a possible mechanism underlying sarcopenia, particularly because protein intake has been reported as inversely proportional to age. Randomized controlled trial data indicate that it is more important to ingest a sufficient amount of high-quality protein (25–30 g) with each meal rather than 1 large bolus, because greater than 30 g in a single meal may not further stimulate muscle protein synthesis [52]. Furthermore, Paddon-Jones reported that aging does not inevitably reduce the anabolic response to a high-quality protein meal, rather it is the presence of carbohydrates that blunts this response due to the effects of insulin resistance on muscle protein synthesis [53]. These data would suggest that high quality protein should be consumed in smaller quantities, but not together with carbohydrates.

Low nutrient intake secondary to the 'anorexia of aging' is considered an important risk factor in the development and progression of sarcopenia [54]. Morley reviewed the

Table 21.4 Nutritional interventions in the prevention strategy for Sarcopenia

Primary prevention
    Level 1
        Balanced Mediterranean type of diet
        High quality protein divided over several meals: 1.0–1.2 g/kg/d protein
        400–1000 IU vit D
    Level 2
        Balanced Mediterranean type of diet
        High quality protein divided over several meals: 1.0–1.2 g/kg/d protein
        800–2000 IU vit D

Secondary prevention
    Level 3
        Dietary history / dietitians advice
        Personalized Mediterranean type of diet
        High quality protein divided over several meals: 1.0–1.2 g/kg/d protein
        800–2000 IU vit D

Tertiary prevention
    Level 4
        Dietary history / dietitians advice
        Personalized Mediterranean type of diet
        High quality protein divided over several meals: 1.2–1.5 g/kg/d protein
        800–2000 IU vit D
    Level 5
        Dietary history / dietitians advice
        Personalized Mediterranean type of diet
        High quality protein divided over several meals: 1.2–1.5 g/kg/d protein
        800–2000 IU vit D
        Nutritional supplements containing essential amino acids, leucine

Quaternary prevention
    Parallel advice together with all preceding levels of prevention

phenomena of the anorexia of aging and reported that early satiety, secondary to decreased relaxation of the fundus, increased the release of cholecystokinin in response to fat intake, and that increased leptin levels and neurotransmitters may all play a role in the anorexia of aging. It is also reported that 15% of those older than 60 years eat less than 75% of the recommended daily allowance for protein [55]. Thus, although poor overall nutritional intake may play a role in sarcopenia, low protein intake appears to be a significant problem for older adults and may be a potential target for an intervention strategy.

In summary, from the nutritional point of view a balanced diet with a protein intake of 0.8 g/kg/d is appropriate for younger and middle-aged adults. However, with the progressive blunting of the anabolic response to a high quality protein meal protein requirements may be higher. In accordance with the clinical situation advice should be given to increase protein intake with aging as suggested in the algorithm (Figure 21.1, Table 21.4).

Vitamin D

Vitamin D has recently received recognition as another potential intervention strategy for sarcopenia. Although our understanding of the relationship between vitamin D and muscle function has advanced over the past decade, a complete understanding of the vitamin D action on muscle tissue and how this translates into improvements in muscular performance are yet to be elucidated. Older adults are at increased risk of developing vitamin D insufficiency and supplementation may be indicated in those older people with low vitamin D levels to combat sarcopenia, functional decline, and falls risk [56]. As people age, skin cannot synthesize vitamin D efficiently and the kidney is less able to convert vitamin D to its active hormone form. The consensus position is that the available evidence of safety and the potential benefits for adults justify recommending that optimal vitamin D status represents a serum 25-hydroxyvitamin D level of at least 75 nmol/L [57]. People may try to meet their vitamin D needs through exposure to sunlight, but exposure to sunlight and dietary intake are insufficient to maintain this level, and use of vitamin D supplementation is therefore indicated for most adults. The clinical approach can take into account three 'settings,' based on suspicion for vitamin D insufficiency [58]. The first group is adults below age 50 years without comorbid conditions affecting vitamin D absorption or action who are at low risk for vitamin D insufficiency. For these people, supplementation at 10–25 μg (400–1000 IU) is appropriate, and serum 25-hydroxyvitamin D should not be measured. People with moderate risk for vitamin D insufficiency are adults 50 years of age or older without comorbid conditions that affect vitamin D absorption or action. For these people, routine supplementation with vitamin D is appropriate, and this should be at a dose of 20–50 μg (800–2000 IU). Serum 25 hydroxyvitamin D should not be measured routinely in initial assessment of these individuals, but if pharmacologic therapy is prescribed, 25-hydroxyvitamin D should be measured after three to four months of an adequate supplementation dose. People at high risk for adverse outcomes from vitamin D insufficiency include those with recurrent fractures, bone loss, sarcopenia and/or comorbid conditions that affect vitamin D absorption or action. In these cases, serum 25-hydroxyvitamin D should be measured as part of the initial assessment, and supplementation with vitamin D should be based on the measured value. Supplementation dose requirements above the current definition of tolerable upper intake level (50 μg [2000 IU]) may be identified by measuring serum 25-hydroxyvitamin D levels. Vitamin D3 is the preferred supplementary form for humans, with vitamin D2 being available for large-dose preparations. Calcitriol and its analogs are prescription products with narrow margins of safety. They are not synonymous with vitamin D and are not advised for prevention or routine treatment of osteoporosis. For most adults given a supplement, an initial dose of vitamin D3 of 20–25 μg (800–1000 IU) daily, is likely to raise serum 25-hydroxyvitamin D by approximately 15–30 nmol/L. To achieve desirable vitamin D status (> 75 nmol/L) many individuals will require doses greater than this minimum dose. A weekly dose of 250 μg (10 000 IU) vitamin D3 may be more convenient for some patients if available.

Quaternary prevention: warning against non-evidence-based interventions

As recently reviewed [23], there is as yet no published evidence justifying any pharmacological intervention to *prevent* sarcopenia. Patients should be warned against the use of anabolic agents (such as testosterone, DHEA and growth hormone), given their risk for harmful side effects. The search for pharmacologic drugs that could prevent sarcopenia is ongoing. The new drugs being studied will have to show their efficacy on physical performance outcomes in addition to muscle mass and strength, and target populations will have to be defined [59]. For the detailed discussion of this topic the reader is referred to the specific chapters in this book dealing with the pharmacologic treatment options of sarcopenia.

REFERENCES

1. Cruz-Jentoft AJ, Baeyens JP, Bauer JM, et al. Sarcopenia: European consensus on definition and diagnosis: Report of the European Working Group on Sarcopenia in Older People. Age Ageing. 2010;39:412–423.

2. Sehl ME, Yates FE. Kinetics of human aging: I. Rates of senescence between ages 30 and 70 years in healthy people. J Gerontol A Biol Sci Med Sci. 2001;56:B198–208.

3. Pollock ML, Mengelkoch LJ, Graves JE, et al. Twenty-year follow-up of aerobic power and body composition of older track athletes. J Appl Physiol. 1997;82:1508–1516.

4. Guo SS, Zeller C, Chumlea WC, Siervogel RM. Aging, body composition, and lifestyle: the Fels Longitudinal Study. Am J Clin Nutr. 1999;70:405–411.

5. Hansen RD, Raja C, Allen BJ. Total body protein in chronic diseases and in aging. Ann N Y Acad Sci. 2000;904:345–352.

6. Genton L, Karsegard VL, Chevalley T, et al. Body composition changes over 9 years in healthy elderly subjects and impact of physical activity. Clin Nutr. 2011;30:436–442.

7. Janssen I, Ross R. Linking age-related changes in skeletal muscle mass and composition with metabolism and disease. J Nutr Health Aging. 2005;9:408–419.

8. Bautmans I, Van Puyvelde K, Mets T. Sarcopenia and functional decline: pathophysiology, prevention and therapy. Acta clinica Belgica. 2009;64:303–316.

9. Fielding RA, Vellas B, Evans WJ, et al. Sarcopenia: an undiagnosed condition in older adults. Current consensus definition: prevalence, etiology, and consequences. International working group on sarcopenia. J Am Med Dir Assoc. 2011;12:249–256.

10. von Haehling S, Morley JE, Anker SD. An overview of sarcopenia: facts and numbers on prevalence and clinical impact. J Cachex Sarcopenia Muscle. 2010;1:129–133.

11. Morley JE. Sarcopenia: diagnosis and treatment. J Nutr Health Aging. 2008;12:452–456.

12. Janssen I. The epidemiology of sarcopenia. Clin Geriatr Med. 2011;27:355–363.

13. Gordon RS, Jr. An operational classification of disease prevention. Public Health Rep. 1983;98:107–109.

14. Merkies IS, Schmitz PI, Samijn JP, et al. Assessing grip strength in healthy individuals and patients with immune-mediated polyneuropathies. Muscle Nerve. 2000;23:1393–1401.

15. Lauretani F, Russo CR, Bandinelli S, et al. Age-associated changes in skeletal muscles and their effect on mobility: an operational diagnosis of sarcopenia. J Appl Physiol. 2003;95:1851–1860.

16. Bautmans I, Onyema O, Van Puyvelde K, et al. Grip work estimation during sustained maximal contraction: validity and relationship with physical dependency & inflammation in elderly persons. The journal of nutrition, health & aging. 2011;15(8):731–6.

17. Bautmans I, Gorus E, Njemini R, Mets T. Handgrip performance in relation to self-perceived fatigue, physical functioning and circulating IL-6 in elderly persons without inflammation. BMC Geriatr. 2007;7:5.

18. Bautmans I, Mets T. A fatigue resistance test for elderly persons based on grip strength: reliability and comparison with healthy young subjects. Aging Clin Exp Res. 2005;17:217–222.

19. Bautmans I, Njemini R, De Backer J, et al. Surgery-Induced Inflammation in Relation to Age, Muscle Endurance, and Self-Perceived Fatigue. J Gerontol A Biol Sci Med Sci. 2010;65:266–273.

20. Bautmans I, Njemini R, Predom H, et al. Muscle endurance in elderly nursing home residents is related to fatigue perception, mobility, and circulating tumor necrosis factor-alpha, interleukin-6, and heat shock protein 70. J Am Geriatr Soc. 2008;56:389–396.

21. Pate RR PM, Blair SN, Haskell WL, Macera CA,, Bouchard C ea. Physical activity and public health. A recommendation from the Centers for Disease Control and Prevention and the American College of Sports Medicine. . JAMA. 1995: 402–407.

22. Vogel T, Brechat PH, Leprêtre PM, et al. Health benefits of physical activity in older patients: a review. International Journal of Clinical Practice. 2009;63:303–320.

23. Visvanathan R, Chapman I. Preventing sarcopaenia in older people. Maturitas. 2010;66:383–8.

24. Landi F, Abbatecola A, Provinciali M, et al. Moving against frailty: does physical activity matter? Biogerontology. 2010;11:537–545.

25. Latham NK, Andersen-Ranberg K, Bennett DA, Stretton CM. Progressive resistance training for physical disability in older people (Cochrane Review). The Cochrane Library. 2003; 2.

26. Saini A, Faulkner S, Al-Shanti N, Stewart C. Powerful signals for weak muscles. Ageing Res Rev. 2009;8:251–267.

27. Nicklas BJ, Brinkley TE. Exercise training as a treatment for chronic inflammation in the elderly. Exercise and sport sciences reviews. 2009;37:165–170.

28. Beavers KM, Brinkley TE, Nicklas BJ. Effect of exercise training on chronic inflammation. Clinica Chimica Acta. 2010;411:785–793.

29. Krabbe KS, Pedersen M, Bruunsgaard H. Inflammatory mediators in the elderly. Exp Gerontol. 2004;39:687–699.

30. Marcell TJ. Review Article: Sarcopenia: Causes, Consequences, and Preventions. J Gerontol A Biol Sci Med Sci. 2003;58:M911–6.

31. Brinkley TE, Leng X, Miller ME, et al. Chronic inflammation is associated with low physical function in older adults across multiple comorbidities. J Gerontol A Biol Sci Med Sci. 2009;64:455–461.

32. Pedersen BK, Steensberg A, Schjerling P. Muscle-derived interleukin-6: possible biological effects. J Physiol. 2001;536:329–337.

33. Bautmans I, Njemini R, Vasseur S, et al. Biochemical changes in response to intensive resistance exercise training in the elderly. Gerontology. 2005;51:253–265.

34. Bruunsgaard H, Pedersen BK. Effects of exercise on the immune system in the elderly population. Immunol Cell Biol. 2000;78:523–531.

35. Minois N. Longevity and aging: beneficial effects of exposure to mild stress. Biogerontology. 2000;1:15–29.

36. Keylock KT, Vieira VJ, Wallig MA, et al. Exercise accelerates cutaneous wound healing and decreases wound inflammation in aged mice. American journal of physiology. 2008;294:R179–84.

37. Emery CF, Kiecolt-Glaser JK, Glaser R, et al. Exercise accelerates wound healing among healthy older adults: a preliminary investigation. J Gerontol A Biol Sci Med Sci. 2005;60:1432–1436.

38. Stewart LK, Flynn MG, Campbell WW, et al. Influence of exercise training and age on CD14+ cell-surface expression of toll-like receptor 2 and 4. Brain, Behavior, and Immunity. 2005;19:389–397.

39. Franceschi C, Capri M, Monti D, et al. Inflammaging and anti-inflammaging: A systemic perspective on aging and longevity emerged from studies in humans. Mechanisms of Ageing and Development. 2007;128:92–105.

40. Bayingana K, Demarest S, Gisle L, et al. Gezondheidsenquête België 2004 Boek III Leefstijl. In: Wetenschappelijk Instituut Volksgezondheid AE, ed., 2006; 1–115.

41. Rütten A, Abu-Omar K. Prevalence of physical activity in the European Union. Soz Praventivmed. 2004;49:281–289.

42. Ewald B, Duke J, Thakkinstian A, et al. Physical activity of older Australians measured by pedometry. Australasian Journal on Ageing. 2009;28:127–133.

43. Allender S, Cowburn G, Foster C. Understanding participation in sport and physical activity among children and adults: a review of qualitative studies. Health Education Research Theory & Practice. 2006;21:826–835.

44. Baert V, Gorus E, Mets T, et al. Motivators and barriers for physical activity in the oldest old: A systematic review. Ageing Res Rev. 2011;10(4):464–74.

45. Bautmans I, Lambert M, Mets T. The six-minute walk test in community dwelling elderly: influence of health status. BMC Geriatr. 2004;4:6.

46. Volpi E, Rasmussen BB. Nutrition and muscle protein metabolism in the elderly. Diabetes Nutr Metab. 2000;13:99–107.

47. Volpi E, Kobayashi H, Sheffield-Moore M, et al. Essential amino acids are primarily responsible for the amino acid stimulation of muscle protein anabolism in healthy elderly adults. Am J Clin Nutr. 2003;78:250–258.

48. Zanchi NE, Nicastro H, Lancha AH, Jr. Potential antiproteolytic effects of L-leucine: observations of in vitro and in vivo studies. Nutr Metab (Lond). 2008;5:20.

49. Campbell WW, Crim MC, Dallal GE, et al. Increased protein requirements in elderly people: new data and retrospective reassessments. Am J Clin Nutr. 1994;60:501–509.

50. Campbell WW, Johnson CA, McCabe GP, Carnell NS. Dietary protein requirements of younger and older adults. Am J Clin Nutr. 2008;88:1322–1329.

51. Rousset S, Patureau Mirand P, Brandolini M, et al. Daily protein intakes and eating patterns in young and elderly French. Br J Nutr. 2003;90:1107–1115.

52. Symons TB, Sheffield-Moore M, Wolfe RR, Paddon-Jones D. A moderate serving of high-quality protein maximally stimulates skeletal muscle protein synthesis in young and elderly subjects. J Am Diet Assoc. 2009;109:1582–1586.

53. Paddon-Jones D, Rasmussen BB. Dietary protein recommendations and the prevention of sarcopenia. Curr Opin Clin Nutr Metab Care. 2009;12:86–90.

54. Morley JE. Anorexia and weight loss in older persons. J Gerontol A Biol Sci Med Sci. 2003;58:131–137.

55. Roubenoff R. Sarcopenia: a major modifiable cause of frailty in the elderly. J Nutr Health Aging. 2000;4:140–142.

56. Dawson-Hughes B. Serum 25-hydroxyvitamin D and functional outcomes in the elderly. Am J Clin Nutr. 2008;88:537S–40S.

57. Bischoff-Ferrari HA, Willett WC, Wong JB, et al. Fracture prevention with vitamin D supplementation: a meta-analysis of randomized controlled trials. JAMA. 2005;293:2257–2264.

58. Hanley DA, Cranney A, Jones G, et al. Vitamin D in adult health and disease: a review and guideline statement from Osteoporosis Canada. CMAJ. 2010;182:E610–8.

59. Vandewoude MF, Cederholm T, Cruz-Jentoft AJ. Relevant Outcomes in Intervention Trials for Sarcopenia. J Am Geriatr Soc. 2011;59:1566–1567.

Index

Sarcopenia, First Edition. Edited by Alfonso J. Cruz-Jentoft and John E. Morley.
© 2012 John Wiley & Sons, Ltd. Published 2012 by John Wiley & Sons, Ltd.